WITHOUT A MANUAL

*The reflections of a woman in her forties
determined to live her fullest life, while facing terminal illness*

SANDY TRUNZER

FriesenPress

Suite 300 - 990 Fort St
Victoria, BC, Canada, V8V 3K2
www.friesenpress.com

Copyright © 2015 by Sandy Trunzer
First Edition — 2015

All rights reserved.

Foreword by Ken Banks.
Introduction by Shannon Delbridge.
Cover image by Sandy Trunzer.

No part of this publication may be reproduced in any form, or by any means, electronic or mechanical, including photocopying, recording, or any information browsing, storage, or retrieval system, without permission in writing from the publisher.

ISBN
978-1-4602-3946-9 (Hardcover)
978-1-4602-3947-6 (Paperback)
978-1-4602-3948-3 (eBook)

1. Medical, Diseases

Distributed to the trade by The Ingram Book Company

For my sweet Suzu; your heart and my heart.

Nothing shall ever break the threads that have bound us together, I love you most of all and forever.

To those who've been supporting me along this difficult journey – thank you. You know who you are (and there are many of you), and you know how much your support has meant to me. I'm grateful beyond words.

INTRODUCTION

We spend much of our lives learning how to live; learning how to ride a bike, how to paint inside the lines, how to balance a checkbook, how to raise our children, how to be kind to one another, and how to chase our dreams.

We draw on our energy, our skills, our past, our fears, and sometimes our sheer grit. But we figure it out ... with support from parents and teachers, guide-books and signposts, lovers and friends. There is a manual for most things in life. There is a place we can go for the answers, and sometimes even the questions.

But there is no manual for this. There is no manual that tells us how to stop living.

This is a story of one woman's journey when hope is lost but there are days yet to come. This is Sandy's story.

***

Sandy felt there was finally space to breathe. Paradoxically, she stepped into her forties with the sure feeling that the most difficult challenges that could fit into one lifetime had already happened.

A tumultuous childhood had forced her to live in an adult world at a very young age; she had spent her youth on her own. She focused on earning money in order to stay in school, while most of her high school peers were preoccupied with whom they would invite to their next party.

Sandy had married relatively young, at twenty four, and learned over the years that she and her husband were far from a good match. The one blessing was the arrival of their daughter, Suzanna, who was six years old at the time the marriage ended. The years that followed were marked by prolonged and onerous conflicts over issues concerning Suzanna's best interests.

Serious, unexplained health challenges plagued Sandy throughout her twenties and thirties. After she saw numerous specialists, it appeared that the riddle had finally been solved. A pacemaker was implanted in 2003, to regulate an unusual cardiac arrhythmia and Sandy's daily life improved dramatically.

Sandy's professional life progressed far more smoothly. She enjoyed the challenges and the rewards as she advanced through various positions in the travel and telecommunications fields, building a comfortable and satisfying life for her and her daughter. A downturn in the telecommunications market was fortuitous as it afforded Sandy a graceful exit. This provided space for her to pursue a passion she'd had since a child; a career in professional photography.

Nearing forty, Sandy was happy with the life she shared with her daughter. Her health had improved; she had financial security and was busy establishing her career as a professional photographer. She was ready to share her life again with a partner, and in keeping with the better luck that life seemed to be delivering, she met a man in a park, at one of her art exhibits. This man would be become her husband a little more than a year later. Sandy was beginning to live the life she had dreamed about; a life she had earned. She felt sincere gratitude to be able to leave the difficult years behind...but this spell of happiness and light was fleeting.

In the summer of 2008, she began to experience leg pain above her right knee after exercise; long walks were a regular part of the week, scouting out locations for photo shoots. During her regular physical exam the following October, Sandy casually mentioned this to her family doctor.

Sandy's blog, *Without a Manual* was never intended to be published in book form. It started out as a way for Sandy to keep friends informed (without repeating the same information over and over again through emails and phone calls). It was a way of updating those closest to her about the progression and treatment of what was, within months of that first doctor's appointment, to be diagnosed as Erdheim-Chester Disease, a very rare illness, which at the time was known to have afflicted only about three hundred patients worldwide. The numbers have grown closer to five hundred cases since Sandy was given her diagnosis, yet ECD holds its place as one of the rarest afflictions with a very poor prognosis. It's a grim statistic and it portends a future that is truly difficult to imagine.

There is no cure for Sandy's disease and eventually, there were no treatments left to bring hope. The outcome of ECD is certain – an envelope of time with the four corners defined. Statistically, time would likely run out within three years.

While Sandy struggled with accepting the enormity of this reality, she was also beginning to understand that it would not be a placid journey. Her journey involved finding ways to manage and cope with intense physical pain and discomfort, largely on her own. This is a story of a young woman forced to overcome much adversity throughout her life, only to be faced with the ultimate challenge. Has life prepared her for this final trial?

Reading the pages from Sandy's blog will elicit many emotions as you walk with her through her personal experiences, observations, and thoughts about facing the end of life. This book, like her blog, will take you through the highs and lows. It will have you laughing out loud and then weeping in empathic sorrow.

It is a powerful read about an inspirational, courageous, and heroic woman who constantly contextualizes her situation with what there is to be thankful for. Despite the grief and sorrow that comes with impending death, Sandy sees the gifts she has been given – including the gift of seeing the best in the friends and strangers around her. She is most thankful for the joy her daughter brings, and for these lessons in kindness that her daughter can carry in her heart long after Sandy has left this world.

The days are growing short, and Sandy marks time by Suzanna's successes and her growth. Sandy is tired. She is tired of fighting.

There are no manuals or FAQs to learn how to die. There are no honed answers to carefully crafted questions. In many ways it can be an isolating journey, but somehow, sharing the path and the pain keeps the tragedy on a human scale that allows us to bear more than we ever thought we could – for and through the love of others.

FOREWORD
by Ken Banks

Courage
Doesn't always roar
Sometimes courage is the quiet voice
at the end of the day saying,
"I will try again tomorrow."
Mary Anne Radmacher

I admire these kinds of very thoughtful, motivational sayings that people create when they are affected and amazed by the perseverance and the sheer strength of those they love, as they sometimes battle conditions, challenges, or illnesses they never thought would cross their paths.

Few of us ever stop for a second to think how quickly our busy lives can change. We all pretend we are infallible.

But! Change they do! Illness, accidents, the loss of a job, the loss of a loved one bound into our lives. Obstacles appear and our loved ones change and adapt in ways that we never expected. And I dare to venture a guess that even they never expected. After all, bad stuff happens to others, it never happens to us.

Once retired, I had time on my hands. I wanted to give back to my community.

Searching through volunteer opportunities, I noticed a need in our local hospice for many dimensions of volunteering within the hospice culture.

My initial placement was in the "Wellness Programme" - a community outreach to provide psychological, emotional and practical support to folks with a life-limiting illness. This is offered in a friendly and caring environment and includes aromatherapy massage, music therapy, reflexology, reiki, restorative yoga and therapeutic touch.

A social time is available to our participants where they can enjoy a lunch and share experiences and offer support to each other and their caregivers.

This was the environment where I first met Sandy, and as we chatted it became clear her illness was very unique and extremely rare. Sandy was receiving one of the hospice treatments that day and I was asked to walk with her to her session.

It was autumn and as we walked she chatted about the colours and what she noticed and recalled from her photography career. I have not, nor will I forget this first time experience.

When Sandy was able, and I happened to be scheduled, she shared the details of her struggle dealing with the many facets caused by and related to the disease that was gradually taking her life.

It is not easy to watch fellow human beings suffer, especially as you grow close to them. You want to do more. You want to see them recover. But you know – and they know – that they are on a journey that will end with their passing. It is not unusual for patients to be able to control their emotions much better than the volunteer caregiver, who often feels helpless and stuck for words, with a big lump in the throat as their patient friends struggle to do many things we all take for granted.

To help us to overcome these natural human feelings, part of the commitment to volunteering is to take a 30-hour course in Palliative Care. Our group was fortunate to be teamed with volunteers from Acclaim Health in Oakville and we had an outstanding instructor who had many years of experience and gave us the courage to keep our commitment to help those who really needed our help.

About two-thirds through the course he explained that we were going to experience something never before done in his many years of teaching. We were having a guest who would share the other side of Palliative Care.

That special guest was Sandy!

An hour-and-a-half later, after allowing us to share her journey, we had a unique glimpse of her world. This is one special lady! An extra-ordinary lady, gracefully battling an extra-ordinary illness.

I remember her later telling me that when she went to hospital appointments, doctors would gather around her to learn from her about Erdheim Chester Disease (ECD). Doctors know very little about the disease – they do not know what causes it . . . they do not know how to treat it. The only thing they do know is that it is going to end the life of anyone who is diagnosed with it.

When she was in hospitals, Sandy at times looked like she was getting the V.I.P. treatment; there were so many doctors eager to talk with her. To this day, ECD still baffles those in the medical field.

Imagine how you would feel, knowing that you had a disease with no known cure. Doctors can't help. Hospital can't help.

ECD patients do not have a chance. Statistically, the diagnosis is death within 36 months, and there is no known treatment at the moment.

Add to this that there are only 300 or 400 people in the world with ECD, and you quickly understand why drug companies are not putting any research funds into developing a drug that may help the ECD patient. Sadly, insurance companies won't cover any drugs that don't carry a notation on the label stating that it is specifically for ECD patients.

It is a horrible, Catch-22 situation. It is a hopeless and helpless situation that would test the psyche of even the strongest. Sandy is one of the rare ones who have carried on in these awful circumstances where doors of hope are slammed shut at every turn.

Some doctors have fought to get some treatments donated – worth thousands of dollars – to help Sandy in her fight. But, often the 'cure' was far worse than doing nothing. But she was – at least in the early stages – willing to gamble that a drug that helped cure one disease might also be helpful in the fight against her disease. No such luck. And those drugs did nothing to ease the pain that she has been constantly under for so many years.

Through her blog she has shared this journey of hope, vision, good times, bad times, smiles, sadness, old friends, new friends, joy, sorrow and every other human emotion known to man.

Sandy shares with her words about healthcare, friends, strangers and others, in the hope of adding to the knowledge of the fight she shares with all those labeled as palliative.

She has talked about her birthdays, her Bucket List, CBC radio, and television interviews examining the rights of the dying patient to be able to die with dignity.

Sandy has used her bed-ridden time to help those who will follow her.

Her blog, *Without a Manual*, captures this. She could have felt sorry for herself and hid away, keeping all her ideas and feelings locked inside of her, upset at the world, and bemoaning her situation.

But she is not a person to moan and groan 'woe is me.' She has long since resigned herself that ECD is going to eventually take her. But she wants to make sure that those who follow her down this painful path at least have the beginnings of a manual to help them.

That's selfless. But that's Sandy. If one person is helped by the hundreds of hours she spent on her blog and putting this book together, then it will all be worth her while.

Sandy's photography is classic. I remember walking with her that bright, autumn day and she was pointing out the beauty all around us. I was seeing the same thing as she was, but it was not registering with me as it was with Sandy.

To me it was there, but I had to be shown the beauty of this earth. My mind simply took it for granted.

I hung on her every word as she put amazing, marvellous, yet sincere and simple words to things that I could only see.

She has a good eye for portrait photography, too, and a growing client base that sadly had to look for another photographer as Sandy slid from being a vibrant, sought-after photographer with so much promise and passion, to a reluctant patient who could not walk to scout out possible photo shoots, to quickly being bed-ridden and not even able to pick-up a camera, much less to push the shutter button.

One of the darkest days during her battle with ECD was the time she had to part with her favourite lens to get some needed cash for necessities. If it had not been evident before, this was the time that Sandy finally acknowledged the disease was winning and was going to claim her body without her taking another photograph.

But even as her days on this earth are drawing to a close, Sandy finds time to have a laugh - as much as it pains her physically. Her make-up is such that life is too short to mope around. She sees the humour in most things. It reflects in her blog. You will recognize this amazing trait in her words. Her humour comes out in every personal visit.

There were times that the average human being would be excused for not wanting to laugh. Sandy drew more short straws in love and life than anyone deserves – yet she always finds a way.

Sandy is also a hugger. She loved a hug at the start and end of every visit. Then, one day, the hugs had to stop.

A doctor, making a house call, was gently examining her when she crushed one of Sandy's ribs. That's how brittle her bones are during the last few weeks.

Sandy leaves us a gift through her words and photographs that will affect all who care to take her hand and walk with her on her special journey.

Sandy,
Thank you for your gift to all of us in sharing *Without a Manual.*

Hugs,
Ken

WITHOUT A
MANUAL

STITCHES COME OUT TOMORROW
Wednesday, June 03, 2009

Really now, why couldn't I have appreciated my body more when it was young, healthy and looked pretty good in a bikini?

Tomorrow I have an appointment to have my stitches taken out, after they were deftly sewn in by a surgeon ten days ago when I had another biopsy done. This time, it was on my back and it was a whole lot easier to recover this time around! The last biopsy (February) was on my femur and had me bound to my bed for the better part of twelve weeks to avoid fracturing my leg.

I look at myself in the mirror in the morning as I dress, and most days don't notice the four large scars that can be found on my chest (two there), leg and back. Not to mention the half-dozen or so from various mishaps growing up. I try to see that for 44 years old, I'm looking pretty good!

Despite that I'd make a decent game board for tic-tac-toe by drawing in just a few more lines at my surgery sites, maybe this summer I'll find the courage to wear a bikini after all!

ANONYMOUSLY YOURS
Sunday, June 07, 2009

I've been asked by a few readers of this blog why I've chosen not to share either my name or the medical condition that I'm dealing with.

First my name – it's primarily economics! I'm self-employed as a photographer and I'm doing my level best to work as much as I can in whatever my current state of health might be. I have to appreciate that a potential client coming upon this blog by searching on my name may hesitate to book me if they have any doubt about my ability to follow through on the job. Without knowing me personally, they wouldn't know just how passionate I am about my work, how dedicated I am to delivering a great customer experience, and how determined I am to keep clicking the shutter.

As for my medical condition (I say "my" as if I own it! I'd gladly sell it to anyone who could dispose of it safely with no harm to others), again it's that beastly on-line search issue. You can scare yourself silly by looking up any medical condition on the Internet, and my experience may be quite different than that of someone else with the same illness.

On the medical side of things...tomorrow I get the preliminary results of a biopsy taken from my back two weeks ago. Stitches are out and the incision is healing well. I'm still dealing with a rather persistent case of pericarditis (an inflammation of the lining of the heart) and will probably need to switch to stronger meds very soon. I detest taking drugs of any sort; this is a rather big obstacle for me to overcome.

WHO'S LOOKING BACK AT ME IN THE MIRROR?
Thursday, June 11, 2009

Admit it. We've all thought about it. What would I do if I were diagnosed with a serious illness and heard that I would have a shorter time on earth than expected? Travel to places I've always wanted to visit? Try daring sports and activities? (Skydiving, anyone?) Meet a person whom I really admire?

There's no right answer of course, and everyone will have their own "bucket list." Maybe you'd be physically limited in some way, maybe finances would be an issue, and maybe you'd just change your mind if this really happened to you (and I pray that you never find yourself in this situation).

Straight up – yes, I hate being in the position where I have to think about this.

It was an acid test. Was I truly as happy as I thought I was before my diagnosis? Did I have regrets; important tasks undone; a life not truly lived? I found myself pleased (after having had time to digest my diagnosis) to find that my bucket list is truly very short. My life was wonderful before the diagnosis, and will continue to be great in many ways. It's not a charmed life in the traditional sense; we struggle with many of the issues that families deal with. But we're a family and I know that through the best and worst of the road ahead, we'll be getting through this together. For that I'm grateful beyond words.

I look in the mirror, and although I sometimes have a hard time taking in what I see happening to my body in the purely physical sense – in my eyes I see who I am. That part hasn't changed, and maybe I see that more clearly than ever.

As for that bucket list? More on that later. Trust me; it's short (but sweet!)

PEERING OUT THE WINDOW
Monday, June 15, 2009

As a landscape photographer, I spend a lot of time outdoors. At least I did before I got sick. Now I spend most of my time indoors because I'm either recovering from a surgery, trying to deal with side effects from various meds that I'm on, or just too darned tired to get myself out the door. And this hurts. Warm weather has finally arrived in my corner of the world and I'm sidelined most days. I'm aching to be outside. Taking walks with my family, tending to the garden (not my favourite job, but the being outside part suits me just fine!) and photographing. I used to think nothing of hauling myself out of bed in the wee hours to arrive at my destination before the sun rose just to get that perfect light for my photograph (and it was usually darned cold too, but totally worth it).

I know this is temporary (no more surgeries scheduled for now, and I'm confident that the next round of meds will finally get rid of a nasty case of pericarditis that's been taunting me) but I can't help think that when I do get outside, I need to make every moment count. I'm hoping it's still quite a few, but I just don't know how many summers are left for me to appreciate. It's ironic that as a child I'd much rather have curled up in my room with a good book – getting outdoors simply didn't interest me. Somewhere along the line, I started to see just how beautiful this world is in its colours, shapes, and textures and felt the pull to capture it all with my camera. And now I just can't get enough.

I'll admit that this has kind of been a "feel sorry for myself" day. They don't happen often, but it happened today. I'm feeling worn out and upset that I'm wasting time doing much of nothing right now. I'll be back out there again soon. Promise.

STARTED ON PREDNISONE
Thursday, June 18, 2009

It's been an eventful week. I can do without eventful weeks like this. In an attempt to clear up this persistent pericarditis that I've been troubled with, my cardiologist had me double up on a med called colchicine this past weekend. Not quite the expected outcome – it actually made the symptoms of pericarditis quite a bit worse (chest pain, difficulty breathing, exhaustion, dizziness, dry cough – I'm adding a bit more medical detail in this post because dear and thoughtful friends let me know that they were looking for updates on my physical status).

A quick call to my diagnostician in the city (have you seen the TV show *House*? His team works in a similar fashion, minus the cranky character that Hugh Laurie plays) and he got me into see the team the next day (yesterday). I'll go further; not only are they minus a cranky doctor, they're an amazing team of caring and dedicated medical professionals who have made me feel like nothing is more important to them than treating my illness as effectively as possible, while taking my comfort and concerns into consideration at all times. I'm truly blessed to be their patient.

It was agreed that it was finally time to try prednisone (a corticosteroid used as a last resort for pericarditis). I'd been dreading this step. I'd heard all kinds of nightmares about this drug (weight gain due to water retention, huge appetite leading to additional pounds piling on, moon face, crankiness, restlessness, bone-density loss, insomnia etc.). Hoping to avoid prednisone, my medical team had me on all sorts of other anti-inflammatory meds prior to now but it appears that if I want rid of this nuisance, it has to be!

I took my first dose this morning, and I'll admit that I raised a bit of a fuss about it. A few tears as I told my husband, "See you on the other side!" meaning nothing more dramatic than hopefully my moods wouldn't change too much and that after the course of treatment I would feel like myself again. Minus the pericarditis of course.

It's been about six hours. Some waves of nausea, a period of fairly intense restlessness (maybe not such a bad thing, I went on a tidying frenzy), and a BIG appetite that I'm trying hard to ignore. Overall not too bad. I'll be cautiously optimistic, I'm aware that side effects can escalate as treatment continues.

I haven't been feeling irritable, thankfully. At least not yet. Because if that happens, my family might be seeking additional meds that will put me to sleep for the duration of my prednisone regimen.

TRYING NOT TO EAT MY CEREAL BAR WRAPPER
Sunday, June 21, 2009

It's day four on prednisone; overall, so far not so bad!

I had a bit of a rough start with a fever on the first night, my doctor had me go for blood tests at the local lab just to make sure all was ok. (Prednisone reduces resistance to infection and any fevers should be investigated.) All was in order, it must have been just one of those things. In fact, the fever has returned a few times since but I don't feel ill with any other symptoms.

Minor side effects have included a touch of nausea and stomach pain, a bit of dizziness, and lack of sleep. (Last night was less than three hours and not much better on the previous nights.) Oh, and the infamous prednisone mood swings kicked in last night for the first time. Bless my family for not slapping me silly for being so weepy and miserable for a few hours there. They know exactly when I need a joke and a hug to feel a bit better.

And now for the good stuff – unbelievable energy (my family hasn't seen me move this fast since pain from the bone tumour started up last summer). No pain in either my chest (from the pericarditis) or in my leg (from the tumour), and I've actually dropped a bit of the weight that I'd put on while taking other meds over the last few months. Normally, prednisone can pack the weight on quickly. I'm prepared that this will likely still happen but for now I don't mind the lower number on the scale.

The hardest part is the intense hunger that kicks in just after lunch and sticks with me until I go to bed. A hunger like I've never experienced before. Really. Don't leave any food lying about, because if you were saving it – it'll be history if I catch sight of it. Closed kitchen cupboards are my friend right now; in fact locks might not be a bad idea. I'm trying very hard though to keep to normal portions and calorie intake, and hopefully I'll be able to keep the expected weight gain from getting out of control.

Off now to put this energy to good use – anyone need their garage cleaned out? Oops, I guess I should start with our own...

IT TOOK ME A WEEK TO FIND THIS FUNNY
Thursday, June 25, 2009

In my last post I mentioned that I'd had a bit of trouble on my first day on prednisone, requiring some quick blood tests to try to explain a fever that cropped up. What I didn't tell you is what a baby I was about one of the tests!

In just one more of the weird coincidences that keep cropping up of late, it turned out that the doctor staffing my local walk-in clinic that evening last week is the wife of my regular cardiologist. (Sad to say, I have several looking after various cardiac complications.)

As required, I gave her a bit of background on my medical status and she mentioned that her husband would find my diagnosis intriguing. We put a few pieces together to realize that not only was I her husband's patient, I'd seen him just a few days before going on the prednisone. She called him to get his slant on what should be done next – my luck in getting amazing medical care continues.

Back to my test. Along with standard blood tests, the doctor said I needed to have a throat swab done, to check for infection. I paled, backed up, and quickly blurted out that I'd pass on that one – thank you very much! With gentle persistence and an explanation of why this test was important (and assurance that she, the clinic doctor, was really good at doing this test) I finally allowed her to quickly swab – with my husband holding my hand (and a tear in my eye).

If you know me well, you'd probably find this as surprising as my husband did at the time. I can be one brave soul. Some pretty tough issues have tested me in this lifetime, and I'm usually able to handle them with a smile on my face. But a silly little throat swab made me want to run!

Thanks to the doctor for not making me feel stupid, and thanks to my sweet husband for holding my hand. For a few minutes I felt like a terrified, wide-eyed, three-year-old. Goodness, I think most three-year-olds would have handled the swab much better! Yes, I'm as quirky as all that...

THOSE AREN'T ACORNS IN MY CHEEKS
Wednesday, July 01, 2009

The good, the bad and the (not yet) ugly....

I've been on steroids now for two weeks. Everyone's experience will be different, but I must say this has been an interesting road.

My skin is smoother and clearer than I ever remember, but I'm also bruising more easily.

I have unbounded energy and strength on most days, but next to no sleep! I'm lucky if I'm getting four hours a night. Getting lots done though (and working a bit too thankfully).

I'm not gaining weight overall, but it's a little disconcerting to see my face expanding every day. My dear husband and daughter tell me they see little difference, but I see it happening.

Most days I have a great sense of elation, but I've had two days of the nasties. Family was warned and I went into seclusion. Tears were cried, vengeance wreaked upon the vacuum cleaner hose. Don't ask (but the vacuum cleaner and I both survived the altercation).

I can finally breathe easily without any chest pain most days. The drugs are working...my heart races a bit throughout the day (but that of course could come from seeing my husband come round the corner).

I had almost two weeks of not feeling any leg pain from the bone tumour, pretty wonderful – I haven't bounced around like this in a long time. Overall muscle and bone pain kicking in now, I understand this is normal at this point in the treatment. Not nearly bad enough to keep me down.

I'm not as hungry as I was during the first week on treatment; I think I've learned just to ignore it for the most part. Although I did get into a box of crackers at 1 a.m. this morning, the first time I've given in to hunger during the night.

More hair seems to coming out in my hands when I shampoo. Thankfully not in patches, it's just thinning out a bit.

We're keeping our fingers crossed that my doctor hears no evidence of pericarditis at my appointment on Monday. If it's still there, the dosage goes up. (Eek!) If not, we start the weaning process. (You can't just quit prednisone, normal adrenal function of the body has been altered and it needs time to produce its own cortisol again.)

The thought of a full eight hours of sleep has me drooling far more than the hunger that comes with this treatment!

IS A PICTURE WORTH A THOUSAND WORDS?
Saturday, July 04, 2009

Over the last months I've had to spend lots of time resting. Not really what I'm good at, to be honest, I'm much happier getting things done; usually multi-tasking. My husband has said that I seem to thrive on organized chaos and he's not far off base.

It's almost impossible for me to just lie there resting, as I had to for almost three months straight following my bone surgery in February. I'm very glad that I invested in a laptop when it was time to replace my computer last year; it was a godsend to be able to continue communicating with family, friends, and clients.

I got hooked on listening to photography-related podcasts; there are several I can recommend if you're interested in this sort of thing. This evening as I was resting (those steroids are taking their toll and I had to slow down a bit today) I caught up on a recent episode of *The Candid Frame*; this one an interview with photographer Douglas Kirkland.

Mr. Kirkland has had a rich and fascinating career, and there was one part of the interview that particularly caught my attention this evening. He was speaking to his process of getting to know his subjects so that he could accurately portray them when he captured their image.

As a portrait photographer myself, I pride myself on getting to know my clients with the same intention – asking lots of questions before the session, trying to get a feel for how they would prefer to be portrayed.

As I listened to this interview, it struck me that in my quest to have another photographer take our family photo (always having camera in hand I'm rarely on the other end of the lens) I wanted to think about this issue. And I'm thrown. How do I want to be remembered when my family looks at these photos after I'm no longer here?

The vain part of me wants to hold off until after steroid treatment; those prednisone-induced chipmunk cheeks are taking over my face.

Despite my husband telling me that they're pinchably cute, I don't want to be photographed right now. But it's not just about what I'll look like. What will my family and loved ones see in my eyes in these photos?

It's not like I've forgotten that this illness doesn't come with a happy ending. I know that unless a wayward bus and a moment of inattention catch me sooner, this illness will take my life.

Today, for the first time, I thought about how people I know might remember me after I'm gone. Will they say I was a loving person? Will they think that I did my best at whatever I attempted? Wishful thinking on my part, certainly not all thoughts will be positive. I'm well aware of my numerous faults and quirks but I'm not done yet trying to be a better person in this lifetime.

How do I ask a photographer to catch the truth of who I am when I'm not sure of the answer to that myself yet?

PHOTOGRAPHING ON A LOVELY AFTERNOON
Tuesday, July 07, 2009

Yesterday I had my weekly check-up at the hospital. Unfortunately the pericarditis is still there; it hasn't improved and that means more drugs (eight different ones now – some to treat the inflammation, others to treat the side effects of those first drugs).

This is overwhelming for me; I pride myself on trying natural approaches to medical issues and prefer to tough it out rather than take even so much as a Tylenol. I feel like a walking chemical soup these days! I'll admit to being a bit down after my appointment; my doctor had been hopeful that almost three weeks of steroids would have knocked my heart back to a healthier state. He isn't crazy about giving me all these meds either but after conferring with several cardiologists, we don't seem to have another option right now if we're to clear out the pericarditis in preparation for the "heavy hitter drugs," to treat my overall systemic illness.

What better way to cheer myself up than to go for a long walk with my camera, through the city in which I used to live? (My hospital appointments are a one-hour train/car ride from where I live now.) It was a spectacular afternoon; perfect strolling weather. While I was photographing, it was easy to forget all about my illness, meds, and pain for a few hours.

Today, I'm in bed. I've overdone it.

Tomorrow will be better. I can feel it...

ERASING THE EVIDENCE
Friday, July 10, 2009

I'm here in bed with my laptop, catching up on this and that as I rest. I look around and today I just don't like what I see.

Across from the bed is a cabinet, and on top you'd see rows of pill bottles, a pill organizer, a pill splitter, a blood pressure cuff, vitamins, and notes written at my doctor and hospital visits. Very organized and neat (this is still me after all!) but today it makes me cringe.

Since early this year, this has been the room where I've spent a great deal of time recovering from surgery, and dealing with the physical limitations that my illness places upon me, as well as those from the side-effects of all these drugs! This week was especially tough and often it felt like even the short walk across the room was too far to go for the next dose of pills.

Enough. I'm reclaiming this bedroom as a sanctuary.

Yes, I do need to spend more time here than I would like – but it has to become a more peaceful place for me. All this medical paraphernalia is going into the cabinet, rather than on top in full view.

There's no chance at all that hiding them away will cause me to forget to take my meds. The simple act of waking up each morning sets off the meds schedule of: "Take upon waking." "Take one hour before first meal." "Take with breakfast," etc. – You get it, I live by the clock and my meal schedule these days.

I'm feeling quite a bit better today than I have in days. So while I have the energy, I'm getting up to put all these reminders of my illness into hiding. I just don't need the evidence staring me in the face!

CONQUERING FEAR
Saturday, July 11, 2009

When I speak with good friends about the prognosis of my illness, I'm always quick to point out that I'm not afraid to die. Hoping, of course, that this outcome is a long way off, but the truth of the matter is that this illness has manifested itself in my heart – and I kind of need that part to keep going!

I'm not sure how I came to have this lack of fear of my life ending, and we could probably speak at length about why someone would or wouldn't be afraid. Maybe the nurturing part of me needs my loved ones to know that I'm not fearful, because it will help them in dealing with this. Maybe I am truly as content with my life as I think I am.

Spirituality can play a big part in this sense of peace but that's a post for another day.

You may come to realize, reading this blog, how important my photography is to me. I immerse myself in learning every day, and one of my favourite resources is *Lenswork* magazine. Every two months I anxiously await delivery of the magazine in DVD version, and spend hours looking at the beautiful images, and listening to interviews with the photographers.

One favourite feature is publisher Brooks Jensen's podcasts, and in the most recent issue he included one called "Managing Fear." The interview was with photographer Camille Seaman; her images of icebergs are absolutely stunning.

This podcast felt particularly poignant today for me. I may not be afraid of dying, but there are still a few things in my life that I want to no longer fear. And just maybe one day you might see my images in *Lenswork*. That short bucket list of mine does include making a submission of my own!

QUESTION OF HEALTH
Tuesday, July 14, 2009

Somehow, I've found myself as a frequent recipient of on-line survey requests. Research companies send me questionnaires, I fill them in and in turn, I sometimes get bonuses as a thank you for my time; often cash bonuses. Given the amount of time that I spent in bed earlier this year, not a bad return for maybe twenty or thirty minutes of my time every week.

I'm completing fewer surveys lately; I just have better things to do with my time now that I'm mobile again. But one survey caught my attention a few days ago; the subject was Emergency Health Care. Interesting enough and I was happy to add my two cents hoping that my responses might end up in the hands of government agencies that might be in a situation to improve my country's emergency care (which I've unfortunately experienced firsthand to be lacking in many respects).

These surveys usually end with a few questions about my personal demographics. Age, marital status etc., but this last survey also asked about my current state of health.

Excellent/ Very Good/ Good/ Fair/ Poor

I answered, and was already a bit farther along in the survey before it hit me that I had answered "Good." If you've been reading this blog, you'll know that "Good" isn't exactly how one would describe my state of health!

I love it when I've forgotten what I'm dealing with. Blessedly, it happens often, but I had to laugh at how I answered that particular question. I'm grateful for the mental holidays I'm able to take from my illness; short or long.

For those kind friends who email us with messages of support and requests for updates, my hospital visit on Monday confirmed what I suspected; the pericarditis is still going strong. Higher doses of the same meds this week – I seem to be tolerating them fairly well, though, except for the steroid "moon face." (I'm afraid my vanity is kicking in a bit and I'm not crazy about going out in public these days.) But...I finally had a decent night of sleep (thanks to a little white pill that my doctor insisted I take so I'd get more than three hours sleep – it was bliss!)

MISSING MY CAMERA
Monday, July 20, 2009

After not working for almost five months (because of my leg surgery and subsequent recovery time) I was gnawing at the bit to get back to photographing. I didn't expect to be further delayed by that still very present case of pericarditis that has required copious amounts of prescription drugs, the side effects of which have further delayed my return to a full work schedule.

I'm beyond pleased these days when I'm feeling well enough to shoot a portrait session, but the reality is that I have to take this very slowly.

Thank goodness I have some very understanding clients! I had a fantastic session this past Sunday and felt on top of my game, and the photos came out really well. I paid for it by being quite tired for a few days afterwards. Totally worth it though for the few hours of bliss!

I'm hard on myself about this light work schedule. I love productive workdays, they give me great satisfaction. When I was well, I was always working on something photographic. Shooting, retouching, preparing images for the galleries that represent my work, and always learning. If I was on my computer, ninety-five percent of the time it had something to do with photography.

A few weeks ago, a good friend to our family called to check in on how we were doing. At the time I was having a rough day, and this sage friend told me that he did understand how much I must miss working, but that dealing with my illness was now my job. At the time I agreed in theory, but it's taken a few weeks for this to sink in. I'm starting to understand that my job now is to take the best possible care of myself that I can; to consult with my doctors, research my illness, and follow through with my treatments. And given how driven I can be with whatever I set my mind to, my current objective is to be the best patient I can be – with the goal of achieving the best possible outcome for this illness.

Hopefully photographing will be a bigger part of my life again soon, I miss it more than I can explain in words.

STEPPING OVER THE EDGE
Monday, July 27, 2009

Last week I was able to meet with a cardiologist who specializes in pericarditis. She's written on the subject for textbooks, medical journals etc., and from what I'm told, she knows pericarditis better than anyone in this country, I'm lucky to have such expertise on my side.

However, it was a bitter pill to swallow (no pun intended, but prednisone does taste AWFUL!) when she told me that five weeks on steroids haven't worked, and are not likely to do so if they haven't improved things by now. Saturday, I started on what's called a prednisone taper; one has to go down very slowly to allow the adrenal glands to start producing the hormone cortisol on their own again. This process will take months – best estimate, if all goes well, it'll be November before I can stop taking them.

I was very surprised that even a small drop from 40mg to 35mg affected me so significantly. It's been a rough few days. I tried a trip to the grocery store yesterday, and after only picking up half a dozen items, I was ready to sit down in the middle of the aisle and beg some strapping young lad to carry me through checkout and to my car. The tumour in my leg is throbbing, and the pericarditis is making sure I don't forget that it's there. I'm anxious that this might herald what the next few months might be like. I've heard that the taper can be worse than the steroid side effects; I'll just have to take this day by day.

This isn't the hardest part for me to digest. My team of doctors agree that it's time to treat my overall illness rather than the pericarditis on its own. Out come the big guns. Next week, I go back to the hospital to get my prescription for a drug called methotrexate. I'm struggling with this a great deal. I had decided early on that I wouldn't put myself through chemo for an incurable illness. Methotrexate, from what I've read, isn't as hard on the system as many other chemo drugs, but it still kills cells and can be unpleasant.

The reality is that in order for our government to fund the interferon (about 30K a year) that has seemed to benefit others with the same illness around the world, I have to try some more commonly used (and far less expensive) options before they'll consider my application.

I'm not entirely sure yet whether I'll agree to take this new drug. I have a lot of questions to ask at my next appointment. Maybe my docs will convince me – maybe they won't.

I value that my team of doctors do their best to educate me on my options, but they've said all along that decisions remain with me. From the very first visit, I was told that their mandate is to research options to slow down the progression of my illness, but above all to make sure that I'm as comfortable as possible.

Just how comfortable do I want to be?

IT HAD TO BE SAID
Friday, July 31, 2009

I hear, "It must be so frustrating that you've gone through four months of all these drugs, including six weeks of steroids that have wrecked up your system – all for nothing. The pericarditis is still there."

All for nothing. I feel like I've been run over by a bus most days (and look like it too), all for nothing. I've tried to remain optimistic throughout this process but when someone close to me pointed out that we're no further ahead four months later (I don't think it's unfair to say that I'm even a few steps further back), it was like a final puzzle piece falling into place. It had to be said, and I hadn't been able to say it to myself yet.

I've gone through the weekly disappointment when my doctor puts his stethoscope to my chest and again hears the squeaking and rubbing. Intellectually, I understand that my treatments have been unsuccessful and, in fact, are in the long term potentially doing more harm than good. It's a series of gambles when dealing with a rare illness, there's just not enough information out there to be able to follow a proven regimen. All of us dealing with this illness have to make the best decision we can, given what our doctors can tell us, what we've researched on our own, and often, listening to what our instinct tells us to do.

Hearing "all for nothing" has caused me to think even harder about upcoming treatment options. I mentioned in my last post that I'm supposed to start methotrexate next week. I still don't know if I'll do it. My body feels beaten up and I feel that I need a rest from all these meds (and I'm stuck with the steroids for at least another few months as the taper continues). We're still trying to address one symptom of my illness (pericarditis) and haven't even yet begun to treat my illness as a whole.

Do I have the luxury of giving myself a rest? Am I weak if I say I need to raise the white flag for a while? Friends and family who know me might say that this doesn't sound like me; they know me as a fighter who can always raise a smile. Right now, I don't even recognize the person I see in the mirror after the effects of steroids. Truth be told, I don't recognize the person inside of me at times either right now. I so desperately need a shred of good news to help boost me along on this journey.

For now, I'm going to step into a long, hot shower. Cleanse my body and my brain, and I'll be ready to face another day. And I will smile because despite "all for nothing" I still have much to be grateful for.

MY "BUCKET LIST" AND NEW FRIENDS
Wednesday, August 05, 2009

In the weeks following my diagnosis earlier this year of a disease that with great likelihood will give me a shorter-than-average life expectancy, I sat down to make my "bucket list." What was it that I most wanted to do while I was still able to do so?

First on my list – a trip to New York City with my husband and daughter. I've been lucky to travel to many major cities around the world, but never to the one that has intrigued me the most. Not just any trip to NYC, but a photographer's jaunt to the neighbourhoods that have come to fill my imagination with colours, sounds, and tastes ever since I can remember.

So, we set about making our plans. My family urged me to dream big. Stay in a nice hotel in Manhattan. Ask friends about great restaurants. Make a list of every spot I wanted to hit in the space of the week we would spend there. We planned to leave right after my daughter's 16th birthday, near the end of this month. This happens to be the same weekend as my birthday. We wanted to be home for both and be back in time for school to start. What a great way it would be to end the summer!

Unfortunately, things haven't worked out as we'd hoped. If you've been reading the posts, I've been dealing with a cardiac issue – but it's the side effects of numerous drugs that have wiped me out and left me unable to travel. Some days I feel lucky to make it to the mailbox around the corner – not quite what I had in mind for my grand adventures this summer.

APPLE TREES AND THE BIG APPLE
Thursday, August 13, 2009

Thank you to all who took time to share my disappointment about postponing our trip to New York. I appreciate the kind wishes. With my medication schedule, our trip won't be an option until sometime next year, at the earliest. I hear that spring in NYC is lovely and maybe we'll aim to be there when the cherry trees are in bloom. I do love cherry trees and get out each spring to our local botanical garden to photograph them; there's a softness to the flurry of light pink petals that captivates me.

It's been a difficult week. I started methotrexate and it's no picnic. On my second round, it knocks me out for about four days with nausea and weakness. I don't want to take this drug anymore, and will call my doctor tomorrow. I have to recognize that this illness has no standard treatment and we're experimenting right now. It's okay for me to say I don't want to partake in this particular experiment anymore, right?

I feel I have so many things to do and can't afford to lose the better part of a week to feeling this bad, when the "T-Trex" (as my husband calls this drug for all the nastiness it attacks me with) is meant to speed up my weaning off the prednisone. I'd rather take the longer wean with all the prednisone side effects than go through this. When I'm feeling poorly I often look out our back window to enjoy the small apple orchard that lies just beyond our yard. There's one large apple tree that's particularly close to our fence, and I've enjoyed watching it going through its seasonal changes.

The stark winter branches give way to fragrant spring blossoms. Then the leaves become thick and lush and then at this point of the summer, I start to see little red apples appearing amongst the greenery. This year is different. Part of the apple tree has died. A good third of the tree didn't produce any leaves this year. It's stark and barren compared to the rest of the tree (which I'm happy to see looks as healthy as ever). Although the owner of this orchard doesn't harvest the apples in the fall (they all fall to the ground, making for some very happy neighbourhood squirrels!) she does do a nice job of pruning all the trees. Why has she left this dead growth? Has she not noticed it yet, or is it not the right time of year to cut down the dead limbs?

Maybe she hopes that the tree will come back next year; that somehow the restorative potential of a winter's rest is just what is needed. The tree and I. Maybe we both just need rest; unfettered by poking, prodding, cutting, and medicating for a while.

I'd like to add some good news. Sick as I'm feeling this week, I wanted to keep my appointment with my orthopaedic surgeon yesterday. The bone tumour in my leg hasn't grown since my last x-rays three months ago. The next step is up to me – if I find the pain intolerable, my surgeon will take out the tumour and do an allograft (cadaver bone, hmmm... probably better if I don't think about the source too much!) with rods/pins/screws (my goodness, the thought of more metal in me!) to keep me mobile. Thankfully I have a high pain tolerance, and I'd much rather take pain meds than have the surgery. I'm grateful to have options.

THE CROWS MUST KNOW A LITTLE SOMETHING ABOUT STORMS
Thursday, August 20, 2009

It's been a summer with lots of rain, and recently, lots of thunderstorms. I love thunderstorms; I can sit and watch them for hours if they stick around that long.

There's a big storm skirting us just to the north with ominous, churning, dark clouds. It doesn't sound like we'll get the brunt of it, but I'm enjoying the skies and hearing the wind blow.

I've mentioned the apple orchard behind our house in a previous post and how much I like looking out my bedroom window at the changing trees. As I was checking out the clouds, I noticed five large crows huddled together on the branch of a dead apple tree. They're close enough that I can see their tail feathers bristling in the wind; they look cold (even though it's very hot and humid right now).

Why situate themselves out in the open, on a dead branch, taking the full force of the wind? There's shelter in the forest a mere ten-second flight away. I would think that the crows would be much better off there.

Maybe they know something that I don't about facing a storm full on.

During the time it took me to write this post, the storm has turned and hit us hard. It looks like those video clips of hurricanes in the tropics. The rain seems to be coming at us horizontally, yet those crows still sit out there (although I can hardly see them in the driving rain).

I think I'd still rather be in the forest. Sometimes it feels good to hide away from whatever onslaught is coming my way – just to get out of the driving rain for a short while. Think about it crows.

ANOTHER YEAR
Saturday, August 22, 2009

It's my birthday today. Forty-five years old. Most days I can't believe that I've spent so much time in this body. (Other days I'm feeling so much older – these drugs that I'm on have a way of making my body feel ancient!)

As people often do around their birthdays, I like to evaluate where I am in my life. Am I where I wanted to be at this age? Have I accomplished what I'd set out to do? When I worked in the corporate sector, we regularly evaluated our short and long-term objectives, and it was a good time to review my personal goals as well.

Short and long-term planning has taken on a whole new meaning for our family in the last year. Really, there is no plan anymore. Appreciate the good days – try to get through the rough ones with grace and good humour.

I woke up this morning feeling very grateful. The two people who mean more to me than I could ever tell you wished me happy birthday with big hugs. They're with me through the best and worst of this illness (and we know that this could be just the tip of the iceberg), celebrating when I feel great and always at my side when I think that I just can't do it alone. And I don't have to. I'm so very blessed.

We spend lots of time at the hospital and often notice how many patients don't have anyone with them. Some have difficulty with mobility, others are obviously distressed, and some just look lonely.

Having had a major health crisis many years ago when I was on my own, I think I can fully appreciate how much it can mean to have someone by your side when ill. I know it means everything to me now to be able to lean on my husband and daughter for support (and best of all to share when I'm feeling pretty good!)

Not that everyone wants to share details of their illness, but if you happen to have a friend who is not well and dealing with hospital visits, uncomfortable tests or treatments, please ask if you can accompany them sometime. I'd bet that in most cases, the patient has just felt too uncomfortable asking for a shoulder to lean on. It can make a bigger difference in their day than you might ever imagine.

FOOD, GLORIOUS FOOD!
Friday, August 28, 2009

I'm grateful for lots of things in my life.

Today I'm especially grateful that my illness generally doesn't affect my appetite – I LOVE good food! Yes, meds over the last few months have taken a toll on my stomach, but when I'm able to eliminate or reduce dosages on some of my meds, I'm so happy to be able to eat normally again. Update – the methotrexate is out of the picture. I was spending three or four days each week feeling very ill – unable to eat – and have decided that it's not an experiment I wish to continue.

This weekend, my niece is visiting and for dinner I made Penne a la Vodka (actually farfalle, I rarely follow recipes exactly). Double bonus – not only have I had more energy the last few days and felt up to cooking a meal, I also was able to enjoy the results with my family. My heart and stomach are both full!

I'll take my achy bones and other pain any day over tummy troubles. It's one wish I often make when thinking about my future – please let me continue to enjoy my meals.

A FAMILY AFFAIR
Thursday, September 03, 2009

At last week's appointment, we (my husband was there too, as always) had a frank discussion with my doctor about other stressors in my life besides my illness. Family issues unrelated to my health have been weighing heavily on me, and certainly aren't helping the situation. My doctor asked me if the usual trials of having a sixteen-year-old daughter added additional stress, and I was proud to say that S. has been the easiest child to raise. She and my husband can lift my spirits like no one else can, just by being in the same room.

Dealing with a serious illness is often said to be something that the whole family suffers, not just the patient. I believe it, and try to respect that at every turn. I realize that this is just as hard on my husband and daughter as it is on me, and felt that it was high time that my doctor and daughter met. There was one other reason to make this happen. As it turns out, my lead doctor and my daughter's grandfather on her dad's side grew up together in another country. Grandpa sadly passed away this spring, making this meeting yesterday more meaningful. I could see in my doctor's eyes how pleased he was to meet the granddaughter of his dear friend.

He had lots of questions for S. about school, future plans etc. Her grandmother had asked for a photo of the two of them together, which he graciously agreed to – and why not include Harvey? Harvey, as I should explain, is a $100K teaching cardiac-dummy donated to my medical team by a former patient, which replicates various cardiac conditions. My doctor cranked up Harvey for S., letting her listen to what a normal heart should sound like, and what my heart sounds like. ("Ooh Mom, that's weird!") S. was blown away – all she kept saying is "That's so cool!" to which he replied that it was indeed cool, and that it might have been the first time he'd used that particular phrase.

It was an important day for me. My interaction with my medical team has become very personal. I know that they care deeply about my wellbeing and are doing everything that they can to make me more comfortable. Having my daughter finally meet my doctor felt right, I know he wants my daughter's mother to be around as long as possible.

As scary as hospitals can be, I'm in a safe place on the 8th floor. I wanted my daughter to see for herself that I'm in very capable hands (and she tells me that this visit did indeed help her a lot with dealing with "our" illness).

PEEK A BOO, I SEE YOU!
Wednesday, September 09, 2009

Just one glance in the mirror this morning, as I brushed my teeth. Yes, I'm sure I saw it. A familiar shadow of cheekbone. After months of looking like I'm collecting acorns for the winter, from the steroids I've been taking, I actually had a moment of recognition for my old self.

Even though it has been months, every glance in the mirror (and I kept those to a minimum of late) had me searching for something more familiar. Not that the change has been that drastic (you'd likely still recognize me), but it has been unsettling. The expansion of my cheeks makes my eyes look so much smaller, and the sparkle in my eyes disappeared. A touch of makeup to disguise the dark circles helps me to feel a little bit better about how I look if I'm going out into the world, but I can't help feeling like I'm adorning someone else's face in the mirror.

And the belly! By early evening my stomach was getting so large that I'd easily pass for six-months pregnant. But the last few days, maybe five – even four months? Very slowly, some of the physical changes that the prednisone brought on are lessening.

Tapering off the prednisone hasn't been easy. Every drop is followed by a few days of unrelenting fatigue, aches, and dizziness. After that however, I enjoy a few days of relative well-being until the next dosage drop.

I'll still be tapering slowly into the New Year, but this morning's moment gives me hope that soon I won't look so ill anymore. I may be dealing with disease, but I don't want to look the part. I don't want the pity of strangers; I don't want anyone assuming that I'm not capable of whatever I set out to do. I want my body to reflect that I'm trying to do all the right things by eating healthfully, sleeping well, and respecting what my body is going through.

If I share the details of my illness with someone, I'll be absolutely delighted if they reply "How can this be? You look so well!" And I'll know that I'm doing the best I can to fight this; physically and emotionally. That's my new job, and I intend to be a stellar performer on this front.

BUT I WAS BEING CAREFUL!
Monday, September 14, 2009

Last February, I had a bone biopsy done on my right femur just above the knee. Then, three months of bed rest and crutches to allow the bone to heal a bit. However, a good portion of the tumour is still there, and I've had my heavy-handed warning from my surgeon – take it easy on that leg! No jumping, running, twisting – the bone is still unstable and a fracture could happen if I'm not careful.

The plan is to stabilize the bone later on with another surgery, and in my quest to keep working through my busy season of September – December, I'm hoping to hold off at least until the new year. (This surgery will keep me off my feet for about five months, I have to get mentally prepared for this!)

I've done a pretty good job of doing as the doctor said. I caught myself running the other day during a photo session (a two-year-old moves so darned fast!) and cursed under my breath – why can't I remember something so simple?

Last night, I wanted to take some laundry detergent to the basement. Two small jugs with handles, and being cautious, I held both in one hand so that I could hold the railing with the other. I have no idea what happened, but I found myself in a heap at the bottom of the stairs. (Only three steps, it could have been worse with all the stairs in our house.) I yelped in pain and both my husband and daughter came running. S. got an icepack and husband sat with me until I could test out my ankle. A bruise quickly appeared on the side of my foot. (I have steroids to thank for that, look at me the wrong way these days and I'm black and blue!)

As the evening progressed, it wasn't so much my ankle that hurt but the area where the tumour sits that was throbbing. Had I jarred my leg enough with the fall to do some damage?

Both ankle and surgery site are better this morning, but on some days I detest living like this; treating my body as if it were made of china; wondering what each day will bring; trying to live a normal life that most days is pretty far removed from normal. I want to be better, but know that I have to appreciate today because we have no idea whether tomorrow, next week, or next year will be any better than right now.

BECAUSE I'M SICK, I GET TO…
Wednesday, September 16, 2009

Buy myself a new lens for my camera.

I'm having a "Damn it, I'm sick" day. Of course I know that every day, but occasionally it hits me upside the head something fierce. Today, it was a good two hours after waking up, taking my first round of pills, looking at my moon face in the mirror as I brushed my teeth, and checking out the bruises on my foot from my fall the other day. (Still ticked off with myself about that!)

What set me off this morning was looking at some photos on another photographer's blog; absolutely lovely portraits of two young sisters. The photographer had written about how lovely these young ladies were, and how beautiful they would be when they grew up. My daughter is a lovely girl (albeit at sixteen more a young woman). What is she going to look like when she's my age? Boom – there it was. Unlikely that I'll be around to see for myself. Self pity ensued.

Around the same time this morning, I received an email from a favourite camera store about a lens that's on my wish list going on sale. Since my diagnosis, my husband has been after me to fulfill any desires on my wish list – and there are several lenses on that list.

On one hand, it seems pretty clear that this is a case of retail therapy. Feel bad – buy something. Not my usual modus operandi. (I'm really not a shopper, the last place I want to be is a mall.) But on the other hand – a new lens is an investment in my photography business, isn't it? That's positive thinking – soon I'll be working much more than I am now.

Negative self-pity and optimism about my capabilities to work in the future have cancelled each other out. New lens wins. Now I just have to wait patiently for my local camera store owner to let me know if he has the lens I want in stock!

EVERYTHING IS DIFFERENT NOW – I AM DIFFERENT NOW
Monday, September 21, 2009

I'm editing an entry that I wrote (but didn't post) a few days ago, and I'm glad that I waited. It's said that when one is writing when upset, it's best to put it aside and re-read before sending. A very wise piece of advice!

My original post came as a result of comments directed at me in the previous days from family members and others. (I'll clarify that they did not come from my immediate household. They ask nothing of me except to tell them what they can do to help me. I'm one lucky woman!) I'm learning that people close to me will deal with my illness in their own way, sometimes in a way that I find very hard to comprehend.

Don't get me wrong, I'm very grateful for all the care and concern that flows my way on a daily basis. As for those close to me – sometimes we may disagree; sometimes we both may say things that the other doesn't want to hear. But my life is not the same anymore. I'm making up new rules along the way that help me deal with what tomorrow brings, and I hope that sharing them brings some insight as to why I may react the way I do.

My New Rules:

I get to say "no" (something I've always had a hard time doing), and I don't need to explain myself. If you know me at all, you know that I want to do everything I could before I became ill, but I just can't. Sometimes I'll have to cancel plans – please don't make me feel bad for doing so. I'm already very unhappy about it.

I want to hear how you and your family are doing, but don't be upset if I don't reply to emails & phone calls as quickly as I used to. Sometimes I don't want you to hear in my words & voice that I'm having a rough day.

I appreciate all the very kind offers of help, and I need to learn to accept that help without feeling like I've failed because I couldn't do it myself. But I will still try to tackle it myself first!

Please don't tell me that you know that the diagnosis is a mistake and that I should see your doctor. This is not a mistake. (I've done my fair share of praying that it was.) I've got a large contingent of exceptional doctors who are working very hard to keep me here (and comfortable and pain-free) for as long as possible. And from my perspective, I'm glad that I know – it's far better than feeling unwell and not knowing why.

Although I've been quite self-conscious some days about the physical changes that prednisone has caused, I'm trying to be more comfortable with seeing friends and family. When you do see me please don't tell me how ill I look, I'm well aware of it. Take notice instead that I'm smiling and laughing. We're still doing a lot of that!

I'm very susceptible to infection as I undergo immunosuppressant therapy. Please don't visit if you're sick – you might get over your cold in a week but I'll likely be down much longer. "Just the sniffles" is too much of a risk right now, and not what I want to deal with on top of the drug side effects.

I've done enough speculating about what might have caused this disease and I'm done. Even if it was an environmental influence over which I might have had some control, I can't do anything about it now (and experts have no idea what caused this, so it's a moot point). Asking me if I ate my veggies as a child (and yes I did) makes me feel like you want to blame me for my illness. I'm not going there.

It's okay with me if you ask about my illness. But let's talk about lots of other things too!

My doctors explain my options, and I decide which drugs & treatments I want to go try. They completely support my decisions, allowing me to weigh the quality of my life against treatment side-effects, and I ask that you support my decisions as well.

My daughter and my husband are my top priorities. Period. They will get "first dibs" on whatever energy I have. I trust that you would make the same decision if you were in my shoes.

GRATITUDE
Monday, September 28, 2009

Despite my health issues, I consider myself a lucky woman and I do hope that comes across as you read my posts (failing the occasional rant like the one I let loose last week!)

Yesterday afternoon I was feeling good. So good that I was out photographing, taking a long walk at one of my favourite parks. So good that I was driving my daughter and her "young man" back and forth from the train station so that they could take in a ball game downtown. So good that I tackled an ambitious menu for dinner.

The train home from the game was running late by about a half hour, although I didn't find that out until I got to the station to pick up the kids. Having forgotten to bring my iPod, I grabbed a piece of scrap paper and a pen and started to scribble out some of the things for which I'm grateful. Here we go!

Although I've had to cut back considerably, I'm still able to get out with my camera. A client told me the other day that she can tell from my images that my work feeds my soul. I can't think of a greater compliment. She's absolutely right, and I'm blessed to be able to do work that I love so much.

I appreciate when I'm feeling good (or at least better than the day before). Those days are certainly not taken for granted.

Prednisone may have puffed up my face – but all my wrinkles disappeared!

I never have to go to a job interview again.

Not much upsets me these days. Not train delays, not broken dishes, not a chipped tub. (I was so proud for not being angry with myself when I took out a large chunk of enamel a few months back – it was my first "standing" shower in almost four months after my surgery and I dropped the shower head. Oh well!)

Thank goodness I was blessed with a very thick head of hair. My drug treatments cause a disturbing amount of hair to fall out when I wash it, but so far it's not been noticeable to anyone but me.

I get lots of hugs. Family, friends, acquaintances, and even the odd stranger who learns of my diagnosis show their support with a squeeze, and I love getting them.

Spending lots of time at home. I'm a homebody through and through; my frequent visits at the hospital make me appreciate our home so much more.

We try to eat healthy meals (my addiction to chocolate notwithstanding). I envision every stalk of broccoli I eat helping to strengthen me. I'm grateful that we can put healthy food in our cupboards and fridge, and that most days I feel well enough to cook for my family.

My car. It's a '97, but keeps going and going. I figure as long as I don't curse at it when it occasionally misbehaves it'll keep chugging along. I hope I didn't jinx it by writing that down!

This list could easily reach into the hundreds of things that I'm grateful for. This is just what came to me as I sat in my car, enjoying the warm sun on my face, listening to a favourite radio station – waiting to see the daughter I adore, taking us both home to the man who means the world to me. Life is good.

GRATITUDE CONTINUED
Wednesday, September 30, 2009

If you've been following my posts for a while, you'll know that it was my intention to remain anonymous for a number of reasons. I'd like to continue to protect the privacy of my family, and I'd rather my clients didn't know about my illness unless necessary, so I don't mention the name of my company.

However, there are two details that I'm ready to share for an important reason, which I'll explain in a moment.

1. I live just outside of Toronto, Canada. I'm being treated by the Toronto University Health Network, a group of hospitals affiliated with the University of Toronto medical school.

2. I've been diagnosed with a rare illness called Erdheim-Chester Disease.

The reason I've chosen to share this information today is gratitude. My lead doctor, Dr. Herbert Ho Ping Kong is being honoured for his exceptional contributions to the medical community, particularly as an educator. He, together with another of my doctors, established The Centre for Excellence in Education and Practice (CEEP) at Toronto Western Hospital; this is the team that takes such great care of me.

As part of the celebration later this month honouring Dr. Ho Ping Kong (referred to as HPK by many of his colleagues), donations are being accepted to fund important projects for his team. (Harvey the cardiac dummy needs skin!) I'm usually uncomfortable soliciting donations, but many of you have asked what you can do to help and unless I mention this, you won't know about it!

Things could have gone so very differently for me after finding the bone tumour almost a year ago. Trust your instincts, and be your own advocate. We all deserve the best medical care that our country has to offer, and I'm grateful to be a recipient.

CONSUMED OR OBLIVIOUS
Thursday, October 15, 2009

I had a good day today physically, which allowed me to go on a drive searching for photo opportunities. The fall colours are coming in nicely and the roads are quiet during the week, which makes pulling over to the side to take photos much easier. These drives usually provide me with an opportunity to forget about my health issues for a few hours. Not so much today.

Not five minutes before finding a delightful gaggle of geese in a farm driveway, I came across at least half a dozen turkey vultures attacking what was left of a raccoon on the side of the road. My mind was going to all the wrong places today from the get-go, and seeing the vultures ravage the carcass caused me to think about how my illness lays little mercy upon me these days.

Then the geese. I've passed this particular farm many times and often hear the geese honking, but this was the first time that they'd put themselves in view. I thought about how much I'd like to fly away and leave my illness behind, if even just for a day, for a most welcome respite. But it's impossible to escape.

Taking meds four times a day sets the tone. I have to eat with this pill, don't eat with that one – don't even think of drinking any alcohol while on the other. I think what set me off today was forgetting my morning pills; the most important ones not to forget. I was an hour late – I had actually forgotten for several hours after waking today that I was ill, and I was simultaneously delighted at having put it out of my mind and at the same time scared. My pharmacist had been so specific about not getting off-track with my morning doses. No harm done, it was only an hour off schedule – but what if I'd gone on my long drive today without having remembered? What if I'd had a reaction when I was on one of those lonely country roads?

It's sometimes just all too much, too complicated, and it at times leaves me resentful.

DOING LAUNDRY – MY BIG ACCOMPLISHMENT
Monday, November 09, 2009

A few weeks back I had a great week. I was able to photograph several families, and got quite a bit of personal shooting in too – during the best week for fall colours no less!

Then I crashed. I hate, hate, and hate prednisone. Did I say how much I hate it? I'm in that phase where my adrenal glands are supposed to kick in and work on their own again to deliver cortisol as required, but they don't seem to want to do that. I'm not a lazy person, but apparently my adrenal system doesn't know that.

I've been grounded. Even taking a shower seems like a monumental task on most days, and my proudest moment has been mustering enough energy to do a few loads of laundry. Although the steroids didn't seem to affect my moods negatively in the first few months, I feel overwhelmed by sadness on some days. This is so very hard on my family and I feel terrible for putting them through all this. This isn't like me, and I'm wondering where I've gone.

I debated this morning whether to call my doctor. I'm pretty sure that he'd tell me to up my dosage and try tapering again in another week or so, but I'm really determined to get off this poison as soon as possible and want to try sticking it out for a few more days.

Please forgive me if I'm being a bit cranky and not replying to emails quickly. I'm feeling sorry for myself and finding it difficult to be happy about anything right now. I'm going to blame the steroids because despite everything we're going through, I know there's a happy person underneath all this – I'm just waiting somewhat impatiently for her to emerge again.

TRYING TO CRAWL BACK
Wednesday, November 25, 2009

I haven't posted here in a while. I wish I could say it's because I've been feeling great, "out and about" (my Canadian is showing!) and living my life.

It's been tough, and when things get tough I get quiet. When I was in the throes of labour, delivering my daughter sixteen years ago, not a peep out of me. Other women delivering that night could be heard yelling and screaming (not to mention cursing!) down the hallway, but I wasn't making a sound. Of course it hurt like nothing else ever had, but the most I could muster was a quick "yup" and "nope" when asked questions by the nurses and doctors. Just the way I operate, like a wounded animal I just want to crawl away when I'm in pain or ill.

The prednisone taper hasn't been going well. I ended up jumping back up on my dosage after a disastrous week. I shouldn't, but I consider it a personal failure when I can't cope with the side effects of this drug. It's become a battle of me against the steroids and I'm determined to win (defined by successfully tapering off this stuff).

I'll keep at this, but I've decided not to taper again for another three or four weeks. I was booked over eighteen months ago to photograph a milestone event for a very dear client in mid-December, and I won't let my illness get in the way. Mind you, I'm not ignorant to the fact that ECD has a mind of its own and I've retained a back-up photographer just in case illness wins on that day. But I've been praying every day that I'll be given a twenty-four hour respite to the worst of the symptoms so that I can capture on film the abounding love that this family shares.

Please keep your fingers crossed for me; I badly need to do this. I'm so very tired of letting family and friends down this last year when I can't follow through with plans because I'm not doing well. It will be the last family event that I photograph; this is tough to accept. Going forward I will only be booking work if the client understands that I may need to reschedule and unfortunately that doesn't work with sessions that must take place on a particular date.

On the hospital front – my doctor was featured in an article in the *Globe and Mail* this past weekend. I'm one lucky gal to be his patient. And he understands and supports my desire to shoot this last "biggie." Together (with my family) we pick my battles.

WHAT NEXT?
Thursday, December 17, 2009

A few weeks ago I wrote about my hopes to be able to photograph a very special event this past weekend. The family booked me eighteen months ago, and at that time I had no idea of the challenges that lay ahead.

I shared the details of my health situation with my client a few months ago, and insisted that they permit me to book another photographer, given that my health was increasingly inconsistent. They'd hear nothing of it, and said that they were confident that I would be feeling great. I did book another photographer on retainer; the thought of letting them down was too uncomfortable.

We worked with my doctor to adjust my meds to give me the best chance of being able to fulfill my commitment, and I'm very happy to report that it worked! I felt in top form last Saturday, and for almost nine hours/3000 shots later – I documented a very special day in this special family's life. I'm truly grateful!

However, I was somewhat surprised to feel quite down the next day. For almost a year I've been focused on being okay for December 12th, discussing it frequently with my doctor (who fully supported the med adjustments), and I had friends and family rooting for me. But now it's over, and I'm feeling a bit lost. What do I work towards now?

There are the milestones such as my daughter's graduation from high school, our five- year wedding anniversary and more – but I need something else that focuses on a personal accomplishment. Not too far off, but further away than the next few months. The rest of my prednisone taper has to happen first. From my experience of the last few months, I know that this could be a rough ride – I've been so happy to stop the taper for a few weeks to feel somewhat normal for a bit.

It definitely won't be photographing an event – I can't go through that stress again of praying to be well enough for a date that can't be rescheduled if I'm ill.

This is going to take some thought. I'm thinking, and I'll let you know what I come up with.

AND WHAT IS NEXT?
Tuesday, January 05, 2010

We got back a few hours ago from a visit to the hospital. Nothing much to report, I'm continuing on the prednisone taper. My third attempt at dropping from 8 to 7 mg actually went quite well over the last few weeks and I'm planning another drop tomorrow to 6 mg! Wish me luck – we're at that crucial stage over the next while to see if my adrenal glands can be cajoled back into action after being suppressed by the steroids.

My doctor said the next visit will include a serious discussion about what comes next in my treatment plan. Likely medication candidates will be Gleevac (chemo) or Interferon Alpha (not chemo, but somewhat similar impact on the system/side effects). It's been a difficult time trying a myriad of treatments over the last nine months, and I'm "side-effected out." It's just felt like too much at times and I need a break. We anticipate another three to four months of steroid tapering – which should end just about the time that the weather starts to get nice again. More than anything I'd like to feel the sun on my face, take long walks with my family (long being a relative term, I'll start with treks around the block – steroid therapy has kicked my behind and I need to build up some strength again), and photograph again! With staying indoors not feeling great, I missed last spring/summer entirely (but apparently so did most of Ontario, it was the summer that wasn't) and I feel that I have lots of catching up to do.

Last post, I wrote about wondering what was next. What could I look forward to? Still working on that, but it's become clear to me – first priority is to enjoy some time with my family. (Hopefully we can take that New York City trip that we had to pass on last August.) Second is one (or several) photography projects. A few ideas are brewing; I'll share once I've decided on what I'd like to do. I miss holding my camera in my hands and can't wait to get out there again.

LETHARGIC
Saturday, January 30, 2010

Fatigued. Spent. Dog-tired. Exhausted. Weary. Sapped. Weakened. Beat. Done for. Petered out. Drained. Languid. Conked out. Shot. Depleted.

And much too tired to alphabetize this list. You know I wanted to.

Down to 5 mg of prednisone, and getting a whole lot of nothing done these days.

AS LONG AS IT'S NOT THE "C" WORD
Wednesday, February 03, 2010

Not quite as tired today as I have been the last week, and getting quite a bit of work done. (It's not the "running after small children taking their picture" kind of work that I would prefer to be doing, it's image retouching on my computer but work nonetheless.)

I had an appointment to have a bone density scan done at a local hospital a few weeks ago, and a comment that the technician offhandedly offered continues to bother me. I was having the scan done to see if the steroids have caused bone density loss, and she asked if my medical status had changed since my last scan two years ago. I briefly updated her on Erdheim-Chester Disease, and mentioned that she might see a bone lesion on my femur on the scan – and not to be alarmed, I was aware of it.

The technician asked if it was cancer. I said no, ECD isn't officially classified as cancer; it's usually described as an auto-immune illness, yet is often treated by oncologists. And it has a poor prognosis. She told me that I should consider myself very lucky that it wasn't cancer, and thank goodness I could look forward to a long life unlike many cancer patients. Hello? Were you listening to me?

I've gotten this reaction a few times. As long as it isn't cancer. How fortunate for you!

Frankly, a fair number of cancers have a much better prognosis than ECD. And most have a course of treatment to follow. ECD doesn't have this yet. Some positive development with some drugs, but it appears to be mostly trials and investigative attempts at this time. Nothing close to a cure (and I'll be happy to correct this should one of the many researchers working on this illness let us know about any new developments!)

When my orthopaedic oncologist first saw my scans last year, his guess was that the lesion was first stage bone cancer. He felt confident that if this were the case it could be successfully and quickly treated. I can't tell you how often in the last year I've wished that this had been the correct diagnosis.

CATCHING UP...AND DOWN AGAIN
Tuesday, February 23, 2010

Last post, I mentioned that I'd had a bone density test, and I'm not at all pleased about the result. The scan indicated that I'd had significant bone density loss since my last test – thank you again steroids! You're the gift that just keeps on giving.

I dropped a few days ago to 4 mg and it's pretty hard to stay awake. I was supposed to go into Toronto to have a check-up on my pacemaker this morning, but there was no way that I would have been capable of manoeuvring myself through the train and subway system today – just that dopey. That's been rescheduled a few weeks out when I hope to be far more coherent again.

I'm getting frustrated with my lack of progression on a number of work and personal projects – I don't understand why I can't just will myself to stay awake, will myself to feel better, will myself to feel less pain. I'm working very hard on my "mind over matter" approach to my illness but there are times I just have to admit that wanting to feel better isn't enough.

MORE DRUGS - ONE I'M ACTUALLY HOPING FOR!
Wednesday, March 10, 2010

I find that I'm fighting an overall sense of dismay with my illness. How dare it not respond to all the meds I've taken so far? What nerve!

A few meds that I know I'll be adding soon:

- A beta blocker. My heart rate has been out of control of late, and yesterday's data download from my pacemaker confirmed it. Over 8,000 episodes of a heart rate over 140 beats per minute over the last six months. Most have no correlation to exercise, stressful situations etc. A good number in the middle of the night – I know my dreams are a little wacky but that's a bit much! Somewhat ironic since I had the pacemaker implanted almost six years ago to deal with bradycardia – a very slow heart rate. That's still happening too, dropping suddenly to below 50 beats per minute on average about 15-20 times a day. My heart is the queen of cardiac roller coaster rides! It's time to exit that amusement park.

- And here's the drug I'm excited about. Kineret. I'm keeping everything crossed that I can cross that I'm given the chance to try it. Several other ECD patients have reported that Kineret has greatly reduced their bone pain, (which for me has been getting significantly worse over the last months). An exciting prospect for this alone, but what really got me hyped was reading about a study whereby three patients who had been dealing with pericarditis had almost immediate resolution after the first dose. I immediately sent off the article to my doctor, who is now discussing the drug with his team. I'm on pins and needles waiting for my appointment next Tuesday to find out if we can go down this path. It would need to be approved for off-label use (it's meant for moderate to severe rheumatoid arthritis), and if approved then we'd need to find funding. (I've read that the cost is between $15-20K per year in Canada.)

Kineret is injected daily; both my husband and daughter are on board to give me an injection when it's time to rotate to a location that I can't reach. I'd be able to do the other spots myself. I'm getting ahead of myself though. It's hard not to, I'm feeling rather beaten down by the pain, fatigue, and general unwellness of late. Just when I'm feeling better for a few days the pericarditis acts up again, letting me know who's boss. Time for a mutiny, don't you think?

PATIENCE, MY DEAR – PATIENCE
Wednesday, March 17, 2010

Last post, I wrote about my hope to be able to try a new drug – an experimental one. I visited the hospital yesterday for one of my very frequent check-ups, and to discuss the possibility of giving Kineret a try. There's more to this process that I had thought!

In theory, my doctors believe that Kineret might be of help with not only reducing my bone pain, but also with slowing down the progression of my illness. However, there are some serious risks with this drug that need to be further investigated. Kineret is an "interleukin-1 receptor antagonist" – part of the "biologic response modifier" family of treatments. This drug increases the risk of infection, and also carries a small risk of causing lymphoma, among other side effects.

Kineret is intended to treat moderate to severe rheumatoid arthritis – and that's where the complication comes in. Researchers don't know what the implications are for Erdheim-Chester Disease, in which white blood cells already don't know how to behave properly, so nobody really knows how they'd react to this treatment. Just a handful of ECD patients have tried this, and only for a short time – far too soon to determine any long-term implications.

My medical team will be doing further research, including consulting with an oncologist at a cancer centre in the United States, who has been doing advanced research on interleukin treatments. If that's a go – then we seek government approval to use this drug for an illness it was otherwise intended for. Then, funding – this isn't cheap!

Am I still on board? Yes. Do I understand that this could go either way? Yes. I know that there's no cure, but I'm desperate for a better quality of life for at least a while. I need to hope for something good, because some nights when I'm feeling quite awful it can be hard to envision a better day tomorrow.

Yesterday was a pretty good day. So is today. I'm feeling greedy; I want more days like these.

TIME FLIES. OR NOT
Thursday, March 25, 2010

Today is the first anniversary of getting my diagnosis of Erdheim-Chester Disease. How clearly I remember our concern of being called back to the orthopaedic oncologist's office after having had an initial all-clear on cancer just a week or so earlier. The relief of the previous week turned to fear – who gets called back after being told that a tumour isn't cancerous? Had the pathologist made an error?

I'm really not sure where my mind is at today. Today is one of my tough days, and even lifting my arm above my head seems like a monumental effort. What will the next year bring? Will I see any improvement – will I have access to the drug that just might improve my quality of life?

The waiting is doing my head in right now.

TOO MUCH EXCITEMENT FOR ONE WEEK
Wednesday, March 31, 2010

To some degree, I measure my health status by the frequency of my visits to the emergency room. I made it to over ten months without, but last Friday broke my streak.

It's been a tough time with pain and breathing problems, but Friday night was different. I'd had a very quiet day, nothing strenuous (my usual trigger). Just hanging out on the couch watching TV.

Suddenly it felt like my chest was freezing up. No air in or out for a few seconds. It passed. This has happened before. It's alarming for a few seconds but then it's over. But this time it happened again a few minutes later. Then again, with less time in between and more forcefully...until I could hardly stand up. When I have an arrhythmia it often helps if I make myself cough, but this wasn't working. Nothing seemed to help, and it felt like I was suffocating. Is this what drowning would feel like?

My husband called 911, and a fabulous group of paramedics and EMTs showed up at our front door within a few minutes. Thankfully, after oxygen, several doses of nitroglycerin, and a few hours in the ER, my breathing was back to usual. Still a bit difficult but nowhere near as frightening as it had been hours earlier.

This episode scared the heck out of us. I don't want to think negatively, but I suspect this might not be the only time this will happen. Having Erdheim-Chester Disease firmly entrenched in my heart is going to cause problems. Lately it's been a wild ride of low to very high heart rates, low to high blood pressure – my heart just can't seem to decide what to do. Can't blame it for having a hissy fit last Friday I suppose.

I talked to my specialist today and he told me that I probably won't be prescribed the drug I'd been hoping to try (Kineret), that the team would rather I try a chemotherapy drug that has been effective for slowing down the progression of lung cancer. (I don't have lung cancer, but then again ECD treatment is hit and miss, maybe it might help to reduce my symptoms.)

I'm just not happy about that prospect. I'm digging up all the info I can find on both drugs so that I can make an informed decision about the chemo option. But I REALLY don't want chemo. Wish me luck over the coming weeks – my doctor today instructed me to go cold turkey on the prednisone. 3 mg to nothing. On one hand, I'm thrilled at the prospect of getting off of this stuff; more side effects than I can count on all fingers and toes. On the other hand, dropping 1 mg at a time had been difficult; the withdrawal process has been rough. But looking at the big picture, I think I'd rather take a big hit of withdrawal symptoms for a few weeks rather than keep dragging this out over the next few months. Plus vanity plays into this a bit – I'm tired of carrying this extra weight – and the last thing I want to do is buy warm weather clothing for this larger size. So here I go.... three, two, one – deflate!

ANXIOUS FOR A DECISION
Monday, April 26, 2010

I've been quiet for the last few weeks, at least as far as posting goes. Truth is, I'm feeling pretty rotten and it's an effort to sit in front of my computer. And I haven't felt like sharing. I'm thrilled to finally be off the steroids (about 2.5 weeks and counting) but as my doctor predicted, the pericarditis is not only acting up – it's screeching at the top of its lungs at me.

Last night was pretty scary. I'd say that it was the worst chest pain so far in the more than two years since the pericarditis was detected. And not just my chest – the pain wraps itself around to my back, my left arm, and up into my neck. I feel like I'm being strangled by a boa constrictor that just won't loosen its grip. And of course it was worst at 2 a.m. - that wicked hour when all is much too quiet, leaving the imagination to run wild. I'd not yet slept, though I'd gone to bed three hours earlier. And then the tears started. And I don't cry easily from pain. Or maybe it was sheer desperation that nothing has eased the pain and the difficulty of breathing. All these drugs and nothing good has come of them.

I have my next hospital visit tomorrow. I spoke with Dr. HPK earlier today to let him know of my discomfort, to see if he wanted to schedule any additional tests. He let me know that the review of meds continues, he's not yet ready to offer the next treatment. His team is leaning towards chemo, and I'm hoping to try one of the new biologic meds. (Kineret, which I mentioned in my last post.) In the meantime, I've doubled up on my current meds to try to ease the pain (and I'm very happy to report that I'm feeling better this evening than I did last night).

This waiting is nearly intolerable. I'm on-line reading up on the results of drug trials of both drugs being reviewed, asking myself which side effects I'm willing to bear. On one hand, I'm grateful that the Internet can offer us so much information, but then again maybe it would be better if I had less to digest at the moment. And I wait.

FINALLY!
Friday, April 30, 2010

Today I finally received the phone call that I've been waiting months for – a decision on which treatment I can try next.

The drug of choice is Enbrel, a biologic medication. It's related to Kineret, but according to my medical team, it's a safer alternative. Not without risks, but my doctors have thoroughly reviewed the pros and cons of several potential meds to find the one that is the best fit for me.

It's likely to be a month or more before I can begin treatment. There'll be appointments with specialists and discussions with our insurance company. (This stuff is REALLY expensive!) Maybe even the chance that the pharmaceutical company can give us a break too. If I ask very nicely? I'm off to start the paperwork!

IN A HOLDING PATTERN
Thursday, May 20, 2010

I love getting mail. Yup, even the bills – crazy me. And there's a letter I'm anxiously awaiting, a decision from our insurance company, letting us know whether they'll cover a portion of the cost of Enbrel.

It's been a busy time. First I met with a new doctor, a rheumatologist who was the one to give the final approval for me to try this drug. Lots of tests afterwards to make sure that I didn't have additional pre-existing conditions that would take me out of the running for this experiment.

Next – a slew of paperwork for the insurance company: The application itself, with supporting letters from my doctors to explain their reasoning for wanting to try this drug on me. The letters were forwarded to me first, and then in turn sent to the insurance company. Not going to lie, those letters were hard to digest. It's one thing to be told you have a serious illness, it's another to see it all spelled out on paper. And I do mean all spelled out – the extent of my illness along with the prognosis. Ouch. Plus we had to attach a list of all the drugs prescribed by my pharmacy over the last year – it was disconcerting to see just how long that list was.

Next, discussions with the pharmaceutical company. They have quite an extensive support program for patients taking Enbrel. Unfortunately

I'm not eligible for many services because I'll be using Enbrel "off-label" (for a condition it's not intended to treat). But, I can speak to a nurse 24/7 if I have any questions or concerns and that's reassuring. Plus, they sent me a pretty neat welcome kit with a travel cooler bag (Enbrel needs to be kept refrigerated), alcohol wipes, and a sharps container for used syringes. And an instructional DVD – but I refuse to watch it until I know for sure that this is a go.

Then today, I received a call from a nurse at my hospital who'll be teaching me how to self-inject, and will supervise my first few shots to ensure that I'm doing it correctly.

And everything now rides on whether my insurance company will help us out. So every day I wait to see what the mail brings. And I have a strong feeling that this drug will do good things. Fingers crossed, toes crossed. I'd even cross my wonky white blood cells if I knew how; that's the least those little devils could do for all the trouble they're causing me!

ENDING UP HAPPY
Tuesday, May 25, 2010

Still waiting on that insurance letter, but in the meantime...

For those of you who know me personally, you're aware that most of my forty-five years have not been easy ones. You'd wonder how so many bad things could happen in one person's life, in fact – my dear friend Deb for years urged me to write a book about my experiences. Childhood traumas that no one should have to endure, leaving home at a very young age to fend for myself, a first marriage that should never have happened (except for the tremendous gift of a daughter whom I treasure), and health issues that never seem to let up.

A frightening path is ahead. If I let myself think about it, I could put myself into a right state, but I try hard not to. I'd like to share with you the thoughts that keep me sane.

I am loved by two people who mean everything to me. Both came to me in the later years of my life, and I truly don't know what I'd do without my husband and daughter. Someone upstairs has been looking out for me in sending me the gift of unconditional love.

I believe in karma. I've tried hard to do the right thing and take the high road and I trust that I will get the odd break. And I do.

I'm getting much better at letting go; not sweating the small stuff. That's all I'll say on that subject right now, but it's been a huge transition for me!

Finally being able to pursue my passion. As I child I was discouraged from following my heart, but almost ten years ago after yet another health crisis, I decided that I could no longer keep plugging away at a career that didn't make my heart sing. My income tanked significantly, and I had numerous setbacks – but I've been able wake up each morning excited about what I'm doing. Even though for the last year and half it's been impossible to photograph as much as I would have wanted to – I can still create images in my head whenever I want. Really, I live and breathe this stuff!

I choose to be happy. Most days. It's really unusual for me not to be happy. I choose to be thankful for the blessings in my life – primarily for those two very special people, and for the chance to follow my heart. I should add that had it not been for giving up my corporate career, I wouldn't have met my husband. It was just meant to be!

Believing that a happy ending is possible. Understanding that a happy ending doesn't have to include a cure for my illness, or living to a ripe old age. I choose to see my happy ending accommodating these challenges.

THE DAY STARTED OFF WELL ENOUGH
Tuesday, June 01, 2010

Insurance application denied.

The reason given is that ECD is not on the list of illnesses that Enbrel has been proven to help. I don't know why they had us (and my medical team) jump through hoops to make a case for this drug, when all along they knew that they wouldn't approve it.

Maybe this isn't completely rational (and I'll admit that I'm not feeling terribly sensible at this moment), I'm feeling that a complete stranger has made a decision as to whether my life is worth investing in. They don't care that I have a teenage daughter I haven't finished raising, that I've only been married just a few short years to a man who has brought such happiness and security to my life, and that I'm getting worse as time goes on and desperate for a chance to be in less pain.

I'm a victim of a set of hard and fast rules that don't make allowances for a very rare illness that doesn't have a set treatment plan. No room to bend for something that falls away from the ordinary. (Not that other serious illnesses are to be taken lightly, just that having more people suffer a particular affliction means a much better opportunity to have outrageously expensive drugs financed.)

I need a good cry and will get ready to look at this with fresh eyes in the morning. But tonight, I need to let myself feel sad.

WAITING AGAIN
Sunday, June 20, 2010

I mentioned a post back that our insurance company had refused coverage for an experimental drug. My husband (not one to give up easily) launched an appeal to have them reconsider their decision. Still a big fat no, despite his rather compelling plea to let me give this a try. They've made it very clear that their company will not fund any treatments for Erdheim-Chester Disease since nothing has been proven to help. Same position coming from our government health agency.

Dr. HPK hasn't given up hope; he's approaching the drug company, as well as seeking out alternate potential donors. I won't be giving up hope either until he raises the white flag.

It makes me wonder however how anyone who isn't wealthy can invest hope in a new treatment. I realize this isn't the case with all diseases, but it comes back again to not having enough ECD patients to make it worth anyone's while. While I say my prayers for anyone who is ill, I'm wishing extra hard for anyone unlucky enough to be dealt a very rare condition. This certainly has been a learning experience in so many ways.

Speaking of learning, I've found it quite difficult to explain exactly what ECD is to people who've not heard of it – which is basically everybody. I dread going to any practitioner who asks if there have been any changes in my health status since my last appointment. Yesterday I came across a description of Erdheim-Chester Disease that is succinct and I believe, fairly clear for the layperson to understand. I think I'm going to take a suggestion from the ECD support group, print this one out and give it to anyone who needs to understand what's happening to my body.

Erdheim-Chester disease is a very rare disorder in which histiocytes, cells that help fight infection, multiply and infiltrate bone marrow and then spread throughout the body.

The disease was first described in 1930 by Jacob Erdheim and William Chester. Since then, about 100 cases have been documented in medical literature. Erdheim-Chester disease most often affects adults in their 40s and 50s and is more common in men than women. There's no known cause.

Erdheim-Chester disease is not a cancer, but histiocytes multiply and spread with the ferocity associated with an aggressive cancer. This progressive disease first affects the skeletal system, causing an abnormal increase in bone density and bone growths called lesions. Bone pain is often the first symptom, usually presenting in lower more often than upper extremities.

As the disease progresses, manifestations can be found in the nervous system, eyes, pulmonary system, heart, lymph nodes and kidneys. Symptoms can include:

- *Changes in gait*
- *Changes in sensory ability*
- *Sleep disturbances*
- *Diabetes insipidus, a disorder characterized by intense thirst and by the excretion of large amounts of urine*
- *Vision problems*
- *Laboured breathing or shortness of breath*
- *Heart failure*
- *Kidney damage*

Given the wide range of symptoms and its rarity, the disease is easily misdiagnosed. Early on, Erdheim-Chester disease can be confused with Paget's disease, a condition that affects how bone breaks down and rebuilds.

A diagnosis of Erdheim-Chester disease can be confirmed with tissue or bone biopsies that show proliferation of histiocytes, cells that are normally inactive and immobile.

Treatment options are somewhat limited. Because the disease is rare, researchers and doctors simply haven't had the experience needed to find effective treatment options. Options used include chemotherapy, immunotherapy and corticosteroids.

Treatment can help delay progression of the disease for a time, but the outlook for patients with Erdheim-Chester disease isn't good. At five years, the overall survival rate is 41 percent.

Thanks to Dr. Castle at the Mayo Clinic for this posting.

A couple of small corrections. To my knowledge, there are closer to 300 known cases (a very select club I belong to), and ECD is as yet unclassified. In the future it may be designated a cancer, or an autoimmune disease (or just as a plain old weird aberration of nature?)

SHARING FANTASTIC NEWS!
Tuesday, July 06, 2010

Thanks to the considerable and determined efforts of my doctors, the drug company has agreed to donate a three-month supply of Enbrel. This news came a few hours ago with a phone call from Dr. HPK (who interrupted his vacation to follow up on the progress of the appeal).

Since hearing the news I've had a huge grin on my face – along with more than a few happy tears. Although I've been trying hard not to think about it, worries about how to finance this drug have dominated my thoughts of late and it's such a huge relief to hear the decision. And of course a much bigger relief that the answer was yes!

We don't know if Enbrel will help, I'll be the very first Erdheim-Chester Disease patient to try it. However, I'm beyond grateful for the opportunity to see if it offers any improvement. If it works to slow down the progression of my illness, we'll need to look at avenues for financing of the drug beyond the next three months. But we can't worry about that right now; we just have to hope that this stuff helps!

I'll hear more next Monday when my doctor is back from vacation, and I'll keep you updated. I know that many of you have offered your good wishes and prayers for good news. I know that they all helped, and I thank you!

SMALL VICTORIES
Sunday, July 11, 2010

In a world where it's mostly one step forward, two steps back I have to revel in every success, no matter how small and seemingly insignificant to most. My health continues to deteriorate slowly but I still to try to keep my chin up and remain optimistic. Tomorrow I'll find out when I can begin my three-month trial with Enbrel (might be as early as this week!) and we have high hopes in this household that it will help with the pain, ease the pericarditis, and let me feel somewhat normal more often.

It's been three months since I stopped taking steroids (huge success on its own there!) and I'm noticing that its effects are starting to wear off. I'm not as fatigued, my muscles ache less, I have lost the "moon face," and have started to lose a bit of the twenty pounds I'd gained.

However, the leg and cardiac pain unfortunately continue to worsen. Weird thoughts enter my mind when I wake from the pain during the night. If I went into the bathroom, couldn't I just cut my leg off with the nail scissors? What if I just willed my heart to stop for a few hours, wouldn't that give it a much needed rest for a few hours? Nights are sometimes just a bit too frightening.

Back to the days – although I'm not allowed to do any aerobic exercises (and me being me, I've had to test that several times – and it does indeed send my heart pattern into a tailspin every time), I've been able, in the last few weeks, to get back to doing Wii Fit a few times a week. The gentle stuff; balance, strength, and yoga. Not only do I enjoy it, it does seem to be helping to tone up all the areas on me that seemed to have gone out of control while on steroids. I don't look six months pregnant anymore – those steroids seem to love settling into the belly!

I'll keep you updated on the Enbrel. Although we're thrilled that I've been given the opportunity to try it – there's a small part of me that jumps ahead to the end of the three-month trial. What if this doesn't help or God forbid – makes things even worse? What next? And I then have to bring my mind back to positive thoughts – this WILL help and I'll be able to get back to doing some of the things I love to do. Keeping everything crossed that is crossable!

NOTHING NEW
Thursday, July 22, 2010

Last week I met with Dr. HPK in Toronto. He let me know that the supply of Enbrel arrived and was in the hands of the doctor who through some pretty deft negotiations, obtained the trial dose for me. I had to repeat a bunch of the baseline tests since a few months had passed since we first set out on this path. Normally I'm fairly patient in the long waits for blood tests, x-rays etc. but that day I seemed to have little tolerance. Maybe all this waiting, testing, and more waiting is getting to me.

Now we wait once again. That drug is sitting in a refrigerator somewhere in the bowels of Mt. Sinai hospital and I await the call that the rheumatologist, my injection instructor, the paperwork etc. are all lined up and I can head into the hospital for my first dose.

Ring, you darned phone – ring.

Update: Fifteen minutes after sending this post out, a call from the hospital came in! Playing telephone tag at the moment, but it's the coordinator of the clinical trial who would like to speak with me. Let's hope we can get things lined up for next week.

DOING A (MODIFIED) HAPPY DANCE!
Wednesday, July 28, 2010

It was two long weeks of knowing that my donated Enbrel was waiting for me at the hospital, numerous unreturned phone calls to the coordinator (and I missed the one call that did come in last week while I was in the shower) – and finally, today I got the call that I'll be starting my clinical trial for Enbrel – tomorrow! (Thanks to my husband who lit a fire under someone's behind this morning. He's great at doing that in a most respectful manner.)

Thank goodness this is finally happening. (I'm very optimistic that this stuff will help!)

I hit a low spot last night that I was unprepared for. My leg pain rose to a level that was close to intolerable – yet I haven't been able to take any stronger pain meds as to keep my body "clean" for the trial.

My neighbour Jennifer came over to our porch last night to check on me (as she often does, I can't imagine a lovelier person to live next to!) and the tears let loose. I'd come on the porch to take my mind off the pain; watching the little kids play in the street always cheers me up. Something about her gentle smile opened the floodgates and she sat for almost an hour with me, encouraging me to vent all this pent-up frustration with the long delays, my pain, and my general sense of being pretty useless to my family of late.

With this good news, I'm doing my Happy Dance – modified, of course, because I'm not supposed to jar, twist, jump on, run with, or otherwise compromise my fragile thigh bone...but a Happy Dance all the same!

DAY SIX ON ENBREL
Tuesday, August 03, 2010

I've been meaning to blog for days about my first injection, but just figured there would be more to tell as the days passed.

First of all, it didn't hurt much. That's where on-line research can get you into trouble! I'd seen so many other patients write on-line about how painful these shots are, but it wasn't bad at all. Burned for a minute or so and then it was over. And I injected myself – pretty easy with the SureClick injector.

So much happened in a few short hours at the hospital, I won't go into detail except to tell you that the nurse who instructed and supervised me was wonderful (as are all of the team members I met that morning) – and to say that the facilities were something else! Beautifully appointed with real wood panelling, lovely lighting, and comfortable furnishings. It felt more a visit to an estate than to a hospital (thanks to a very generous donor who wanted to make the patients going through clinical trials feel more comfortable – and it works!)

My first (almost) week on Enbrel has been up and down. At the end of the first day, I was completely without any pain. Something that hasn't happened in a very long time!

Second day was unexpected. I'm usually upbeat and optimistic, and I was a depressed, weepy, glop of a girl who couldn't shut up about all things sad and grim. I have no idea where that came from. I'm blaming the drugs, but sure hope that it doesn't happen again.

Third day was the toughest so far. I woke during the night with bad stomach cramps, nausea, fever, and wondering why I had done this to myself. I called into the Enbrel hotline around lunchtime. (They want to hear about pre-specified side effects, fever being one of them.) They suggested going to a walk-in clinic to see if I'd picked up an infection at the hospital. (Enbrel greatly reduces my immunity.) I decided to wait it out, and sure enough, by evening I felt a bit better. Even ate a little, but that day sure helped with dropping off a bit of the steroid weight.

Since then it's been easier, but I can't say that my ECD symptoms have eased at all. The bone and chest pain returned after that wonderful first day, but I do realize it can take a few weeks for any benefit of the drug to make itself known. I don't think that I've been having any side effects from the drugs since Saturday, except maybe being a wee bit sleepier than my already frequently napping self.

I'm so used to taking an assortment of pills daily that it feels a little odd to be waiting for my next injection on Thursday. Every night I dream that I've gone to the fridge for the next dose of my liquid gold (given its cost), and awaken quite relieved that I've not jumped the gun accidentally!

BEING FIRST IS NOT ALWAYS A GOOD THING
Thursday, August 19, 2010

You haven't heard from me in awhile, and I'll tell you that this isn't an easy post to write.

Our experiment with Enbrel has failed. Miserably.

There will be people who search on-line for "Enbrel" and will be led to this blog, so I want to quickly say that I understand that this drug has been a godsend for many patients who have conditions that Enbrel is meant to treat. My use was "off-label," and we had no prior use of this drug for Erdheim-Chester Disease to use as a reference. And maybe it might even help others with ECD, but it just wasn't a good match for my particular set of cardiac ailments.

The side-effects of the first injection were unpleasant but tolerable. The second shot was another story altogether. I won't bore you with all the details but it's been quite the nightmare. Two weeks later, I'm still dealing with a number of issues that weren't present before starting Enbrel.

My doctor wanted me to keep going; to have the next dose administered during a hospital stay of a few days in the cardiac ward. I was told that if I went into cardiac arrest, they could be there right away for me. (That statement was a wee bit intimidating just on its own.)

I mulled over this option for a few days but my heart continued (and continues) to act up. Every ounce of me is saying this just isn't right and I've chosen to trust my gut instinct.

Despite some very dear and wise friends gently and lovingly telling me that I shouldn't feel this way, I'm feeling like I've failed. That I've done something to cause such a violent reaction to the drug, that I haven't been tough enough, or didn't want this to succeed enough.

I have ten weeks worth of this drug safely stored in my fridge at home and it taunts me every time open it. I think about how hard everyone worked to get me this drug and how long I waited for that lucky break of a donation. I feel like I've failed my medical team and that I've disappointed them.

Deep down I know I have to do what I think is right. But these feelings of guilt are difficult to shake. I worry that my doctors won't be willing to try other treatments on me. On the other hand, I worry that this experiment may have shortened my time. My heart is doing back flips and just doesn't seem to want to fall into a regular pattern. I get two-minute breaks whenever the pacemaker kicks in, but the rest of the time it's annoying the heck out of me with the pain, weird sensations, and strange rhythms.

And sometimes I'm just not sure I have it in me to keep fighting this battle as hard as I have been.

AFTER TEN LONG, LONG DAYS
Saturday, September 11, 2010

Sometimes I think I should have called this blog "Up the Creek without a Paddle."

It's been a trying time over the last while. Today is the first day in a week and a half that I've not had a fever or significant chest pain. I'm not sure what my body is trying to tell me but I'm really not getting the message. Well, maybe that's not entirely true.

Eleven days ago, I felt well enough to go to my hospital appointment on my own on the train. My husband dropped me off at the station so that I didn't have to deal with that long walk from the end of the parking lot. It was a pleasant ride; lots of families going into the city for the day to visit the CNE (the annual end of summer Canadian National Exhibition). From there, I took the streetcar to the hospital. Lots of Torontonians detest the city's streetcars; they're slow, noisy, and can be unbearably hot in the summer if you happen to land on an older, un-air-conditioned car. But I love them. I've always loved this city, and the streetcar shows me a slice of this city that many who rely solely on their cars miss altogether.

Dr. HPK and I discussed our revised plan of action after the disappointing Enbrel trial. We decided to let me have a break from the "more serious" drugs and let me stay on maintenance meds for a month, to let my system calm down. I had sent him some info on Kineret (a drug I mentioned in a post early in the year). A study of Kineret has produced some promising results. The clinical trial documented its use for two ECD patients in Europe. Yes, I said two. That's what happens with extremely rare diseases, but I'll take whatever hope I can grab onto. Kineret was initially dismissed by my team of doctors but I'm keeping my fingers crossed that we can start this whole approval/insurance application/beg for a drug donation circus all over again.

After my appointment, I still felt fairly energized and decided to again tackle the streetcar, this time with a pit stop for some people-watching on Yonge Street. A visit to a favourite store, and then feeling still pretty awake (rare for me!) I decided to walk down to the train station.

I hadn't had that much fun in a long time. I felt normal. Years ago, I worked in the financial district, facing these crowds every day. Although

I love my new career, at that moment I missed the normalcy of that life so far away – busy, productive, somewhat predictable. Travelling often to some fascinating cities (and some really not so fascinating!) I regularly updated my five-year plan, and it all seemed feasible – and for a few years afterwards, it was.

I came home with a big smile. No one who'd seen me that day in the city would have guessed that I'm ill, other than maybe noticing that I walk a bit awkwardly and slower than I used to. Maybe she has a twisted ankle? Sore from an extra tough workout at the gym?

The next morning, I awoke with a fever and excruciating chest pain. And I don't use that word lightly. And for the next ten days it didn't let up, except for a few brief hours every few days. No appetite, the most I could stomach was a few crackers to take with my pills. After a week, I called Dr. HPK who asked me to double all my meds, and add one more to try to get on top of this flare of pericarditis. He suggested that I might have picked up a virus on my trip to the hospital/downtown – after all my immune system isn't very strong right now. Maybe I just exerted myself far too much on my downtown trip and my heart was rebelling.

I've been feeling defeated – that I will pay each time for a small bit of freedom. It just seems too coincidental that every time I do something a bit more strenuous that a virus is the cause.

And I'm simply amazed that despite the daily gymnastics going on in my chest, my heart still keeps going. One truly amazing example of the resiliency of the human body. But for how long?

Today I'm eating again, working a bit in my office and I even managed a quick trip to the grocery store. These better days are essential to my mental health and I treasure them.

NOT A NO
Wednesday, October 06, 2010

Yesterday was hospital day. It was the longest I'd gone between appointments in two years, and I'd had high hopes that there would have been a significant move forward towards the next treatment.

No such luck, but in all it was still a pretty good meeting with Dr. HPK. We're in agreement that my health is declining and that we have to come up with some sort of treatment plan. My wish to try Kineret hasn't been shot down, it's still being considered, but we're going to take a different path. I'll be meeting with the doctor/researcher who obtained the Enbrel donation for me – and have him assess me in person and decide on the next step together.

He is however, renowned in his field and lectures around the world frequently – so getting in to see him might take a while. That's the hard part to swallow – as I get weaker and the "good days" become less frequent, it's sometimes difficult to be optimistic about the road ahead. I can't help but hope that the Kineret (or something else that is prescribed) just might be the miracle treatment that improves my quality of life. So I'm not wallowing, right? Still looking forward. Most days.

Yesterday's appointment felt far less clinical than usual. It was an honest discussion about how frustrating it is to treat an illness about which so little is known, and how treatment options have so far been hit and miss with the small number of patients around the world.

I felt that we were skating just above the admission that we seem to dip towards at some appointments. Unless I'm careless crossing a busy street, this illness is what will end my life. Dr. HPK has a way of asking questions of the two of us (my husband is almost always with me at these appointments) to see where I'm at mentally with all of this. Actually where all three of us are at; my husband and daughter suffer through this just as much as I do in their own ways.

Yesterday I felt emotionally strong and I hoped it came across that way to Dr. HPK. I sometimes think about the stages of grief – and believe that I tend to bounce quite a bit between them. Up a step, down two, and back up again on the ladder. Yet I think that he could read between the lines; the only change to my prescriptions was to make sure that I get outside for ten minutes a day. Drive (or get driven as is the case most days now) to a park, sit on a bench, or walk if I'm up to it – but get outside of the house.

I've learned much about myself in the last two years. I'm as human as everyone else. And I have to forgive myself for not always being Miss Optimistic and Strong. Bad things happen and I'm not weak for sometimes thinking that I got a raw deal in all of this.

THE MIRROR IS NOT MY FRIEND
Friday, October 08, 2010

However, my husband and daughter most definitely are.

I'm looking pretty haggard these days. Lack of sleep and everything else going nuts in my body have me hardly recognizing myself these days. I've lost the steroid chipmunk cheeks and about half of the steroid weight so far – but all I see are sunken eyes and a rather unhealthy looking tint to my skin. Yesterday I came across a photo of myself taken about two years ago and I seem to have aged at least ten years since then.

But every single day, both of my sweeties tell me that I look beautiful. I'm grateful that they can see past what I'm seeing in the mirror. Or they've both become great fibbers.

One upside – every year I dress up as a witch at Halloween to dish out the treats; this year I won't need much make-up to look convincing!

THE VIEW FROM THE BOTTOM STEP
Sunday, October 31, 2010

I'm raising my white flag.

I sit at the bottom step, looking up at where I came from. I didn't arrive here with a thud. Nor did I arrive at the bottom. I got here as I would have expected, with a slow, careful descent; step by step.

It's taken a few weeks to get here, feeling as if I've been tripping my way down the stairs clawing to grab onto a rail, a step or by some miracle a tremendous gust of wind to nudge me back up a step or two.

The quick decline in my health has been horrifying to me. I've tried to keep some normalcy; cooking a couple of meals a week, keeping up with the laundry, even driving my daughter to school once in a while. At my very best I've even been able to do two photo sessions with clients.

At its worst, I realize that this is all slipping away from me very quickly right now. Most days are spent in bed lately, trying to keep my mind off of the pain that seems to be settling into other bones with a burn that at times is nearly intolerable. Trying to save up enough energy to do a few simple tasks each day. Trying to ignore that my pacemaker kicks in all day long to correct a heartbeat that refuses to keep steady. Trying to keep the relentless fever under control. Watching so much slip away from me.

October was especially hard to deal with. It's the month that as a photographer I would have been out in nearly every kind of weather, either photographing families for their holiday pictures, or capturing the fall colours in their glory for the galleries that sell my work. Although most of them have dropped me in the last year because I've not been able to honour my obligations to regularly provide new images.

Last night, Dr. HPK called (yes, a Saturday night) to check on me. We're back in to see him tomorrow and by the sounds of it he's ready to try to help me pull out the big guns. Enough of this being stoic and trying to handle the pain and discomfort with a brave face. It's time to admit that I need more help than perhaps I've been letting on.

Within minutes after the call, I received some very sad news. One of the members of our ECD support group passed on this week. She was only thirty-three and left behind a young daughter. My heart goes out to her loving, and beloved family.

This really is an evil disease.

JUST DON'T GET ME STARTED
Thursday, November 04, 2010

This afternoon, I had an annual appointment with my local family doctor, I don't think I've mentioned him before in a post. One of these female check-ups; not my favourite things to do but I have to suck it up and get it done. Or do I?

I'm at that age when a few extra tests are requisitioned at the annual check-up. None are terribly pleasant; parts get squished, prodded, palpated and swabbed. But lately I wonder why I'm getting them done. If I'm being honest with myself, I believe that at this stage, it's highly unlikely that if cancer was detected I'd do anything about. I realize I might raise an eyebrow or two out there, but really – I'm already dealing with a serious illness that has no cure. Would I subject myself to more surgery/treatments than what I'm already prepared (or not prepared) to do to deal with the ECD? And really, could anyone have that much bad luck with his or her health?

This doctor has been getting updates on my condition from the hospital in Toronto. As he started our conversation he already had tears in his eyes, confirming that what he'd read was not good news. I'm not sure how I feel about his reaction. On one hand I recognize that he's a kind, compassionate man; isn't that what we'd all want in a doctor? On the other hand, his reaction brings out something in me that I don't recognize. It's not self-pity; after all it was me reassuring him at the end of my appointment that I felt quite optimistic about the next drug trial.

I'm used to emotional outpourings when sharing details of my illness with others. It's not something I spend a lot of time talking about, but I try to be forthright when people care enough to ask about the progression of my illness.

Today's appointment? I think I can best describe my reaction as fear. I try so hard not to be overwhelmed by my illness but his tears make me feel like I ought to be more frightened.

I know my doctor's heart is in the right place, but it makes me need my husband to hurry home for one of his wonderful hugs that make the rest of the world disappear for just a little while.

WE'RE STILL GIGGLING!
Saturday, November 06, 2010

Despite the somewhat more sombre mood in our household, we're still trying to hang on to our sense of humour.

A few days ago, my daughter got a call from her dad's house (she splits her time between two households), asking if there was any particular reason why her school uniform was strewn across the front lawn. Turns out she had stuffed her clothes into her school bag as she ran out to the driveway where her driving instructor was waiting. (He was going to drop her off at our house afterward and she needed her uniform for the next school day.) The clothes had fallen out as she swung her bag over her shoulder. Easily solved, my husband picked up the clothes that evening. No worse for their public airing.

The next morning, I felt well enough to drive my daughter to school. (She otherwise takes two buses, which don't always connect as scheduled due to lots of local road construction.) We leave pretty early and I didn't feel like showering and dressing for the half-hour round trip. The sweatpants I'd been wearing the previous evening were handy and I pulled them over my pyjama bottoms so the neighbours wouldn't be able to see that I hadn't bothered to dress properly.

My daughter got in the driver's seat, and I climbed in beside her. (She's getting to be quite a good driver. We're keeping our fingers crossed that she passes her next exam to allow her to drive on her own.)

An uneventful trip and I was soon back on our street. *What the heck is in the driveway? Can't be...*

I hurried over to the side of the drive where I'd climbed into the car thirty minutes earlier. A wee bit embarrassing – but it was my panties. In plain view.

They must have slipped out of the leg of the sweatpants; in my exhausted state the night before, I hadn't separated my laundry.

How many of my neighbours saw, and how many are wondering what kind of drugs I'm on these days? And why can't the women in our family keep track of their clothes?

We truly are still finding lots to laugh about. And my latest comedic indulgence? *Modern Family*. Did you catch the episode about Gloria's accent and mispronunciations? That brought back memories of growing up with a mother with a strong German accent. I can't tell you how many times my friends would look at me with alarm, clearly misunderstanding what my mom had just said.

I don't think my husband and daughter can understand just how much it helps when they get me laughing. And they do, every single day (especially when I keep inadvertently providing the fodder!)

TOO MUCH TIME, YET NOT ENOUGH
Tuesday, November 23, 2010

I feel like I'm spending months inside of much shorter time frames. Now that I've written that, it doesn't seem to make much sense, but there's too much going on to have logically fit into the last two weeks and that's the only way I can describe it.

Two weeks ago, I got a long-awaited call from the hospital. The researcher had decided, that no – I was not going to be taking Kineret.

For a reason that floored me, he told my doctor that the shots are too painful and patients tend not to comply for that reason. Just one sec here, has a word I've said even been heard? What about short-term pain for possible long-term gain? Doesn't he know that I'm one tough cookie?

I went to bed that night completely dejected. After all these long months of lobbying, the answer wasn't at all what I had expected. Despite taking my nightly sleeping pill (my leg and chest pain has gotten a bit much at nights lately, and it helps to take the edge off so I can get to sleep), I found myself staring at the clock at 4 a.m. not having slept a wink. I quietly crept downstairs to my office and spent the next two hours composing a letter to my doctors – a rational, unemotional plea to reconsider. What other options do I have right now? So many of the other drugs used for ECD can further complicate my cardiac condition so I really don't have much else to try.

When my husband woke up a few hours later, I asked him to read the letter to make sure I was as lucid in the wee hours as I thought I had been. He encouraged me, in fact, to put a bit more emotion in my words; to get across how devastating this decision felt.

A few hours after emailing my letter, I got a call from Dr. HPK. He'd spoken to the researcher and Kineret was back on the table. We're still waiting to hear if this is going to happen, but at least we don't have a definite no to deal with. And now it's back to being about funding.

YAYS AND BOOS
Thursday, December 02, 2010

Just a quick post, I'm on way to the hospital. For once not for me – Dr. Ho Ping Kong is being honoured tonight and we're invited guests. (A photography project that I worked on for the hospital is being unveiled tonight.) Yay for HPK!

Dr. HPK managed to get me a three-month trial supply of Kineret. A very persuasive man is he; we got the phone call late yesterday. Waiting now for a shipment to arrive from Sweden, and then I start my injections.

Boo to my hip. It's been causing me quite a bit of pain, and the results of an x-ray came in yesterday. Doesn't sound like good news, but I'll have a bone scan to confirm exactly what's happening there.

Boo to my jaw. I get so tired of bad news that I neglected to have it checked out when my teeth started not fitting together about six weeks ago. And then it became difficult to eat (which has certainly helped me dump some of this last steroid weight, so that's a yay). While I was on a heavy dose of prednisone for almost a year I was warned that bone problems can develop in the jaw and hip. Am I lucky enough to have gotten both?

Yay to my husband and daughter. I've been a major grump this week. They forgive all; I'm one lucky wife and mom.

HANGING WITH "MY PEOPLE"
Friday, December 03, 2010

Last night I was able to make it to the hospital in Toronto to attend the dedication ceremony for my doctor, with the help of a family friend who drove me to the train station and my husband who "caught" me on the other end.

What an evening it was. Maybe eighty people were there; mostly doctors, a very generous philanthropist who has donated millions over time to the division that takes care of me, and one patient. Me.

I can't tell you what an honour it was to be there. I had a special role – it was the unveiling of a painting/portrait of my doctor for which I had taken the original photograph earlier this year as a special request. (It even has my husband and daughter in it too!) The painting will hang in the newly renamed wing, in honour of Dr. HPK; the one I frequent so often that many of the doctors passing through will wave in recognition when we catch sight of each other.

I was among "my people." Certainly not as a peer, this was a gathering of some of the most respected doctors in this city. But I was among people who get what this battle is all about. Who have great respect for this amazing doctor that cares for me, but also respect me for trying to beat this with a smile on my face.

They understood that it was hard to physically get there last night. They get that this disease has a poor prognosis, yet applaud my efforts to keep a brave face.

I'd also mentioned in yesterday's blog that I would be going to the dentist today to check on my painful jaw. Not good news I'm afraid, it would appear that ECD has asserted itself there as well. But in need of a "yay," this household is glad that that I've kicked my recent grumpiness aside!

ON CLOUD NINE!
Friday, December 10, 2010

Kineret. Arriving by Wednesday at the latest.

I just had a conversation with the drug company liaison. (Am I ever glad I picked up the call coming from an unidentified telephone number at 9 p.m. on a Friday night, something at times I'd let go to voicemail, suspecting a telemarketer).

I can't believe this is actually going to happen after a wait of almost a year. I can't tell you how badly I needed this news; it's been a tough few weeks. I'd made the decision to (hopefully temporarily) shut down my portrait photography business, and had let my clients know about two weeks ago.

Some very thoughtful clients sent wonderfully supportive notes, but I must say – there were a few responses that really soured what was already quite a painful exercise for me. Several organizations to which I'd donated portrait packages annually, to support their fundraising, tried really hard to make me feel bad for not being able to donate another package this season. Couldn't I commit to mustering the energy to do just one session in the spring? For just a few hours? (My photographer friends would cringe, no session is just a few hours – most of the work comes afterwards.)

My photography means everything to me; I hope that has come across in previous posts. It had just become too hard to hold my camera to my eye for any length of time, and a session would wipe me out for days afterwards. And I'd become so unreliable for a booking, resting up for a few days prior just wasn't working anymore. And I detest being unreliable, but that's my story these days.

But there's hope. I really believe that Kineret will do wonders for me. That I'll be able to work again in a few months. That I'll be able to walk farther than a half a block again.

That I'll start sleeping again without pain waking me up in the wee hours. That I just might feel a little more like my old self again. Because these days, I often lose sight of what normal felt like. I know I'm asking for the world, but just maybe I might get a slice of something great coming my way.

MAKING MY DAUGHTER'S BOYFRIEND FEEL AT HOME
Monday, December 13, 2010

Still waiting on info about starting my Kineret. I'll need to be monitored at the hospital when I take my first injection or two (in case of allergic reaction), but Dr. HPK is leaving on vacation for two weeks on Wednesday. My Kineret arrives that afternoon and we're hoping to line up another doctor who's around over the holiday break but so far no luck. So it looks like there's a possibility I won't start until the New Year.

We can't have many visitors here at home, especially at this time of year when the flu is rampant. I pick up colds and infections too easily (and this will be even more the case when I start Kineret). So anyone coming over has to assure us that they're feeling well and the first place they head coming in the door is the bathroom to wash up. Just the way it has to be.

Most of my socializing is done over the phone, on Facebook or on email because of these restrictions but there is one visitor who comes by quite often – my daughter's boyfriend James. They've been together nine months. He knows the drill and takes the necessary precautions to not expose me to illness. I'm delighted that this doesn't faze him. And we love having him around!

James has become quite familiar with the odd sense of humour that resides in this household. (He's very sweetly told us this is the weirdest family he knows!)

Here's an exchange from a few nights ago.

Me to my daughter and James: "Thanks so much for picking up my prescription at the pharmacy this afternoon after school." (She's driving now!) "Now that I think about it, I should have had you drive me over there to get it myself. Did the pharmacist explain how to use it? She usually takes me aside for a consultation for new meds."

Daughter: "No, Mom. Why?"

Me: "Actually, I'm a little surprised that she didn't insist that I come in personally given what it is."

Daughter: "Really? What is it?"

Me: "Um...medical marijuana."

I couldn't have timed it better. James was taking a long sip from a water bottle for that last bit, of which most ended up being sprayed across the room. My daughter caught on right away, she knows that I've never had an illicit drug in my life, and don't drink alcohol either. It would take some pretty heavy convincing from my doctor to have me smoking up, even for medical reasons!

We may at times be totally inappropriate, sometimes morbid, and almost always a bit goofy in this home – but humour is what's getting us through this together. I'm relieved that James fits right in!

TOMORROW
Tuesday, December 14, 2010

I have my Kineret.

And tomorrow morning I go to the hospital for my first injection. Quite a few people have worked very hard to have this happen before Dr. HPK and his team go on holidays. (They leave tomorrow afternoon.) The stars have been shining on us over this last week!

A BREEZE
Thursday, December 16, 2010

Yesterday, I was at the hospital learning how to give myself the Kineret injection. I'm really not nervous about needles and such, but I'll admit the idea of giving myself a shot in the stomach did give me a slight case of the creeps. (The injections should be rotated between a few different areas in the body, to lessen the skin irritation; the stomach being one site.)

My nurse was so helpful and calming and before I knew it, I'd stuck that sucker into my stomach and pumped my precious Kineret in. Next stop was back to my doctor's clinic upstairs to watch for any reaction. At first there was a wee bit of blotchy redness about two inches across, but that was gone within an hour. After that, clear. Two hours later, clear. THREE hours later, clear.

Shortly afterwards, my doctor came in to review how I was feeling. Any concerns about an allergic reaction were calmed; I was doing just fine and able to go home.

Honestly, I think my doctor is far more nervous that I am about this. He's leaving today on two weeks' vacation and wishes I had waited until his return to start the Kineret. I explained that I really appreciated everyone moving heaven and earth to make this happen THIS week – emotionally I needed to be on more solid ground going into 2011, feeling more hopeful about the year ahead. The last two holiday seasons were quite difficult – the first was a diagnosis of a leg tumour of (at the time) unknown cause and possibly cancerous, and then last year I was in the middle of weaning off prednisone, which took yet another four months to do successfully, and feeling quite horrible day in and day out.

This year I'm hopeful. I know it's way too early to predict anything after just one injection, but I feel very positive that this drug will improve upon my current quality of life (which to be perfectly blunt has really sucked the last few months).

So, yes – I did push my doctor into starting Kineret before his vacation. He's prepared me well with the pager number for the chief resident at the hospital (who's been prepped on what to do in case I get into trouble), we have antibiotics on hand in case of infection, and drugs to help lessen the expected injection site reactions due to come along in a week or so. And I'm good with this. My doctor not so much, but he respects and understands how much I needed to do this now before a new year begins. How could I let the opportunity for three months of free access to the drug wait any longer than necessary, after we've been hoping for this for so long?

So upstairs I go now, for my husband to take his first stab (!) at this in my arm. He practiced this morning with an empty syringe on an orange. He's concerned about hurting me, but I know there's nobody who cares more about whether I feel pain – I know he'll do just fine.

SEVEN INJECTIONS AND DOING JUST FINE
Tuesday, December 21, 2010

I'm getting used to the shots. Really.

After seven of them I find it easy to quickly poke the needle in, push the syringe and before I know it I'm done. Yes, it does hurt a wee bit for about ten minutes but given the improvement, I'm already seeing the small amount of discomfort is well worth it.

It's way too early to say if this experiment is a success. (I'm still experiencing some bone pain and my local cardiologist heard the pericarditis still active at yesterday's appointment.) But I'm quite impressed for what the Kineret has done so far.

For the last year, I'd become increasingly arthritic. I was avoiding stairs whenever possible, and walking even short distances was taking me much longer. Plus I'd be paying for it afterwards with significant joint pain and stiffness, especially the last few months when that first swing of my legs out of bed in the morning told me that I was in for a painful day.

Perhaps I'm exaggerating when I say this – but it does feel like I'm bounding about the last few days. I'm easily tackling the stairs with armloads of laundry, even getting some holiday shopping done with my daughter yesterday – and she didn't have to walk at a snail's pace for me to keep up with her!

I'm feeling "normal-ish". I can't tell you the last time that I felt so able. I'm certainly not up to the pace of a few years ago but not being reminded that I'm ill every time I move has been a tremendous blessing.

I've yet to experience the injection site reaction that is very common with Kineret but the nurse at the hospital told me it's likely to start up within a week or so. Just hang in there for that first month when things can get a bit nasty and I should be in for an easier time after that.

Time to just enjoy what's happening right now. We don't know if this will get rid of the pericarditis or help with the bone pain; only time will tell. But I'm feeling very optimistic! What a tremendous Christmas present that's been given to me – to the three of us.

TWO WEEKS IN
Tuesday, December 28, 2010

What can I say? I feel better.

Walking has become so much easier, I'm not cringing anymore as I make my way up and down the stairs (and we have lots in our home).

My almost constant fever of the last year has all but disappeared. Just one day last week and even then it was quite mild.

I'm still having cardiac episodes, but they're happening infrequently and don't knock me down as hard as before. Still having shortness of breath, but hey – we're only two weeks into this treatment!

The bone pain is still there, but I'd say that it's becoming less frequent. Sharper pain when it does happen – but I'm being optimistic that it means that the Kineret is doing something. And by something, I mean something good.

As predicted by the nurse at the hospital, I've started in the last two days to break out in some unsightly (and fairly itchy!) skin reactions at current and previous injection sites. Tolerable so far, they seem to be under control with oral allergy medication – I'm saving the corticosteroid creams for when the itching is driving me totally crazy! And as I've been told – just hang in there for that first month to six weeks and this phase should pass.

The injections are getting much easier – just part of my daily routine now, no stressing about them. Yes, they still hurt a bit, but I suspect being relaxed about the shots makes them easier than they might otherwise be. Finding a spot that isn't inflamed might be a challenge for the next while though. We'll make it a party game – help me find a spot that doesn't look like I had a fight with a patch of poison ivy and you win a prize – I'll run up the stairs to fetch anything you need. Because now I can!

GOING STRONG!
Saturday, January 08, 2011

What an amazing week.

A few days ago I had my first check-up with my doctor since starting Kineret. (I should say doctors, there was a quite a parade of them coming in to see how I was doing.)

Although my pericarditis can still be heard through the stethoscope, it was generally agreed that it has become quieter. One cardiologist who's listened several times was sure that it was even undetectable every few heartbeats.

Less bone pain every day. I've even had some completely pain-free days, and I've dropped my pain meds by half – and intend to drop down further over the next week.

The rashes are tolerable, and I've stopped my oral antihistamines. I was given a stronger topical ointment and that seems to be enough.

I can't tell you just how much better I'm feeling as each day goes on. The odd day I've had a setback; it seems that increased sodium intake really doesn't agree with me especially since I've been on Kineret. It throws my heart into an arrhythmia for about twenty-four hours but that's fairly easy.

This is all great stuff but the real measure of how well I'm doing is what activities I can do now that weren't possible before. Let me sum it up. I shovelled the driveway. Twice this week. And this morning was a pretty heavy snowfall! And not one single twinge from my heart. This may not seem like a huge deal, but for someone who most days had quite a bit of trouble getting up two flights of stairs at once this is of enormous relevance.

Although my doctor is very cautiously optimistic about what Kineret will do, I can't help but be pretty darned excited about how I'm feeling. And I'm feeling hope.

TOO STUBBORN FOR MY OWN GOOD
Thursday, January 13, 2011

In my last post, I was boasting about how I had shovelled the driveway twice over the weekend when we got a good dumping of snow. I tell you, sometimes I really ought to be more careful – I'm often pushing my limits a bit more than I ought to. Despite my husband asking me to take it easy and offering to do these more vigorous chores instead – there I go and try and do it myself.

After having a great week, I think I undid my progress; I ended up in bed for a few days trying not to get my heart too agitated – it really let me know that I had overdone it.

Lesson learned. For now.

Next obstacle was my flu shot. I should have gotten it a couple of months ago but there never seemed to be a clinic date that worked. At an appointment with our new family doctor a couple of days ago (we had to find a new local doctor, it's a long and boring story) she suggested that we get our shots, especially given that Kineret plays havoc with the immune system. She had the vaccine on hand and my daughter and I got our shots at long last.

Another setback. I've gotten my flu shot annually since my daughter was born. (I'd been a single mom much of that time and wouldn't have been much use to her if I'd been sick.) I never had more of a reaction that a bit of soreness in the arm and a slight fever the next day. This time was quite different (and I can't blame the Kineret, my daughter had a similar reaction and wasn't able to go to school yesterday because of it). This time, we both were lightheaded (to the point of having difficulty standing), nauseated, and generally feeling pretty icky. We're both starting to feel better today, and appreciate this is still much better than having the flu for a week or more.

So after a difficult week, I say the same thing that I say to my husband at the end of every challenging day. Tomorrow will be better.

NEW FRIENDS
Sunday, January 23, 2011

Bad things happen. And not that we want bad things to happen to others but there is some comfort to be found in knowing that you're not the only person facing a particular challenge.

Finding the Erdheim-Chester Global Alliance has allowed me to connect with other ECD patients around the world, and for this I've been grateful. And I'm very thankful for the efforts of the Alliance volunteers who maintain the website, raise funds for further studies, and provide us with a forum to communicate and much more. Especially the "much more" part – a special thanks to Kathy who is always there to listen and offer suggestions as we navigate the maze of dealing with a rare illness.

Here comes what could be a very long story, but I'll keep this short. In the last week, I've connected with two ECD families; one about a five-hour drive away and one about a ten-minute drive away. The first was diagnosed in the last couple of months and the latter in the last two weeks.

I was floored. Here are two families that face the same Ontario health system, and in some cases the same hospitals. (However, not the same doctors, but we'll be working on making some connections between our medical teams.)

Of course I wouldn't wish this illness on anyone, but there was elation in finding nearby "teammates" in this challenge. Last weekend I even met the wife of the patient who lives very close by and we hope to get our families together soon. (And the one farther away promises to be in this area later this year.)

I'm excited about connecting with these two families, and we've committed to working together towards getting drug funding (we're all facing the challenge of getting help paying for Kineret) and other issues that might be unique to furthering the cause for ECD for patients in Canada.

On the subject of Kineret, I'm well used to the shots now. A nurse from Biovitrum (the maker of Kineret) called this week to check on me and gave me some very useful suggestions for making the injections a little less painful.

Here's the dirt. After six weeks of treatment my joint pain has greatly diminished, to the point that I'm walking quite normally again. Bone pain is still there, but less frequent. When it does come it seems sharper, but I'm concentrating on the "less frequent" part! The cardiac pain has still been a bit of a challenge. Today is the first day in about two weeks where I've not felt it. (I hope I haven't jinxed myself, still about six hours to go!) The pericardial rub is still going strong, although my doctors feel that it's less widespread across the heart and concentrated more in one area.

Still very optimistic about this trial!

SELF ADMISSIONS
Thursday, February 03, 2011

I detest admitting that I'm sick. But ECD has slapped me around a bit the last few weeks, and just maybe it's time to realize that I shouldn't push myself so hard. I think I've said this before but maybe it's high time I had a serious chat with myself. And actually followed through.

I'm eight weeks into my twelve-week Kineret trial, and decided today that I definitely want to keep taking it beyond the trial period. Now comes the funding nightmare, but the upside is that the drug company is helping me this time. I suspect that its voice is much louder than mine.

Kineret has helped greatly with my mobility, and now with the bone pain. (I've hardly had any the past week.) The cardiac issues are something else, but maybe Kineret needs more time. Or I need to stop pushing those boundaries so hard.

Although it felt great at the time, shovelling the snow a few weeks back seems to have set off weeks of misery. What the heck did I do to myself? I'd been doing so well in the first few weeks of Kineret; did I undo all that in just one hour?

I've made a promise to my family. No more lifting, no more, "Let me do it!" and most definitely no more shovelling. No more of anything that feels like it just might be more than I should be doing.

Give the inflammation in my heart a chance to settle down; to let Kineret do its thing. To hopefully breathe more normally again. Talking on most days this past week sets off a round of coughing that leaves me gasping for air. Not to mention the tremors that have kicked in too. What an adventure one night last week, trying to get food on my fork, and then fork to mouth. I came way too close to asking someone else at the table to feed me so I didn't leave the table hungry.

Dr. HPK called this morning (on his day off no less) to let me know I'd be at the hospital longer than usual tomorrow. He didn't want to say just yet what tests were being lined up, but I'm ready to know more about the extent of the ECD in my body.

Not only ready, I need to know.

WHERE TO LAY BLAME
Tuesday, February 15, 2011

I feel as if I've been hit by a bus the last few weeks. What did I do to myself to set off this latest round? That shovelling from a few weeks back? One of my meds? Something I've been eating?

It's natural to search for a reason when things change. I have a difficult time admitting that it might simply be the natural progression of my illness; that I have to be more accepting of how I'm feeling and the limitations that my health places upon me.

I'm not quite ready to blame Kineret, however. I'm nine weeks into this trial and it's still helping greatly with my mobility and to some degree with my bone pain. My heart, on the other hand, has been misbehaving. Badly.

It's been rounds of scans and other tests to see what might be going on besides the pericarditis. We're waiting for results of the latest CAT scans to see if my lungs and brain might have developed any problems. Nothing seems to be working right, from the weird tremors that shake my hands, the numbness in my foot, and the continued breathing difficulties.

And I discovered yet one more medication that I'm allergic to – Pulmicort. I was put on this steroid inhaler to see if it would help with my breathing but all I got was a lovely rash from neck to knees for a few days.

It's hard not to feel beaten down and trodden upon by ECD when it's hard to do anything more than lie on the couch, occasionally getting up to do something useful around the house that doesn't require a lot of exertion. Every action is measured – is it worth how it's likely to make me feel afterwards?

Yes, I'm feeling sorry for myself right now. This just isn't me. It's me with ECD tugging at me every single moment until I want to kick it clear across Lake Ontario. If only I could muster enough energy to at least get it to the curb for a few days.

LET'S PLAY THE GOOD NEWS/BAD NEWS GAME
Thursday, February 17, 2011

The Good News:

Last week I went back on some heart meds that didn't work out well for me last year, but in combination with Kineret, things are looking up. It's taken some experimenting with dosages and the time of day that I take this new drug but I've had two good days in a row. I even felt well enough today to drive for the first time in about a month. Just to the pharmacy to pick up more drugs, mind you, but it felt wonderful to get out of the house.

The Bad News:

On the way back from the pharmacy this morning, I picked up the mail. I didn't expect to hear back from the insurance company so soon – the application for Kineret coverage only reached them Thursday evening. But I could have waited a bit longer for this news. No, no, and absolutely no. No coverage for ANYTHING that doesn't specifically state that it's for the treatment of Erdheim-Chester Disease. But there's no such thing. There's not one drug in existence that states that it's for the treatment of ECD. For the icing on the cake, the letter was unsigned without a printed name of the bottom – an anonymous slap in the face.

So despite the fact that medical teams around the world are investing heavily in research to improve the quality of life, and hopefully the lifespan of ECD patients – their findings are dismissed by our insurance company. And our government also declines to help. A fellow ECD patient in Ontario already had to find this out the hard way, and I've been advised that it's not worth the effort to apply to the government after another patient has been refused coverage. Again because it's "off-label."

I have two and half weeks worth of Kineret left in my fridge. I try really hard not to dwell on this point, but the stats tell us that 60% of ECD patients die within 32 months of diagnosis. I'm at month-25. And I'm in the group (cardiac involvement) that usually lands in the 60%.

So I play that stupid mind game of, "What would you do if you were told that you had six months to live?" Fight like hell with our insurance company and government for a drug that might improve those odds? Or save whatever energy I have to spend time with my family? There is no right answer to this one.

I'm not the only ECD patient (or person with a rare and serious illness) out there and many of us are dealing with this issue. Things have to change. Change so that we can stop wishing that we instead had a "common" serious illness for which drugs would be handed out without a blink of an eye because of what is printed on the drug label.

TIME TO BUST OUT
Saturday, February 26, 2011

Yesterday was a tough day.

Our appeal to the insurance company went down in flames, refused once again.

We're hoping that the manufacturer of Kineret will help us out, but I'm not terribly optimistic since they made it very clear at the beginning of my three-month trial that it wouldn't be extended.

I have just a few vials of Kineret left, and have started alternating my shots every other day, in order to stretch it out. I wonder how soon after that last vial I'll be again hobbling around and in significant pain? The thought scares me silly. Although I still don't have a lot of energy, being able to sleep (mostly) pain-free and being able to get up and down the stairs for the last couple of months has been a huge blessing. Just being able to go to another floor of our home has helped me to stay positive.

The sad thing is that if we (myself and the other Ontario ECD patients) had cancer or other prevalent serious illness this wouldn't be an issue. This denial of treatment is down to one thing and one thing only. There is no drug anywhere that lists on its label: "For the treatment of Erdheim-Chester Disease." A few words keep us from getting treatment coverage.

When I first started this blog almost two years ago, I explained why I was using a pseudonym. Being self-employed, I didn't want to scare away clientele. The reality is that it looks far less likely that I'll ever get back to work and all I'm looking for now is a bit of mobility and pain relief for whatever time I have left.

So we launched one of our big guns yesterday. A letter was sent to a reporter of a major Toronto newspaper who had recently written a series of articles about a young patient refused access to an expensive drug that was provided to another patient elsewhere in Ontario at no charge. We're hoping that International Rare Disease Day falling on Monday will open the door to conversations about treatment coverage for rare illnesses. At the very least it might shame our insurance company and the government into helping us.

We're well aware that the prognosis for ECD is not good. Kineret and other drugs being prescribed around the world for ECD are not a cure. I'm just looking to spend the rest of my life in a bit more comfort rather than constantly be battling for the opportunity to get some relief.

MOVING FORWARD
Tuesday, March 01, 2011

What a whirlwind the last few days have been.

First of all, I must say what incredibly supportive friends we have. I put a request out on Facebook, asking if anyone had contacts in the media to help spread the word about the issue of drug funding for rare diseases here in Ontario and didn't they just go all out! I don't want to jinx anything by being too specific just yet, but we're hopeful that we'll be able to share our story as part of the big picture of the challenges that patients with rare diseases face. Keeping our fingers crossed!

A bit of good news today at my oncology appointment. My leg tumour is the same size as it was this time last year. I'm not sure if we have ten months of prednisone to thank for that. (For all the nasty side effects it had better have done something positive!) It's been over two years since I had a full-body bone scan, and I must admit even with today's good news I'm a little anxious about what that might show. It's unusual for an Erdheim-Chester patient to have the bone involvement on only one side; it's most often mirrored on the other half of the body.

It's funny how things come around in life. When we first moved to Burlington almost six years ago, I wanted to jump into being a part of my new community. A local clothing store was holding a fundraiser for the Juravinski Cancer Centre in Hamilton and asked if I'd be willing to donate a portrait package as one of the silent auction items. I happily did so, and through this donation met a wonderful family who subsequently referred me to several of their friends for portrait sessions. I count several of these families as good friends today. (And they bring tears to my eyes when they tell me to hurry up and get well so that I can photograph them again!)

Today I was able to see the Juravinski Cancer Centre today for the first time as a patient. (Even though ECD is not classified as a cancer, an oncologist is often part of the patient's medical team.) My oncologist had transferred from Mt. Sinai in Toronto, and I happily followed him to his new hospital. After all, he was the one who had diagnosed ECD and for that we share a special connection. I'm his first ECD case and I do hope his last.

And lastly, it would appear that our insurance company may have caught wind of our efforts to contact the media. I received a call yesterday asking for proof that the pharmaceutical company had indeed limited my trial to three months. I was able to get that document from my doctor in Toronto, and was told they were willing to reconsider their decision. Hmmm, let's see what the next few days bring!

WHAT WAS I AFRAID OF?
Thursday, March 03, 2011

When I began writing this blog, almost two years ago, I'd decided to keep it anonymous. I feared that I would lose clients; that I'd be looked at differently if people knew that I was ill, and worst of all, that I'd be pitied.

I feared that friends, colleagues from the past, acquaintances, and neighbours would all give up on me and leave me to survive the rest of my illness alone.

Little did I anticipate how things would go.

Little did I realize that it would actually be clients who would be among my strongest supporters. There have been cards and email messages of support that have reduced me to a puddle of happy tears. I didn't know that clients I'd photographed would become close friends, who over and over again, ask if they can do anything to help. That they'd tell me that they look forward to me getting back behind my camera to photograph their families. This belief in me getting better has helped more than they'll ever know.

I didn't know that friends (and even more so my husband's friends) would be in frequent contact to ask how they could help us out. That they would feel as helpless as we often do in our trek through our medical system.

That a neighbour would become the person that I felt I could be most honest with when it came to talking about how scary this all can be. (A huge hug for you Jennifer, I don't know if you realize how much you mean to me.)

That Larry, a dear friend of my husband's, who has also become my dear friend, would offer to ride his bike across the province to raise funds for my drugs.

That a client, now a friend, would realize that I need some stress relief despite me insisting that I'm fine. (Truth be told, I'm not always upfront about how I'm really doing.) We have a date when the weather improves to do some paintballing in her backyard – guess what three letters will be written across the target. Thank you Sandra, I can't wait to pummel the heck out of ECD!

That a dear friend, who used to be our family doctor when we lived in the city, would help me get through this with her loving and supportive words of advice to help my amazing daughter find some sense in all of this. Donna can always be depended upon for thoughtful and sage observations.

That my dear friend Sue, whom I needed more than just about anyone else to stay in my life, would continue to be there for me without question and always without judgement. The many miles between us have never mattered, and she will always be there for my daughter after I can't be anymore.

It's been a polarizing experience. There are those dear friends who have rallied around, but there have also been those that I've not heard from in quite some time. I do understand. Really. This all sucks and I'm not very exciting to be around. I wish that I could go to dinner with the girls, meet up for coffee, or have you over for dinner – but that isn't my reality anymore and those invitations have long since dwindled away. I've come to terms with it.

My status as an "ill person" is very likely to soon become public. This is a good thing; it looks promising that I'll have a chance to speak up on behalf of Canadians with rare illnesses and I'm proud of this opportunity.

So I make the leap to letting you know who is behind "Sessa," the pseudonym I've been using for this blog for the past (almost!) two years. My name is Sandy. Sandy Trunzer– an ordinary forty-six-year-old wife and mother with an extraordinary illness. The names of my husband and daughter remain private. (They both have different last names than me.) You know how much they mean to me and they deserve whatever privacy that they wish to maintain.

The photography business that I've mentioned numerous times in this blog is "The Intrepid Lens."

This wasn't so painful after all.

And I'd also like to thank you for reading my blog. This blog gives me an outlet when I feel like talking, and I thank you for listening! (And for contributing with comments – I love getting them!)

With warm regards, and the knowledge that I have blessings in my life beyond what I ever thought possible,

Sandy

ONE LAST KICK AT THE CAN
Monday, March 07, 2011

Thank you for the wonderful outpouring of support after I put my last post out there! It wasn't an easy one to write, but now I'm certain that it was the right thing for me to do.

We're waiting on the REALLY final decision from the insurance company. They themselves initiated an appeal on their decision last week and the final piece of information that they were seeking was sent to them late this afternoon. Keeping our fingers crossed for a positive reply tomorrow. We did go ahead and bite the bullet, purchasing a one-week supply of Kineret today. (I have two days left of my donated stock, and I didn't want to miss any doses with a special event happening later this week!)

We've noticed a correlation between my diet and my "bad days," maybe it's just a coincidence but it would appear that perhaps I have sensitivity to gluten. It seems that every Saturday night lately, I've been awake all night with bad chest pains and trouble breathing – but I couldn't understand how the pericarditis could tell which day of the week it was.

For the last few months we've usually had company on Saturday night. Nothing fancy, usually just an extra setting at the table – but being one who loves to cook, I can't help myself from trying to cook something a little different than the everyday fare. And lately I've been turning to some sort of pasta dish on these Saturday nights. This is something we don't normally eat, it's mostly salads, veggies and fish around here. And then hours later, I'm in bad shape. I'm not lifting anything especially heavy; I'm not missing my naps, not doing much out of the ordinary for which I could otherwise blame the added discomfort.

It finally occurred to me that it might be gluten; after all I was supposed to be tested for celiac disease a few years ago and just put it on the back burner when I got my ECD diagnosis. So, I'm going gluten-free this week to see if it does indeed help. I had no idea that gluten was found in many foods beyond the pasta, bread, and baked products you might think of first.

I have lots of cookbooks but none that feature gluten-free recipes, so I'll need to hunt around a bit on the Internet. Oh, and one complication – no poultry or egg for me – I'm allergic (anaphylactic shock for the poultry, I always have my Epi-Pen with me). Not much left for me to eat, eh?

GOING PUBLIC IN A BIG WAY! AND SHARING GREAT NEWS...
Thursday, March 10, 2011

I'm at my desk in my basement office, looking at a white mug with the words, "CBC Radio," on one side, and *The Current,* on the other. And the big deal? At this moment it's my only souvenir of a radio interview I did this morning for *The Current,* the national (and very popular!) radio show that will air tomorrow morning, Friday, March 11th across Canada.

I'm very grateful and proud to be a part of bringing awareness to the challenges of diagnosing and treating rare illness across my country. And this is huge; the program has an audience of one million listeners!

Also on the program will be a fellow ECD patient from Ontario, a representative from the Canadian Organization of Rare Disorders (CORD), and the doctor that I often mention on this blog and who I admire more than I can ever say; the incredible Dr. Ho Ping Kong.

And I was able to share some really wonderful news during the program recording. Late yesterday, we received the call that we've been anxiously awaiting for weeks. The insurance company WILL fund Kineret on a compassionate basis for one year. Nothing like leaving it to the eleventh hour to add some stress – I was an hour away from my very last Kineret syringe when the call came in!

Thank you to CBC Radio for picking up this story. In particular, thanks to; Hana Gartner, our very gracious on-air host who made my nervousness disappear immediately; Anna Maria Tremonti, *The Current's* regular host who brought this story idea to the show producers; Ellen Saenger, producer for our segment, who pulled all the pieces together, and who helped immensely to give me confidence in going on air; Lara, who coordinated the morning's activities flawlessly; and to all the other behind-the-scenes staff whom I didn't have a chance to meet. What a great experience!

OUR THANKS
Saturday, March 12, 2011

My family and I cannot thank all of you enough for your overwhelming support after taking time to listen to the CBC interview. We're reeling from the huge number of emails that have arrived in the last twenty-four hours, every last one of them positive, encouraging and uplifting!

I've spent a good amount of time teary-eyed, reading your generous offers to help in any way you can.

If you'd like to help directly fund research for Erdheim-Chester Disease, please visit the ECD Global Alliance website.

In the broadcast, you heard the representative from CORD eloquently explain one of the challenges that rare-disease patients face in needing to visit their local emergency department when their disease places them in crisis. Doctors and nurses often have never heard of the patient's condition and in turn, the patient may not get the appropriate care. I can't think of a better reason for computerized health records for Canadians! I'd like to share one of my own experiences from this past year.

Last March, I wrote about an experience of visiting our local emergency department when I was having trouble breathing. Wonderful care from the paramedics at home and on the way to the hospital.

However, at the hospital, it was unfortunately a different story. I was quickly taken into the cardiac room in the ER, and things started off well. My husband was trying to explain what my illness is about, and that the problem quite likely was fluid accumulation in the heart or lungs; something we're constantly on watch for.

When the doctor arrived, he asked my husband to leave the room. He very abruptly turned to me (on oxygen but still somewhat struggling for air) and asked if I had searched on-line for my symptoms and self-diagnosed myself with Erdheim-Chester Disease. "See this sort of thing all the time," he says. Then he proceeded to write an order to the nurse for morphine, with me insisting all the while that I didn't want narcotics. (Nor could I take them, I have a severe allergy to opiates – my issue was breathing difficulty that night, not pain.)

I felt embarrassed at being labeled a hypochondriac. If you know me, you already get that I'm much quicker to downplay my pain and discomfort rather than use if for attention. I felt that I'd done something wrong, and it's been bothering me ever since. I should have spoken up to the doctor and stood up for myself, but when you're feeling as scared and ill as I felt that night, relief is the only thing on your mind.

Things need to change. And I'm excited about the possibility that I might be able to help in some small way with the CBC interview.

THE PROCESS OF "UN-BLAHHING" MYSELF
Friday, April 01, 2011

Ok, I know – a totally made-up word this "un-blahhing," but it's the best way to describe what I've been trying to accomplish over the last few weeks. It's been a little while since I've posted, and I'm pleased to report that for the most part, I've been physically feeling much better. Very little pain and that heart of mine seems to be listening to my requests to please just settle down!

If I'm feeling physically better, then why I have I been feeling a bit down? I ask myself that and the best answer I can come up with is that I'm not close enough to either side – well or sick. Not that I want to be anywhere near the sick side, but it's easier to define what I can and can't do. I'm not well enough to do many things I'd like to...yet! (My optimism hasn't escaped me completely.) I'm still lacking in strength and very tired much of time. I think if I'm not in much pain and my heart isn't acting up too badly surely I can resume working occasionally (or participate in any number of activities that I enjoy that are currently off the table). Not quite as easy as that, I'm finding.

Just let it be said that I'm trying hard to lift my spirits up. The CBC radio interview was a wonderful experience and it looks like some very good things (re: rare disease awareness in Canada) could arise from the contacts I've made. I'm delighted to have reconnected with a few old friends recently, in my very weird "this can't be a coincidence" kind of way that seems the norm for our household. And various scans and tests at the hospital over the last few weeks show that my current meds seem to be keeping my illness in check.

Is it wrong to want more? It's this in-between space where I've landed that makes me feel like I'm hanging precariously between good and bad... wondering more than ever after a good day how the next morning will look. I'm looking for consistency that will likely never be there again with this unforgiving illness. And after all this time, shouldn't I be used to this roller coaster ride?

THAT WHICH KEEPS ME SANE/MY FAVOURITE THINGS
Sunday, April 03, 2011

If you follow this blog, you'll know that I spend a lot of time at home. If I leave the house, it's almost always for a visit to the hospital or some other medical appointment or test. On the rare occasion, I might be up to a short trip to the grocery store, or if I'm having an exceptionally good day, we might even go out for a meal together. In any case, right now I need someone to drive me so that limits my options as well.

Thankfully I'm a bit of homebody so I don't feel like a shut-in too often, but it helps that I'm able to keep myself busy within these four walls. I'm often asked how I keep myself from going stir-crazy so I thought I'd share a little of what I do here at home – which translated into My Favourite Things!

My iPad. My husband had to talk me into getting one last summer and now I truly don't know what I would have done without it. It's been great for keeping my mind busy when I've had trouble moving around and it also gives me something to do between appointments on those longer hospital visits. And I'm addicted to Angry Birds and Epicurious!

My kitchen. Yes, there are three of us living here in this house, but it's really MY kitchen. I love my collection of gadgets, the well-stocked spice cupboard, and my Paderno pots and pans. Feeding my favourite people gives me so much pleasure. It's an activity that unless I'm really badly off, I manage to save energy for at the end of the day. Current favourite recipe? Curried basmati rice with cashews. With thanks to my husband and daughter who happily fetch whatever ingredients I need, and always eagerly eat up whatever I serve them.

The dishwasher. I wouldn't be so enthusiastic about cooking if I didn't have the dishwasher to do the bulk of the washing up!

Meyer lemons. Sadly gone for the season, they'll be available again at the end of the year. I'm going to miss those sweetly tart fruits that added so much to my meal repertoire over the last few months.

Now to veer from the kitchen – my hot-pink blanket. Not just any hot-pink blanket, a thoughtful gift last summer from my daughter who knows that I'm almost always feeling cold, and it's got "One Tough Cookie" written across it. I do try to live up to that title!

Crossword Puzzles. The really hard ones, I prefer puzzles that I'm not able to finish. Just what I need before bed to calm my mind.

And a recent addition to my list; MAC makeup. I'm not a cosmetics fanatic, but putting on a face just makes me feel more human these days. I'm fitting back into most of my old clothes again after my steroid adventure (good riddance black stretchy pants!) and I needed to feel more feminine again, and less "patient-y"!

MY APPLE TREE AND OTHER BROKEN STUFF
Sunday, April 17, 2011

Almost two years ago, I wrote a post about the apple tree that sits not far from my bedroom window. A tree that's special to me, it's also had its share of indignities cast upon it during the few years we've been living here.

I've been looking forward to the luscious aroma of apple blossoms that comes forth every April, telling me that spring is truly here. Time to throw the windows open and welcome the freshness indoors. Well, it isn't that kind of spring this year! It's snowed twice today. Nothing that sticks to the ground, but enough that we're all moaning that, instead, we should be getting out the short-sleeved shirts and shorts – not hanging on to our parkas and turtlenecks.

It's also been very windy over the last week, gusts that make the house moan and creak. On one especially windy night earlier this week I heard a large crackle just as my husband was coming up the stairs to bed. I called out to make sure he was okay. He'd not taken a tumble down the steps thankfully and I chalked the noise up to a garbage can blowing around outside.

The next morning as I was looking out at my apple tree as I always do, I was shocked to view what must have been the source of the noise the previous night. A couple of substantial limbs had been sheared off and lay close to the trunk.

Normally I'd just think this quite sad that such a beautiful tree had been damaged – but this is MY tree. The tree that I'd hoped would recover from previous damage, just as I had hoped at the time I wrote my earlier post that I would recover from the damage to my body. We were in this together!

The timing of this really hit me hard; it was just a day after we'd been to the hospital to review the results of tests and scans that I've undergone over the last few weeks. My illness is advancing. The bone lesions are spreading up my leg and into my hip, and my aorta now has involvement as well.

My tree and I are both not doing well. And in that same post of almost two years ago, I wrote about having to postpone my dream trip to the

Big Apple. And finally I must accept that it'll likely never happen. But sometimes, when you can't have something, it seems like it's all you can think about.

And as I finish up this post, it's snowing again. Not just snow, it's almost blizzard-ish. I think I'll just go back to bed and pull the sheets up over my head. Because it's just that kind of a week.

DARE I DREAM? NOT!
Tuesday, May 10, 2011

I was like most kids at bedtime, not wanting to go to sleep for fear that I might miss something exciting. And I was also an avid reader who hated to put a book down until I'd turned over the last page. It wasn't unusual to find me still awake far later than I should be with a flashlight and my newest novel under the sheets.

It's usually much later that we truly appreciate what a gift a good night of sleep can be. For most of my adulthood, it was something I took for granted; my head hit the pillow and I was out for a good seven or eight hours. And aside from a pretty rough first six months with colic, my daughter also joined the league of good sleepers.

During the ten months I was on steroids, my need for sleep diminished significantly, a very common side effect during prednisone treatment. But during that time, I didn't feel the need to catch up with naps – steroids put me into overdrive. My family were probably secretly begging for a pause switch to be installed!

As my dosages dropped over the months, my regular sleep pattern returned. And then some. It seemed like all I could do was sleep all night and nap most of the day, getting absolutely nothing productive accomplished besides keeping the bed and couch warm.

And then something happened about five weeks ago that I'm at a loss to explain. Within a few days, I went from sleeping excessive amounts to hardly sleeping at all. Hard to believe, but over the past few weeks I've slept on average about three hours a night, and up to five hours on the best night in the last month.

I'm not fretting, I'm not worrying, and it's not stress that keeps me alert every night. Just a complete inability to drift off. It's actually a bit alarming just how chipper I am at

3 a.m. Even annoyingly so, I'd venture.

My days however are long, and I'm feeling physically spent but unable to nap. Like there's a brilliant light shining into my eyes that I can't turn off or dim. Every single night it's the same routine, I lay awake until about 4 a.m., and wake up just a few short hours later to a day that drags on, seemingly forever.

Why didn't I appreciate it more when a good night of sleep took no effort whatsoever? And why do my most alert hours have to happen when I can't use them to best advantage? I'd love to spend time with my family, catch up with friends, and enjoy meals with loved ones. (I'm as hungry as all get-out when I'm so awake!) No takers I'm afraid, I'm on my own.

Sleep, please find me again. I promise I'll appreciate you more this time around.

SLEEP, GLORIOUS SLEEP!
Thursday, May 19, 2011

I don't always listen to my doctor, and at tomorrow's hospital appointment I'm going to explain why.

A post ago, I wrote about my inability to sleep. After night after night of just two or three hours, I was wearing thin after weeks of this pattern. Feeling the kind of exhaustion that you know just isn't good for you at all, I could feel myself losing whatever fragile grip I might have on my health. My appetite had gone wacky and I was feeling hungry all the time, unable to make decisions because the brain fog was so thick, and my sense of humour was obviously going out the window as my husband's attempts at getting me to laugh fell flat (and he's pretty darned funny).

I would take sleeping pills for a few nights in a row, but unfortunately they did absolutely nothing (whereas half a dose would usually have me out cold within half an hour when I was having a bad bout of pain). I tried most nights without pills, finding myself ever so alert at 3 a.m. and the opposite at 3 p.m. the next day.

In a call to Dr. HPK about ten days ago, he informed me that there was nothing else he could prescribe – and to just relax. Relaxing was not my problem, just NOT SLEEPING was my problem!

I felt that somehow I needed to break the pattern, and it was time to get creative. Everything that is normally suggested for insomnia just wasn't working. I took a trip through my extensive collection of prescription meds and came across an antihistamine that was prescribed when I had my injection site reactions to Kineret. What had the doctor told me? Be careful with these Sandy, they'll knock you sideways with drowsiness! Hmmmm...Do I see a rash coming on?

When I did have the site reactions, I'd not taken the prescription med (do you see a trend here?), relying instead on topical lotions. So I had no idea how I'd react to them.

Out in ten minutes. And I stayed asleep for six hours. Absolute heaven. Tried again the next night – eight uninterrupted hours. And then twelve hours, a bit too much sleep but I was feeling energized again, and certainly more clear-headed. One more night of almost twelve hours and I felt that I'd broken that nasty cycle of insomnia.

Time to try without anything to help me sleep, and I've had a fantastic last three nights. Eight hours, waking fully rested – and back to my regular afternoon nap as well to reenergize when I start to sag.

Never have I been so pleased to realize that I was out like a light for the whole night. Bliss! And no rash either!

TAKING A BREAK
Saturday, July 09, 2011

It's been over six weeks since I've posted here, and I see from the daily stats that many of you are still checking in regularly despite my inactivity. And I thank you for your continued interest, concern and sweet notes of encouragement.

However it's time to take a break from writing *Without a Manual*. There have been some significant changes in my life over the last months and I just don't have it in me to share with the world at large right now. I've been told that occasionally past posts have been helpful to others seeking info about the treatment of Erdheim-Chester Disease, and for that reason I'll keep the blog up for now.

For those of you interested in how my meds are working out – I couldn't be happier with my Kineret treatment. Pain is infrequent, and when it does occur it's much milder than it had been before starting treatment in December. There's been talk at a recent hospital appointment about a new IL-1 inhibitor type drug that is administered less frequently. (These once-a-day shots are becoming more difficult as scar tissue builds in the allowed injection areas.) It's reassuring to know that my medical team continues to investigate other treatment options.

I thank you with all my heart for the amazing support I've received from so many since starting this blog two years ago.

With my gratitude, Sandy

STILL HERE...
Friday, April 06, 2012

I apologize. There are so many of you who were following my journey with ECD on this blog and I let you down.

Half jokingly, I said to my friend Sue a few weeks ago, that followers who aren't in direct contact with me might have believed that ECD had finished me off. You'll gather now of course that this isn't the case, and I'm sorry for leaving you wondering for so many months.

This will be a very short post to let you know I'm still here. For readers with whom I've been in contact, you know it's been quite a year. My illness continues to progress and I'm on another new, experimental treatment.

A little older, maybe a little wiser, and still trying to get through this with a brave face and a sense of humour in a life that is very different from one short year ago.

To those who've been supporting me along this difficult journey, thank you. You know who are (and there are many of you), and you know how much your support has meant to me. I'm grateful beyond words.

Saturday, May 26, 2012

Today is the first anniversary of a day that I never thought possible. My husband told me he was leaving our marriage. Not in my worst nightmare did I see it coming, and it continues to change the expectations I've had for every day since. The physical pain of my illness continues to increase, but over the last twelve months, the emotional pain far outweighed it.

Through this experience, I've seen the worst of the people around me, but also the best. I live by a "there are no coincidences" philosophy, and it's been proven over and over again in spades over the last year. As recently as this week, when I went to go choose my cemetery plot, I got a good old slap upside the head. "Sandy – listen to what the universe is whispering to you." (Or shouting in some cases.) Faith continues to be on my side and all will be explained in due time.

For the privacy of those involved, I choose not to go into details other than to let you know that my communication on this blog may be sporadic for a time. (I should say for a bit longer if I'm being honest, I sure haven't done a good job of keeping up here over the last year.) In one week, my daughter and I have to leave our home without a fixed address to go to. The implications are far reaching, emotionally, medically and practically. I'll soon find myself without a home to call our own, without professional nursing care, without the personal care workers who have made certain that I can remain independent for as long as possible as this illness progresses. And progress it does – I can see it in the eyes of friends who've not seen me for a few months. They can see that the essence of the person they know is still in there, but its physical housing deteriorates as the weeks and months pass.

To my friends, I keep saying if I can just reach the finish line of the closing date for the house I'll be at peace. Trying to move mountains when you're not even strong enough anymore to cut meat on your plate requires a special kind of fortitude. I thank God every day for the strength I still seem to be able to find, and for the endless support of dear friends who lift me up. I'm blessed beyond words.

I leave you with this quote:

"The truth is the truth even if no one believes it and a lie is a lie even if everyone believes it."

This is what gets me out of bed each day. I'm deeply saddened that people in my life whom I care a great deal about are no longer around because they've either believed lies, or chosen to put the truth into a corner.

I'm beyond grateful for those who can see truth and love, and know that this past year has not tarnished my capacity to love with every ounce of my being. If anything, it's been increased exponentially. I look back on this past year and know that what I've learned is that unconditional love does indeed exist in the hearts of many...but also not in all of them. This is one of the sad realities I've come to learn, along with many other lessons I've been given an opportunity to learn in this lifetime.

PACKING, WITH PLEASANT DIVERSIONS
Tuesday, May 29, 2012

A friend put it quite succinctly last night – this move is like no other I've experienced. Not only do I have no idea where I'm eventually moving to (which complicates what should be kept, sold or donated) but it's also like packing at the same time for a trip that I don't know how long will last. Do I pack for a week, a month, six months?

I've spent weeks trying to decide if each item is to go into storage (becoming somewhat inaccessible) or should be with me. (Is more than a couple of suitcases too much to bring?) Labelling has been a long and tedious process – what if I need something in a hurry? Will I find it quickly enough? More to the point, if I'm not mobile – have I labelled everything clearly enough that someone else can find it for me amongst the many boxes?

Every turn brings a new challenge. I'm finding out that lots of government departments don't accept a PO Box as a legal address. And that you can't do a Canada Post mail redirection from a PO Box to a new address when I have one. Frustration after frustration.

With losing my email addresses, my phone number, and my home address I've been feeling like I'm falling off the grid on Sunday. And then I get the most pleasant reminders that there are lots of people who won't let me.

This week I heard from several colleagues from my pre-Intrepid Lens days. News is travelling that I'm not well, and I'm touched that many have taken time to write lovely notes of encouragement.

One in particular shared a sentiment that touched me more than he probably realizes. He thanked me for giving him his first big chance. Many years back, I was in a position to hire several associates for a new team and his resume had caught my attention. He, along with several others at the time, joined the team I was assembling for the telecom company I worked for. We were making it up as we went along, trying to fill a void in looking after the needs of our customers. Quite the ride!

If I can give myself credit for anything, it's for being a pretty good judge of character. I've hired many employees over the years in different companies – and never regretted one. Some working relationships may have been more challenging than others, but everyone brought something valuable to the table. And it's never been about technical skills – those can be taught – it's been about who each of them was as a person.

To hear that my decision to hire this gentleman so many years back made a difference in his life put a grin on my face yesterday. We all want to feel like we've made a difference. And I have my lovely daughter as living testament to having done at least a few things right during my time here.

I know by now that I left a footprint. Good or bad experiences, I was here. A very dear friend pointed out to me that none of us are forgotten until the very last person that each of us knew leaves this earth.

"HOW LOW CAN YOU GO?" AND OTHER ACTEMRA PARTY TRICKS
Wednesday, June 13, 2012

Round three of my experimental treatment complete. And a complete failure. As grateful as I was to have the opportunity to try this treatment (it had been financed by a very generous anonymous donor through Toronto Western Hospital after the government and private insurance refused to fund it), it wasn't a lot of fun and I'm relieved that it's over.

One of the common side effects listed on the Actemra website/monograph is high blood pressure. Of course my body decided to do the complete opposite – the nurses who visited for the days following each treatment would get a look of shock in their eyes when taking my blood pressure. "How the heck are you still conscious, Sandy?" That low. "Let's get you to the hospital if it drops one number lower," kind of low.

I had started fainting again before the treatment, and this certainly wasn't helping. I'd scared my poor daughter out of her wits when she found me at the bottom of the staircase in the middle of the night a few months ago. I almost didn't even get the third infusion last week. The nurse took my blood pressure. And again. And a third time. It had dropped during the hour-long infusion twice before and she was quite hesitant to continue. I however, wanted to at least see the three-month trial continued to the end – maybe we'd be third-time lucky?

I asked my daughter, who'd driven me for this infusion, to say something that was sure to get me riled up – and she quickly piped up that there was something she'd been hiding from me. She'd gone ahead with the tattoo she'd previously promised to not get while I was still here. Sure enough, my blood pressure went up just enough to proceed. (And for the record – no tattoo as yet, but her quick thinking was quite helpful!) What other delights were in store?

Third day in, after each of the first two doses, I clogged up the shower drain when a good handful of hair fell out. That was accompanied by a heart rate that was even more irregular than usual. Then came the 5-10 days of mouth ulcers each month – making eating and talking quite uncomfortable. Fevers, flu-like symptoms, blurred vision, fatigue – all especially not welcome as I was trying to pack our home for the move last week.

And still no home to go to – we're in temporary quarters (very welcoming quarters at the home of my daughter's boyfriend's family). Bet you're begging to trade places with me at this point! And NO pain relief – which was the objective of this experiment. I'd hazard to say it might even have worsened over the last months. So came the expected decision Monday at the hospital. And where do we go from here?

A CHANGE OF HEART
Friday, June 15, 2012

I'm grateful to hear that my writing has been of some help to others (and their caregivers) facing illness. And that you give a darn about what's happening in my corner. I'm deeply thankful for your concern and good wishes.

Over time, I've come to know some fascinating people – who've connected me to other fascinating people – who've connected...you get the idea. However fascinating they are on own, several have shared with me writings, teachings, and concepts that have been meaningful to them.

Not a week has gone by in the last few months when I've not been given/sent/loaned/smoke-signalled books, articles, quotes by authors that I've never heard of – or in some cases had heard about but had never invested time in learning more about.

A big thank-you to the kind and generous souls who've sent audio books. With my vision declining, they've been a welcome respite from the printed word. But I do need to invest in a new CD player. My decades-old one makes me start from the beginning again of each new chapter whenever I pause it – but maybe that's a blessing in disguise in listening to interesting ideas more than once.

Yesterday afternoon I had one of my scheduled nurse visits (which will disappear soon if I don't find a fixed address in the next weeks, but that's out of my control at the moment). At every visit, the nurse takes my vitals, asks me questions about my pain, appetite etc. and evaluates my overall health. You might be familiar with (but I'd be pleased to know you don't have a reason to be) the Palliative Performance Scale. I've slid several notches in the last months, another one yesterday. It was recommended that I have the nurse and personal care workers come by more often too. That will have to wait until I find a home, hopefully that won't be too long a wait.

That spurred me to crack open a book that was loaned to me weeks ago (actually to us, this kind friend thought this book might be helpful to my daughter) called *The Needs of the Dying – A Guide for Bringing Hope, Comfort, and Love to Life's Final Chapter*, by David Kessler. Maybe not the sort of thing you want to get into on a sunny Thursday afternoon but I was pleasantly surprised as to how much I looked forward to reading it to its end. My goodness, I'm human!!! All these feelings and concerns I'm experiencing are normal and pretty much par for the course it would appear.

THE SUM OF CONSEQUENCE
Saturday, June 16, 2012

As a child, I was an avid reader. Undoubtedly, for the better part of my free time I'd be found with my nose in a book – lost in another world for hours at a time. (My daughter comes by the same obsession honestly.) My favourite Easter Hunt find ever was discovering a copy of *The Wizard of Oz* tucked on my bedroom window ledge behind the curtains. My parents understood that I'd get far more pleasure from a good read than from a basketful of chocolate (although they're very close and as an adult I'd say chocolate wins most days!)

My favourite Mother Goose nursery rhyme was "The House That Jack Built," as for most kids, the repetition was comforting. This rhyme has been on my mind a lot lately. The line about the cow with the crumpled horn can still produce a vivid image to this day, as to how that horn might have come to be crumpled. I don't claim to be any good at figuring out hidden meaning in literature – but this rhyme speaks to me about the layering of experiences (both in and out of one's control), to arrive at the place you may currently rest at.

Today I had a truly uplifting few hours with two people who without doubt (and we're going back thirty-five years on this one!) had a hand in shaping how I think and act as an adult.

They say that having a serious illness can be a blessing in disguise (there's no way I'm ready to declare that as my truth!) but my diagnosis has brought me to a place where I want the people who brought something positive to my life to know that I appreciate the gifts they've given me. I was very lucky to have been able to do that today. Thank you Arlene and Fred for teaching me about family, faith, and so much more. But most of all about trust; a lesson I wouldn't fully comprehend until I had a child of my own. Thank you for entrusting me with all that was and is most precious to you.

And let's not wait another twenty-eight or so years before we meet again!

BY GOSH, I THINK I'VE GOT IT!
Tuesday, June 19, 2012

I often think about why some of us have to follow a more difficult path than others on this earth. Many wonder, under the cloak of various faiths, if there's a higher purpose to suffering; something that will be explained on the other side. I think I may have found a use for some of the trials I've experienced in this lifetime.

It would seem that I'm to experience the full range of medical tests, treatments (and indignities) that can be foisted upon the human body. I've had scopes, biopsies, toxic chemicals running through my veins, implants (an internal loop monitor and my pacemaker), steroids, surgeries, scans, more meds than you can count, etc. etc. etc...With more on the way.

Perhaps after I leave for the hereafter, my job is to get inside the heads and dreams of those who have some control over the health care system. With a gentle whisper I'm to remind them of how hard it is to manoeuvre through the system when you're already behind the eight ball. To re-think that refusal to cover an expensive experimental treatment that might help the pain. To suggest that they offer a kind hello on the phone instead of a growl that makes the caller wonder if they're about to get a boatload of attitude for having had the nerve to call for an appointment.

Don't get me wrong. I've seen much of the good that happens in our healthcare system. Some really wonderful people who continue to provide me with excellent care on this journey – and who look at me as a person rather than as a patient file. Good people who often don't get the recognition they deserve. My family doctor right through to my specialists at several downtown hospitals, and the staff who support them. But in between, there are some mighty big gullies to fall into – especially if you're on your own without an advocate watching out for you.

My physical pain has delivered me to a point that I just don't think I can take much more without considering drastic measures. The last few days I've taken over five times the dosage of pain meds each day that the average grown adult should take and it's hardly making a dent (and yes, my doctor is aware of this). All non-narcotic – unfortunately I'm allergic to the whole family of opiates so they're out.

I finally gave in and placed the call to my orthopaedic oncologist this morning. Tell me doctor what you've got on offer – Bone graft? Chemo? Radiation? Let's think of something quick because I've been checking out chainsaws on the Home Depot website – I swear, if something doesn't give soon I'm going to tear that leg of mine off. Add to that, letting myself get a decent case of dehydration and I'm one miserable puppy today.

So, on a more serene note: Please God, let me get through this with grace, a smile, and a kind word for all I meet on the next part of the journey (I was going to say leg, but that's just too lame a pun!)...and humour. And let me feel the all the care and love that flows my way in abundance.

BY THE SKIN OF MY TEETH
Monday, June 25, 2012

I'm not a big Twitterer myself, but do enjoy following a number of people. My daughter for one, who can sum up quite a lot in only one hundred and forty characters. She often posts with courage that I lack, in admitting her struggles with what she/we have been going through. You're right my sweetheart, a lot of this really, really sucks. You may put it in different words, but know that I hear you. For the beautiful, honest, loving, smart, courageous (and often hilarious) person you've always been. I'm so proud to share you with others in your life who love and care for you. This post is dedicated to you.

I recently started following a gentleman by the name of David Roads (Motivational Quotes.) A few hours ago he posted the following:

"We all, at certain times in our lives, find ourselves broken. True strength is found in picking up the pieces".

Broken. This is a word that has come up a lot in conversations over the last year and some. Broken. What does that mean? I've said I feel broken. My physical body is surely broken, and my spirit at times has been broken. Almost as palpable as if my spine had been snapped in two.

By admitting that I've felt broken, I've had others share that they too have felt broken at times in their life. We have words for this emotional pain; shattered, torn apart, ripped open, stabbed in the heart, crushed. All physical descriptions for that which has devastated one's very soul and not left a single mark of evidence on the outside of what has happened on the inside.

I'm not alone. Having felt broken doesn't make me less of a person. It doesn't make me irrational, unbalanced, or immature. It doesn't make me undeserving of respect and compassion. It makes me human. And if you've been there, welcome to the clan – you're human too.

I'm picking up the pieces...by the skin of my teeth. With the love and support of friends, family, and even lots of people I hardly know. (Since starting this blog three years ago, I'm astounded as to how many strangers have taken the time to write to me with words of encouragement, faith, and stories of their own to share.)

Major obstacles keep being thrown in my way and sometimes I do feel myself nearing the lip of the Pit of Despair. (*Princess Bride* reference – one of my all time favourite movies. I could use a Westley of my own right about now!)

But I pick up the pieces. And try to pick up my daughter's pieces. True strength...or is it having just enough optimism to hope that tomorrow will be better?

WHEN ONE DOOR CLOSES, ANOTHER DOOR...
Monday, July 02, 2012

Can't even be nudged open a tiny crack. I had mistakenly believed that the Ontarians with Disabilities Act meant that any building erected after a certain date had to be handicapped accessible. Sadly I'm learning that term usually means only if one has additional persons to help.

In an attempt to be somewhat optimistic that I'd soon be able to find a home for myself and my daughter, I accepted the offer of our good friend Janet, to take me to view a few apartments. I was dropped off at the front door to avoid the painful walk through the parking lot. It being a crisp morning, I thought I'd go into the entry foyer to warm up and wait for my Janet to join me.

A harsh reality hit me. The doors were just too heavy for me to budge. My increasing weakness prevents me from doing lots of things for myself these days, but having relied on automated doors at my usual haunts of hospitals and clinics, I hadn't even attempted a non-automated door in quite a while. This was simply not an option for accommodation if I couldn't get the front door open by myself.

And so the morning continued in much the same manner. Each entry door was simply too heavy for me to manage on my own. We thought we got lucky with one building that had a handicapped entry button – but it proved to be out of order. And the apartment, once we got in to see it, was simply disgusting. Even the agent agreed that it needed a total overhaul to make it liveable. I was already looking at the top end of what I'd been counselled I might be able to afford, once all the legal separation details are at long last settled, and this was unnerving to see what was on offer.

I've since learned that newer buildings meet Disability Code by having doors wide enough for a wheelchair, but that only works if you have two people with you. One to push the wheelchair, the other to hold the door open. This wasn't coming together at all in the way we had hoped and prayed for, under already trying circumstances. So many apartments that had seemed like they would meet our very basic requirements for an affordable apartment in a safe neighbourhood were no longer options. Ninety percent, or more, of potential housing off the list in one fell swoop – and I'm only on crutches at this point. It will be totally out of the question when a wheelchair is required.

As you might know from previous posts, my daughter and are currently without a home. The very wonderful Miele family (Tony and Janet, and their three sons Joseph, Thomas, and James – my daughter's boyfriend) have rescued us from the disheartening alternative of a homeless shelter offered by social services. But "couch-surfing," in my condition, is far from ideal. My daughter and I currently share a small room, and share a bathroom with others. Those of you who are familiar with my susceptibility to infection will understand the concerns there. And we have to deal with stairs – lots of them. And we're relying on the Miele family to feed us – and I'm surely driving them up the wall with the restricted diet I have to adhere to avoid the dreaded Epi-Pen.

Living out of suitcases for the last four weeks is taking its toll. I end up resting in bed for most of the day, in an attempt to take the pressure off my leg and hip. Talk about a serious case of cabin fever! No TV in there, limited Internet access, and a computer that shuts down from overheating after just ten minutes of use. And almost invariably, I've forgotten my towel or toiletries after making the trek down the hall to the bathroom.

Don't mistake me, I'm so very grateful for the friends who have given us shelter when there wasn't any other viable option – but we all recognize that this was meant to be a temporary fix to a larger problem that should have been solved long ago.

This goal of a fixed address slides further and further away. Landlords turn me down immediately for rental units – I have no income and insufficient liquid assets to assure them that I can pay out for a full year of a lease. (A good portion of my retirement savings was depleted over the last three years and most of what's left is locked into a pension fund that I can't access.) And no landlord will allow me to alter a rental unit with the mobility aids required to allow me to remain independent as long as possible.

Nor can I buy a small condo because the portion of the house proceeds that I'm entitled to stay in trust until legalities of my separation are worked out. Buying a condo would be the ideal scenario so that I could make alterations (for example replacing a bathtub with a shower/seat) as my illness progresses. Then I could stay as long as possible in a home of my own before moving to a nursing home or into hospice care. If you know me personally, you know how doggedly determined I am to be independent and do as much for myself as possible.

Over the last few months, I've checked the real estate listings first thing upon waking; they will have been updated overnight. There are only a few complexes in Burlington with that precious handicapped button that even come close to my very meagre budget. Apartments are listed, and disappear almost as quickly. And now that we're into summer, hardly any appear at all.

The thought of further imposing on our dear friends deeply concerns us; my daughter and I are both anxious to find a place of our own. In two short months, she heads back to university and for her own peace of mind, she wants to see for herself that I've been ensconced in a safe environment and that the nurses and personal care workers are in place. And that care too is at risk right now without proof of permanent residency in Burlington.

Hopefully you never find a need to impose on anyone in this way that we have had to, but we certainly count ourselves very blessed to have the kind of friends who would welcome us in the way they have. However, it's difficult to accept that my health issues create a burden on others, especially knowing that there's a window of independence left for me that I've not been able to take advantage of.

And c'mon builders – how much more can it cost to install automated doors on the front door of an apartment building?

R U KIDDING?
Thursday, July 12, 2012

My daughter tells me that I'm a really cool mom. High praise coming from an eighteen-year-old! But of course by using this title for my post, I've just made myself totally uncool. Does not caring that it might appear uncool make me cool again? You'll have to ask her yourself.

Really though, a week we could have done without.

I'll start off with my daughter's car accident on Saturday. She'll be fine but it was quite a scare for us. Whiplash and her body reacted to the jostling with a fever that went over 104 degrees...several times. Her first ride in an ambulance ensued. (Can we make that the last one too honey?) Lots of physio and massage therapy and she's on the mend. As for the car, it really didn't take it well either. Or rather my Visa didn't. Less than a week later and we can (sort of) laugh about it. But only a little bit.

Then there was my cardiac assessment today at Toronto Western; the news was not welcomed with open arms. I need to undergo an emergency, specialized, cardiac CT scan on Monday, and I have to forego chocolate in the meantime – simply unacceptable! This will be followed by a decision as to whether surgery is required. Those of us familiar with Erdheim-Chester Disease might know the term "coated aorta," and it's not a good thing. The only thing I want coated these days is the outside of me – with all this weight loss due to stress, I'm shivering half the time, even in the heat southern Ontario is dealing with.

But on the upside – a roomful of doctors agreed that I'm just about ready to take the medical school entrance exam with all that I've learned during my many, many hospital visits. I speak English, some French and

German and enough medical jargon to impress the chief resident. C'mon – for a lark let me just see how high I can score!

Almost six weeks now without a home. It's getting quite tiresome living out of a suitcase. At least once a day I think to myself, "I'll go get my....oh, yeah – it's in storage." My daughter is being such a trouper over this situation but it weighs heavily on both of us. And although I know she loves me very much, sharing a small room and a bed with your mom isn't the most fun. One of us likes things quite neat, the other not so much. You might envision how I'm dropping down on the cool-mom scale as each day passes.

This weekend, I'll be trying to figure out how I'll kill lots of waiting time in hospitals next week. (Thursday will be spent at the cancer centre assessing surgery/radiation for pain management.) There's only so much of Words with Friends, Angry Birds, Plants vs. Zombies, Facebook, and Twitter a girl can take.

Bring on tomorrow...but I won't turn down a completely boring day where my biggest concern is pondering whether my daughter thinks that the title to this post was indeed completely uncool.

RESURRECTING THE "NEW YORK PROJECT"
Saturday, July 14, 2012

When I was diagnosed three years ago with Erdheim-Chester Disease, my then-husband asked me to think about my bucket list. What would I want to do, see, experience, taste, feel, or own before it would become too late? One thing on my list was easy and it never felt like it actually needed to be written down. I'll let you figure that one out – let's just say that my family situation couldn't be further from what I'd envisioned or had been promised would be there for me unconditionally when I was first told that I was facing a daunting future.

The first thing on my bucket list was a trip to New York City. I'd been privileged to travel a fair amount in my twenties – visiting wonderful cities around the world but somehow never made it to the Big Apple. To be clear, I had been in NYC airspace many times in my frequent commute to a second office in Princeton, New Jersey in the mid-90's – always hoping for clear weather for a good view of Manhattan and the Statue of Liberty as the plane made its descent into Newark Airport.

When I imagined visiting the city on my first and likely only trip, I saw myself enraptured by all that my senses could take in. We'd be trying new flavours offered up by street food vendors, I'd be walking through Central Park, hand in hand with my sweetheart, visiting MOMA trying to understand what the artist was trying to convey as we viewed some abstract piece of work, checking out the creativity of the High Line Park … the list goes on. As I planned my trip, it became apparent I'd have to trim down my wish list – a week wouldn't be nearly enough time!

And by some miracle, my leg pain would subside just enough to do the walking that would be required to really experience New York. And of course I'd have my camera around my neck the entire time – except for the times that it would be raised to my eye to capture what I would interpret as the essence of the city. The people, the architecture, the sights. (The sounds and smells however would have to be committed to memory rather than a digital file!)

The trip never happened. The risk of going across the border without medical insurance was too high and even walking half a city block was now out of the question. When we realized about a year and a half ago that this trip wasn't going to happen, my ex made a lovely suggestion. Why not go to New York virtually? He immediately went to work contacting friends and family asking them to share their experiences, and a few did before our marriage suddenly took a very different direction and my bucket list had no importance to me at all anymore.

I recognize that I still very much want to go, but it's truly not an option. A dear friend took me on a virtual trip to NYC last November; it's a gift that I'll treasure always. If you're visiting me, I'd be happy to share the experience with you – it was a gift put together with forethought, ingenuity, a bit of gumption and most of all lots of love.

And now I reach out to all of you to help me fill "my week" in New York City. If you've had the opportunity to visit, or live, or if you dream of going there yourself, I'd be most grateful if you'd share your experiences (or anticipated ones if you, like me, would love the chance to see it for yourself but haven't). Please share your funny stories about a wild cab ride, a fantastic meal, a sight you'll never forget, a description of a New Yorker who was imprinted in your memory.

Please share photos, quotes, and tales of adventure (or misadventure)! Even if it's just a quick sentence – or more if you've got a great story to share, I'd be honoured if you'd send me your version of what New York is to you. With Google Streetview, I love looking up the locations that are mentioned to me so please include street addresses, it certainly enhances the experience!

With that, I thank you in advance for your contributions – and thanks to those of you who contributed when this project had been initiated last year. It's time for me to pick it up again on my own now.

It's not the same as being in New York, but it feels like with your help it could get very close.

CAN'T THINK OF A BETTER PROBLEM TO HAVE
Monday, July 16, 2012

The view is pretty astounding from where I am at the moment. The majestic New York City skyline spreads out before me as I look out from midtown Manhattan down towards the Financial District. I'm straining to pick out the neighbourhoods I've familiarized myself with over the years as I've researched my trip to the Big Apple. It's a beautiful day and I've let myself get lost in the wondrous scene in front of me.

All this from the comfort of my bed. Across the room sits a most spectacular (and huge!) photo canvas, in a style of how I would likely have photographed the view had I been there to do it myself. With a fish eye lens, printed in black and white, capturing the wispy clouds as they waft by on an otherwise clear day.

The canvas, along with a beautiful note and an inspiring book for my daughter (with a heartfelt inscription) were waiting at the entrance of our temporary home when I came home from the hospital today. The note and inscription...unsigned.

Here's the wonderful problem. Although I think I might have narrowed the suspects down a bit by the handwriting and phrasing, I can't be certain of who presented us with these amazing gifts. It could be one of several women I'm so very lucky to count as my friends. (Not that a man wouldn't be this thoughtful, but I suspect the lavender ribbon around the canvas and the smiley faces in the note were the work of the fairer sex.)

Just when I think I'm pretty sure it's one friend, I allow myself to reconsider that it might be another. At first I thought it must be a local friend, but then again I have some pretty darned ingenious friends who live far away who could have pulled off a surprise like this too.

Over the last hours, I've let myself ponder over who this very thoughtful soul might be but instead I'm going to marvel in the fact that I'm blessed to be in the position of wondering at all.

Whoever you are, thank you. You must have your reasons for leaving these wonderful gifts anonymously, and I'll respect that. But know that when we have a place to call home, I'll be watching the faces of all those who visit me to see if you're scanning the apartment to see where I've hung this gorgeous photo. I promise you won't have to search very long at all, New York will be there for me to enjoy anytime I like. And thank you for including my daughter in your generosity (and by the inscription there was a solid clue that you've met her!)

To anyone else who contributes to the "New York Project", I do hope that you'll give me a chance to thank you directly. Friends (and friends-to-be) have gone to much trouble to launch my virtual adventure. Dear readers – please know that every contribution, however brief, is much appreciated. It all adds up to one heck of a collection of New York experiences that I'll treasure.

A BIT OF LEVITY
Thursday, August 02, 2012

I'll soon explain in another post why I was there today (and for me, it's significant ECD related news!), but I wanted to share the following conversation overheard in my oncologist's waiting room this afternoon.

Envision three elderly women, seated with walkers at their side. Very animated as they speak, and apparently unaware that everyone else could hear them.

"What's your favourite ice cream flavour?" They exchange replies. "How about the best burger place?" again, answering each other. "Did you know that bar food is better than anything else?" Oh really? "Have you ever boiled lettuce by accident, thinking you were making cabbage soup?"

By this time, I look up from my iPad to realize that these women had the rapt attention (yet the pretence of not paying heed) of all the other patients in the room. "Have you ever tooted on a bus and pretended that someone else did it?"

And with that, I got called into my appointment so I'll never know if it's just something that elderly ladies in general try to get away with.

WHAT GOES AROUND, COMES AROUND
Friday, August 03, 2012

A dear friend recently gave me the gift of some downloadable university lectures and another friend kindly provided the bandwidth for me to transfer them to my laptop. The course that I selected was *Great World Religions*; it's been absolutely fascinating and what I've heard has led to some truly amazing conversations with friends.

Normally I'd consider religion to be a sensitive subject to address, but these are friends whom I trust to converse about these issues without judgement. The subject of karma is often brought up. Many of you may understand why I struggle with this. Over the last year and a half I've faced the end of my marriage/loss of my partner and most avid supporter, the loss of our home, the shutdown of my business, and my only child leaving for university. Not to mention that whole serious illness business. All of these falling into the category of the top stressors one can face in life. And all at once.

I've tried very hard to be a loving, honest, and kind person and like most people, at times I've had my failures in my attempts to be the best person I can be. Asking "Why me?" seems a natural question to ask. As I go through my course, one message seems to be abundantly clear. All religions, however differently worded seem to attempt to follow a version of the Golden Rule. Treat others as you wish to be treated. Karma, as I understand it, follows a similar basic concept. What you give out comes back to you. The religions vary as to whether one might expect the repercussions to occur in this lifetime or another; but it all comes down to doing the right thing.

Seven years ago when we moved to Burlington, I was trying to gain a foothold locally for my portrait photography business. It's often suggested to photographers starting out in a new market to donate one's services to a local charity, and a local clothing store mentioned that they'd gladly accept a portrait package to be auctioned off in support of the Juravinski Cancer Centre in Hamilton.

It didn't go without notice and a smile that yesterday I sat in an examination room at that same hospital, the Juravinksi Cancer Centre. I was hearing the news that upon review of the pathology of my bone tumours (I'm the first case of ECD that they've seen) – they'd be happy to give radiation a try. In their opinion, I had a about an 80% chance of pain reduction.

We'd start on both legs. (I received confirmation that the tumours have spread to the left side, in addition to the right). If radiation was successful, we'd move to where other bone tumours have grown and cause me significant pain. The doctors had clearly done their research. The few ECD patients elsewhere in the world who'd tried radiation treatment for pain had been administered a lower dose, and in these cases it appears that pain returned fairly soon after completion of the treatment.

With my permission, they were proposing high doses of radiation in hopes that pain relief would be longer lasting. In the next week or so I'll be heading over to the hospital to get my marker tattoos, to accurately guide the radiation beams. My vanity disappeared long ago; I'm so marked up by surgery and accident scars I'm not the least bit bothered by the permanent markings. Heck, we can even have a bit of fun playing connect the dots to see who comes up with the most creative design!

The treatment schedule unfortunately is likely to be delayed; two months out and my daughter and I are still without a home or financial support of any kind. The last thing I need is to be packing up again (albeit on a much smaller scale this time), moving and unpacking, during the rigors and side effects of treatment. But there is one huge bonus in this. For once, funding of treatment is not an issue, all radiation treatments are going to be taken care of. Bless you karma. I'd like to believe this has come my way because the owner of a lovely little shop in Burlington gave me the chance to give so many years ago.

P.S. My mail was just picked up, my first opportunity in the last week. Nine more anonymous NYC postcards. Thank you, whoever you are! I promise that once I'm in my own place, I'll make every effort to watch all of your favourite NYC-themed movies that you listed. Some of which I've seen (and will happily watch again) and others will be new for me. What a delightful surprise to distract me on a day full of calls and paperwork I'd rather not be tackling!

A CASE OF MISTAKEN IDENTITY
Saturday, August 04, 2012

One step forward, three steps back. Usually the pattern seems to be two steps back, but it's just been that kind of a week. And month. And year. Upon hearing the news on Thursday that I'm eligible for radiation therapy for pain management, yesterday took another downward turn. After pleading my case for the last week, the CCAC is recalling the wheelchair pad that many of you have seen me hauling around to doctors' appointments and for the rare outing.

That thing had truly been a blessing for the last six months. Most of my day is spent in bed, trying to take pressure off of my hips and legs. Hence the addiction to Words with Friends, on-line courses, and whatever it takes to occupy my mind in a semi-productive way on my iPad. As for Angry Birds, I'm going with the excuse that it's good for my manual dexterity! For car rides to the hospital or for longer periods of time visiting with friends, the wheelchair pad allowed me to sit with considerably less pain. Instead of trying to contort myself to shift weight from my hips, I could get away with appearing to be a healthy person for a good half-hour or more.

To put it bluntly – I've not expired quickly enough. My allotment of time for use of the pad as a palliative patient has passed, but they can put me in touch with the manufacturer to purchase one for about $750. As if I have that kind of money floating around – they're well aware of my situation of being without a home and financial support. This "expiring not quickly enough" concept is wearing a bit thin in my world right now.

I know the direction that this is heading. The disease is spreading, and I'm getting worse. There is no question about that. In the last forty-eight hours, I've had the following conversation three times with specialists (various phrasings, but you'll get the drift). "Sandy, you do understand that the radiation is only meant for palliative treatment to try to decrease your pain. Right? There's no reason to believe that it'll slow down the progression, and we need you to understand that." I'm sorry, but at what point did I express that I had any hope whatsoever that I was going to get better with any of these experimental treatments?

I may be a "glass half-full" kind of gal in many ways but I do understand the prognosis. I just want less pain! And most certainly the physical challenges and test results indicate what is going on. It's pretty amazing that my heart hasn't imploded yet, according to the data downloaded from my pacemaker. The Energizer Bunny just keeps on going!

Back to this issue of qualifying my treatment expectations. My presentation as a generally happy person is confusing the heck out of many. Because I'm in their office with a smile on my face and an occasional joke, I fear that they sometimes believe that I'm not taking this seriously. But this is the way that I'm choosing to come to terms with my various challenges. I pick my battles, because I don't have the energy to fight them all (and there are some really crucial ones on my plate right now that suck every ounce out of me on a regular basis).

There are many aspects of my life that are out of my control, but I do get to choose my attitude every day. I want to be the person that others still enjoy being around (and to my friends, I thank you for letting me know in so many ways that you think that I'm worth spending time with in person, on the phone, on e-mail or Facebook). Heck, I just want to like myself when I'm on my own! Being cranky just doesn't feel pleasant at all. Don't let the failing body fool you. I'm still in here. No false hopes, just a strong desire to spend the rest of the time that's left with a smile on my face far more frequently than you'll find a frown or tears.

I still want to enjoy what I can with abandon, love the people I love, and graciously accept kindness and love in return. Lie that it may be, sometimes I just need to hear that everything will be okay – to keep me going, even though as every day passes it becomes less of a truth.

AN UNDOING
Saturday, August 11, 2012

Dr. HPK called me a week ago last Friday; it was a chance to update him on how things had gone at the cancer centre the afternoon before. At the end of our call that morning, he quickly added "CBC. Watch at 5 p.m. on Monday. A film crew has been here with my team for the last few days and I'd like you to catch it if you can."

There's no DVR machine where I'm staying, and didn't have any luck finding anyone who'd be able to record the program for me. But I was able to watch a TV for the hour- long program that afternoon, and I was thrilled to learn that Dr. HPK (and a primary benefactor for his team as well) were both to be featured on a documentary highlighting the accomplishments of Jamaican-Canadians in a wide array of fields.

My heart filled with gratitude and warm memories as the program included an interview with Dr. HPK, showed many of his associates whom I've come to meet, and panned the lobby of the hospital wing that was named after him in a ceremony almost two years ago. I had been at that ceremony. It took quite a bit of effort physically to be there, coming from our home about an hour from downtown on a blustery November evening. It was arranged that a friend drive me to the train, I met my husband at the station in the city, and we proceeded by cab to the hospital.

As the only patient invited, I felt so honoured to be there and nothing was going to stop me from attending. My husband so carefully held my hand as we made our way up and down staircases; and as was his habit he'd invisibly form a circle around me that no one could enter lest they bump me and break one of my fragile bones or cause me any pain. My reason for holding the honour as the sole patient in attendance was because in the months prior, my doctor had given me the privilege of photographing him for a project to be entitled "Empathy."

It was his idea to include my husband and daughter in the photo session, and from those photographs, a beautiful painting was created (by a doctor who happens to be multi-talented), which was used in a campaign for 3M. I'm also told that sometime in the future it will hang in the National Gallery of Canada in Ottawa as part of an exhibit honouring outstanding Canadian doctors. Postcards of the image hang on bulletin boards around the hospital; it always makes me smile when other doctors point out that they know my photographs inspired the painting. And they know because my doctor will tell anyone who'll listen about how this all came about. His humility is astounding; he finds any way he can to give credit to others. We all know the truth of what an incredible man he is and I couldn't be prouder to have contributed in a small way to recognizing what he does for his patients and the medical students/doctors who have the phenomenal opportunity to learn from him. I watched his segment of the program with tears in my eyes, thinking about all that he, his team, and the benefactors have done for me over the last three plus years.

But then it flashed on the screen. I knew in my gut it was going to appear in the program, and there it was. The painting. On the big screen, I was seeing my husband and my daughter interpreted in a lovely piece of artwork that sums up so much to me about empathy. When we did the photo shoot I was so grateful to my family for agreeing to take part. At that time all three featured in the photograph conveyed what was desired. Empathy. The three of them were doing everything possible to support me as patient, a wife, and a mother, and I was beyond grateful to have so much love around me.

It felt like a punch to the gut. Here I was on what would have been our seventh wedding anniversary, looking at my ex-husband on TV (or more accurately the back of him). Remembering the ceremony at which he kept telling me how proud he was of me. To anyone who would listen, he would say how grateful he was to be by my side, proud of my courage in fighting my illness – that I was his hero, that we made a fantastic team. That it was so easy to forget I was sick because our house was always full of laughter, affection, and love. Hadn't Sandy done a wonderful job of portraying the intended emotional response?

A few short months later (incidentally soon after I did a radio interview for CBC radio, in which I praised his unrelenting support) he told me that he wanted out of the marriage (or at least wanted a version of marriage that turned my stomach). That he hadn't loved me for years, didn't like me anymore, and at times even hated me. And vehemently, at that.

A punch to the gut. Trying, on one hand, to share in the thrill that my doctor, his family, and his staunch supporters might be feeling after watching the program but reeling from the reminder of what used to be. I was told that when the exhibit opens in Ottawa, I'll be invited. I'll move heaven and earth to be there to support my dear doctor, but I don't imagine at this moment that I'll have it in me to ever look at that painting again.

LOCATION, LOCATION, LOCATION...
Monday, August 13, 2012

To say that that the last eighteen months have been challenging is about as deep an understatement as I could possibly make. There are many of you who are aware of my personal and medical struggles, and nothing hit them home quite as sharply as taking notice of where I was on the occasion of my ex-husband and me respectively signing our separation agreement. Yes, friends, as of this afternoon that particular struggle is at long last put to rest. As one astute observer put it, this experience was like having my arm cut off and then being asked to be thankful for being given back a finger.

On Friday afternoon as my ex signed off, I was having my legs permanently tattooed in preparation for high dose radiation treatment at the Juravinski Cancer Centre, in hopes that this experiment offers a smidgen of pain relief. Its treatment I must defer because I don't yet have a place in which I can properly recover from side effects, nor should I be traipsing around during treatment looking for an apartment.

And note I said legs in plural – the bone tumours, as I had suspected, have spread to my left leg and to other bones as well. They've gotten away with having a party in my body without my permission! And not just spread, the little beast on the left leg arrived and outgrew the tumour on the right leg in one short year. No wonder I walk as if I have lead sewn into the hems of my pants.

Today it was my turn to sign the paperwork. My lawyer came to meet me; and where was I? Again at the hospital, of course. Waiting to discuss how the results from a barrage of tests (with more to come) affect my prognosis and what my quality of life might look like during the time that's left. Signing the paperwork in a room in which I've received a great deal of bad news over the last few years, I can't help but remember a video I found on YouTube when I was first diagnosed with ECD. A doctor specializing in hystiocytic disease said, of all the nasty diseases under this umbrella – "...ECD is not a particularly good disease to have." Isn't that the truth. Especially when you face it on your own.

WHERE DID I FILE THAT GANTT CHART?
Wednesday, August 15, 2012

There are the rare days when the realization that I'm seriously ill hits me particularly hard. Strangely, it's not the "procedure" days; an all-purpose way of stating that I'm to be poked, prodded, scanned, sliced, tattooed, injected, sampled, radiated, operated on – or anything else they can throw at me. It's also not the appointments in which I hear evidence presented to me that the illness has spread or that my "numbers" are up/down (or just not where they should be).

It's not even the days when I feel so physically beat up and exhausted that it's hard to think about moving my limbs, much less use them to lift myself out of bed. It's days like today, right after I'd finished a phone call with a friend I'd not spoken to in quite some time. Neither of us have had it easy over the last years; there were many points on which we could relate and commiserate. I'd say we both have a positive view on our challenges, and can see what needs to be done and we do it. Probably the reason why years ago, while employed at the same telecom company, we worked well together when on the same project team.

What left me unnerved afterwards was how indifferent I've become to discussing my illness and prognosis. And my death. To a great degree, my illness is my life. It has to be. It's a succession of appointments, tests, treatments, side effects, and symptoms. Absolutely every move I make has to take my condition into consideration. Are there stairs to contend with? Should I expect to be sitting up for a long period of time? Are there doors I'll need to try to open on my own? I was taken aback when I realized afterwards that I'd discussed my disease, prognosis, and my plans for the future with as much ease as I would have years ago, working out the details of a project at a conference table with my colleagues.

Here's what needs to be done; let's figure out who does what and then get the show on the road! Good old reliable Sandy, right to the end. Except some days it hits me exceptionally hard that this is the last project

I'll be working on. It's not a business objective that I'm plotting; I'm planning the project completion of me.

WHEN WE COULD FLY
Thursday, August 16, 2012

I can think back on the moment as if it were yesterday. It's a summer day in our old neighbourhood in Scarborough. I'm hot, sweat beading down my neck and chest, and so full of bliss I imagine the neighbours around me can see sunbeams shining out of my pores.

I'm telling myself to remember this moment, to treasure it. That one day, I may not have what I have right now. Almost reprimanding myself, *Sandy – you must remember what you're thinking, feeling, and most of all are doing.*

I'm running. I'm running foot races up and down our street with the neighbourhood children. My daughter running beside me, so are my niece and nephew who live two doors down. I'm at the time probably thirty-seven or thirty-eight years old and running faster even than some of the pre-teen boys. We run over and over again, to the point of sheer exhaustion. I suspect that some of the neighbours may think I've lost my marbles; why is she not joining the other grownups on the porch for a relaxing glass of wine?

Why I consciously decided to hold that moment in my memory I'll never understand. Probably at the time I was envisioning myself in my eighties or nineties, thinking that I'd be lucky to walk without a cane. Never imagining that walking just a short distance at age forty-seven would be as challenging and painful as it is.

I wasn't sick then (not entirely true, I've spent most of my adult life with health complications that might well have been the sprouting of ECD). But I wasn't hurting at that moment. I just was. Appreciating a gift that some never have a chance to know. I was going to take this moment, store it away, and one day recall it and be very grateful that at one time I could run. Fast, strong, and with joy in my heart.

That memory comes back to me frequently. What blows me away is that I'm not feeling sad that I can't run any more, it's a sense of overwhelming gratitude that I had consciously, deliberately appreciated the chance to run when I could.

WHAT AM I MADE OF?
Tuesday, August 21, 2012

I've been on one heck of a wild rollercoaster the last months, but the last few weeks have been beyond the scope of anything I could have imagined. I shared last week that our separation agreement was at long last signed (tens of thousands of dollars in legal fees later; the delays and arguments defying to me, and many others, any reasonable explanation).

The good news is that my daughter and I can finally look for a home; a very modest one but a place to call our own. A mission to find two homes actually, some pretty weird goings-on at the house in which she'd rented a room at university resulted in a mad search this past week for new accommodation for her. It's a long story – but I'll let your imagination run when I tell you a pig was involved. As in a farm animal, and that's far from the worst of it.

We were successful in one search, and hoping for good news soon on the other. A dear friend said to me that it seems like I'm trying to squeeze three months' worth of tasks into the next two weeks and I don't think that's at all far from the truth. Between coordinating efforts with social services, doctors, hospitals, lawyers, insurance companies, movers, superintendents, contractors (though let me not forget the efforts of friends to make this all a bit easier); I'm trying to keep my head from spinning off.

In the past, I've seemed to always be able to juggle and orchestrate myself through any difficult situation. This set of circumstances however, takes the prize. Everything that is in or out of my control is sucking every ounce of energy from me. What was it that I was told about taking it easy before I start high-dose radiation treatment in less than three weeks? What I'm trying to accomplish is beyond reason for even a healthy person, and to go it alone in this state of poor health is even more of an outrageous challenge.

As I scrolled through my to-do list on my iPad (over thirty phone calls alone in the last two days) I sat back and wondered to myself where I'm to find the stamina and strength to pull this all off successfully. What are my limits? When is enough, enough?

As it happens often with me, coincidences occur that seem as if they are only puzzle pieces falling into the place that they were meant to land. Within hours of having that chat with myself to take stock of how I'm to attack the weeks ahead, a Facebook friend posted quotes from various authors, with advice on how to write effectively. The following from Kurt Vonnegut caught my attention. Be a sadist. No matter how sweet and innocent your leading characters, make awful things happen to them—in order that the reader may see what they are made of. Who knows if our life plan is predetermined or bound by fate (I've been reading up quite a bit on Buddhism and Hinduism these days), but if there's any truth to those concepts – it's quite the sadist who wrote my life story out for me. And is this my chance to prove what I'm truly made of?

WILL I BE ASLEEP BEFORE I FINISH THIS POST?
Thursday, August 23, 2012

Tonight is the first night trying out another new drug; this time it's Pregabalin, which is typically used for the nerve pain of Fibromyalgia and Multiple Sclerosis. The hope is that some of my pain is caused by pressure exerted on the nerves by the tumours and not necessarily 100% coming from within the bones directly. Although it's not "on label" for ECD, the insurance covered the majority of the cost thankfully. But those deductibles are killing me on my extremely tight budget.

As an added bonus, I'm told that this drug may make me feel quite drowsy and I might have a better chance of sleeping through the pain that always wakes me up a few times each night. My friend Sandra, who joined me at that doctor's appointment, shared in my excitement at that prospect, knowing how difficult my nights can be. (We take our "high-fives" where we can get them!) Sometimes I'm lucky enough to drift back to sleep after a bit of meditation (or pain medication depending on how bad it gets). Other times it's game-over for the night and I have that unnerving time between 2-5 a.m. to contend with, when I feel more alone that at any other hours of the day or night.

There's always a wee bit of nervousness trying out a new med. I have a talent for having some odd side-effects. Being alone and trying new drugs makes me even more ill at ease. There's no one to check on me, to make sure I'm okay, to hold my hand when the side effects are uncomfortable or disconcerting.

I'm still awake. I was really hoping that I'd fall asleep in the middle of typing this post but no such luck.

Still here...playing Words with Friends.

Still here...playing soothing music.

Still here...thinking lovely thoughts about my beautiful daughter who turned nineteen today.

Still here...but getting too tired to worry about the fact that my right leg has gone numb.

Still here...barely...

Keeping my fingers crossed that I don't wake up for at least four or five hours. What's it come to when that's the best possible gift I can think of at this moment?

WELL BEYOND A GAME OF BROKEN TELEPHONE
Sunday, August 26, 2012

It's high time a few misconceptions were cleared up. Yesterday, for the umpteenth time (and I'm praying it's the last) I had an interaction with someone who expressed surprise that I was out in public – and miraculously able to string two words together. One more person who had been led to believe that I had lost all control of my mental faculties and was no longer making sense at all due to the brain tumours that supposedly had invaded my brain. My brain is just fine, thank you very much.

My body may be falling apart, but I consider myself incredibly blessed to be spared the tumours that can infiltrate the brain of ECD patients and cause numerous troubles. My faculties are intact, as the many people I frequently interact with, have lived with, and continue to laugh with can attest to.

Last year I went through a tragic grief process akin to dealing with the death of a dearly loved one; and it wouldn't be unfair to look at our situation from that perspective. I hit rock bottom with the loss of my marriage, my home, my business, and my health. I'm not ashamed to admit that. But lose my sanity? I did not. Mental health professionals whose support I sought as I went through my grieving process applauded the strength that I demonstrated under tragic circumstances. And continue to do so.

For those of you who've heard or read wild stories that I know are being shared, I can most confidently assure you that I'm still the same loving , serene, and gentle woman; a person who despite all that has happened can find plenty of humour under incredibly trying circumstances. My daughter and I are moving on. We're done with the turmoil, the wild accusations, and the unconscionable name-calling that continues to revisit me through the gossip mill. Done with living with the anxiety of what the next day would bring during the outrageously expensive legal proceedings.

We're pleased that this weekend we finalized the deal on an apartment that we will call our own, after three months of being without a home. Trust me – if I was in the state that may have been described to you, it would have become quickly apparent to those whom we've lived with in tight quarters. We were welcomed with open arms when we had nowhere to go, and now my daughter and I leave these dear friends who have become our family. The Miele family will continue to hold a very special place in our hearts and lives.

We're okay. We're not in great shape financially; we'll be sharing a small, one-bedroom apartment when my daughter is visiting from school, trying to keep my very old car glued together so that my daughter has transportation to her part-time job, and counting every last penny. We'll have to do without a lot; my budget doesn't allow for the cleaning ladies who've made my life much easier over the last year.

Even basic cable TV had to be cut with the realization that I just can't afford the deductibles on my pain and cardiac medications without resorting to limiting ourselves to the very barest of necessities. (This shall be an interesting experiment given that I'm pretty much housebound.)

My health continues to decline; the measures being taken at this time are palliative and on some days that's hard to swallow. (Perhaps the decision to move into an apartment by myself isn't the best decision, given my physical disability, but I've been left with no other options due to financial constraints.) The new place will be ours and we're at peace with our decision to leave the memories of the last two years behind us. But that's all they'll be – sad memories that we're choosing to bury.

But for goodness sake, if you're going to partake in the string of gossip surrounding the circumstances of my ex-husband's decision to walk out on me – try to remember who you knew me to be before. Whether you liked me or not, I'm still me. I'm done trying to understand how someone, who when handed an option to leave when I was first diagnosed (a very difficult offer for me to extend three years ago, but thought fair, given my prognosis) assured me with a loving heart that I would never be left to deal with this burden alone, could have adopted such a drastically different perspective in a very short time frame.

Before sharing the tales you may have heard, please take a moment to consider how it affects my daughter when derogatory comments reach her. Do you know these stories to be true without doubt? If you're not sure, just ask me. I'll be candid about the challenges I went through during this time; others have told me that they've been of some value in facing their own difficulties in life. My daughter's not in the dark to the fact that I have my faults; you'd never hear me say that I'm without them. She's already dealing with the fear (and not an unreasonable one) of losing me to this devastating disease. Isn't that more than enough for a nineteen-year-old to deal with?

A THOUGHTFUL GESTURE STRETCHES A VERY LONG WAY
Monday, September 03, 2012

Sometimes the most amazing things happen when you least expect them. Today so far had been a tough one, in bed and feeling run down from the move prep over the last few days. Not to mention the prospect of starting radiation in one week with the knowledge that I'll be dealing with the side-effects alone. It's scaring me silly at this moment.

I just got a call from the owner of the pharmacy near our old place. She'd remembered that I'd inquired many months ago about the cost of a nutritional supplement that I'm supposed to start my day with. (The meds make it hard to tolerate a proper breakfast.) I'd thanked her for checking, but it was unfortunately way out of my budget. (I'd received generous samples from social services prior to that, but had run out.) The pharmacist had several cases come her way today due to a cancelled special order and she called to offer them to me as a donation.

The funny thing is that I was going to call her tomorrow anyway to ask if my new place would be within her delivery area; they'd given me fantastic service over the years and I'd hoped that I could continue to give them the business for my numerous meds. (The answer is yes, they'd be happy to include me in their deliveries even though out of the official boundaries.)

It blows me away over and over again just how kind people can be.

REVELATIONS PART I
Wednesday, September 05, 2012

This is moving week, and it's been a week of moving revelations. Not to mean revelations that are moving, there's nothing at all touching to be found in this process.

I detest moving. Twice in just over three months. Never again. And I mean it. Please remind me of this week if I ever mention moving again. If it doesn't work, hit me over the head with something heavy.

I hate Styrofoam, and Styrofoam hates me. Hours that should have been spent unpacking tonight were instead spent vacuuming up and picking off those annoying bits that fly everywhere when you try to break it up into smaller pieces for the garbage. Please explain how Styrofoam found its way under my clothes, as I found the case to be a short time ago when getting ready for bed. The stuff is evil.

I'm shorter than I thought I was. Or they're making kitchen cupboards taller. In any case, I can't reach many of them in my new kitchen. Why did I not notice this before committing? It must have been those beautiful countertops – true love blinded me. It's happened before; apparently I'm a slow learner.

Cheesies (which to my delight were discovered to be gluten-free by my daughter last week) make a perfectly sensible dinner all on their own. My new home – new rules.

It's okay to enjoy the eye candy that was my telephone and Internet installer tonight. Good Lord, I'd forgotten that sometimes men come in arrestingly adorable packages. Who am I kidding? Have I forgotten that I watched a Bradley Cooper movie the other night? Just his dimples alone can put a silly grin on my face.

There was a time that I loved to map out room dimensions and furniture sizes/placement onto graph paper. Not so much anymore. Furniture lands where it lands on Saturday and I'll deal with it then. In our wildest dreams there's no way to squish half the contents of a four-bedroom, plus finished-basement house into a one-bedroom apartment. And I'm no hoarder, it's just the detritus of almost fifty years, a photography business, and the raising of one terrific daughter who LOVES books (who starts her second year of university tomorrow!) Stay tuned for the sale, it's going to be big and it's going to hurt. Whatever photo equipment I'd said I could never part with when you offered to buy it, it's time to ask me again.

No matter how lovely the kitchen, there's just no hiding the Do Not Resuscitate order that has to hang on the fridge. Which by the way isn't magnetic on the front as I tonight discovered; it's stainless steel that is just pretending.

I've just realized that I forgot to ask the telephone installer how to access my voicemail. Or he forgot to tell me, in which case he's completely forgiven. Adorableness gives him a free pass. Completely unlike me to let a detail like that slide for several hours, however, it's been a very unusual day.

REVELATIONS PART II
Thursday, September 06, 2012

I still hate moving – nothing's changed since yesterday.

You really need to listen to me on this point, I beg of you. If I ever give you the slightest impression that I'm considering changing abodes again in the future, you can not only hit me with the heavy object I mentioned in yesterday's post, you have permission to take my iPad away from me. Now you know that I really, really mean business.

I've lived out of a suitcase for over three months. How is it feasible that in transferring this small amount of clothing to the new place, I've lost one of the three pairs of pants that come close to fitting me?

Furniture can hide a multitude of sins; the carpet is in awful shape! I wish I'd checked it out before committing to this apartment.

Who manufactures a fan with a light so dim that even the moths take a pass? Another lamp is added to the list of things I need to get tomorrow.

I've always been against the idea of a TV in my bedroom, but I think that's the room that's going to win. If you're coming to visit and suggest that we rent a movie to take my mind off things, you've been forewarned. You'll be watching from under the duvet, but I'll lighten up on the no-snacking-in-bed rule.

I think I have a screw loose in booking high-dose radiation two days after a move to a new home. Yes, I'm that darned desperate for pain relief. But that badly needed to be in a one-story home before I did anything about it.

My biggest revelation today is that although I'm one tough cookie, this is seriously deep mud that I'm wading into on my own. Despite trying to keep a sense of humour about myself throughout this latest in a long string of challenges, I have to stop sweeping the gravity of what I'm facing under the rug. For at least a little while, I'm giving myself permission to be as frightened as others who care about me say I have the right to be.

REVELATIONS PART III
Tuesday, September 11, 2012

Move accomplished, however the unpacking part is far from over – there's just not enough space to put our things. I'm going to have to deal with it slowly over the next few weeks and months. Just look past the wall of boxes if you come to visit, I'm in there somewhere! Two days into radiation and I'm already beyond exhausted – but I'll take a few minutes to offer up my third and final set of moving revelations. I would have offered them up earlier but the Internet installation last week didn't stick. And I've been told that this building has unreliable connectivity; the joys of an old building.

There's something you should know about the paper that's used to wrap dishes and other breakables. It comes in a reasonably-sized (albeit very heavy!) package, yet by some miracle once it's been used, it explodes to a gazillion times its original volume. And it keeps growing! I'm hopeful that sometime tomorrow I'll find the kitchen.

Rolls of toilet paper made wonderful padding when packing fragile items – but when you unpack, what you have left over is a heck of a lot of toilet paper. Maybe I'll make a dividing wall with it, to give my daughter some privacy when she's home from school. I'll bet that I'll be the only one in the building with anything like it!

I came this close to not keeping the bed that I love so much; by some miracle our movers were able to get the headboard around a tight corner into the bedroom after forty-five minutes of most strenuous effort and trying every conceivable angle. They deserved a big hug for persevering, and they each got that along with a big kiss on the cheek to boot. I love my bed that much. (And the fact that they're handsome young men whom I adore took away any hesitation in showing my appreciation!)

Thankfully, a friend reminded me that she needed moving boxes – I got out of the job of cutting up lots of cardboard into 2 x 2-foot pieces. I suspect that they would have sat there in my hallway for a very long time had she not rescued them today.

I have friends who love to see me eat, and eat well at that. Two deliveries today of delicious goodies and one yesterday – maybe I should go through radiation more often!

Feeling very retro. The super in my building hooked me up to the antenna today so that I could get a few TV channels. Out of 158 units, only ten of us don't have cable, and I got the last port. So anyone else who moves into this building – sorry, it was me who kept you from the experience that is antenna TV.

I wish I'd visited my new place during a weekday before committing to it. For the last two days there's been the screeching squeal of metal on metal, hour upon hour – I need someone to help me find the nearby source so I'll at least know what led me to drive spikes into my eardrums. However difficult it might be to get on my knees, I'll be down there praying tonight that this is a temporary assault to the senses.

The recycling room in the basement of the building gives me an uneasy feeling. (Or as my daughter says, it's so sketchy!) But I do go down there alone with little hesitation – after all, what else could possibly happen to me? It's already been a life beyond the scope of what seems possible

– wouldn't it make quite a story to hear of me murdered while attempting to be ecologically responsible?

HALFWAY THERE (OR 1/4TH OR AN 1/8TH?)
Saturday, September 15, 2012

Officially, I'm halfway through my two weeks of high-dose radiation treatments, but having had the chance to meet many other patients over the last week, I'm coming to understand that there's a long way to go. I'm told that treatments tend to make themselves felt more afterwards; if I'm feeling tired now – just wait.

Thanks to the friends who've checked on me regularly this week. (And for the wonderful meals, snacks, diversions and encouragement too!) I'm holding up. As warned, the pain did increase sharply over the last few days (radiation pain flare) and I'm getting more fatigued as the days go on. The nausea is occasional and tolerable. When it hits, soon afterwards I get a craving for potato chips (which happily I had on hand but need to find more tomorrow). I was a little nervous to eat them on an angry stomach but weirdly, they do settle the nausea quite a bit. A few have commented that it sounds like morning sickness; thankfully I'm feeling nowhere near as queasy as I did when I was pregnant!

The nurses are coming daily right now to check on me. I pointed out today that I'm breaking out in bruises all over – not just on the irradiated sites. Hopefully it's not a sign of trouble with my blood cells; it's a good thing that I see my radiation oncologist on Monday so that he can see them for himself.

The irradiated skin is getting a bit pinkish; I'm diligently applying the Glaxal Base cream to minimize the anticipated skin burn. And forgive me for looking forward to one of the potential side effects of hair loss, I wouldn't mind a bit if I never needed to shave my legs again!

For those who have been wondering, the radiation treatments are themselves completely painless – and they come with a great team of technicians whom I look forward to seeing every visit.

I'm grateful for a weekend break from treatment; it's a chance to get myself mentally prepared for what's to come. The logistics and practicalities have been taken care of; the cupboards are full, the volunteer drivers from the Cancer Society booked – and phone numbers of friends who've insisted that they're available 24/7 for me are close by.

The tough part of this is coming home to an empty apartment, knowing that two things that were always guaranteed to soothe me and help more than any pain medication ever could – a loving hug and a head rub, aren't waiting for me anymore.

So much for "in sickness and in health," when there are greener pastures to be pursued. Yeah, I'm feeling a little bitter this week, especially after hearing that my ex landed himself a luxury apartment in an expensive neighbourhood when I've had to settle for something a distant throw from that description. One of us ended up in a far better financial position than before we married, the other far worse. You know which end I got.

LOOKING IN THE MIRROR. OH DEAR.
Sunday, September 16, 2012

A very busy week indeed between unpacking and radiation treatments. In preparation for the weeks ahead, I've spent the last few hours moving a few things around the apartment to make it easier on myself. I'd put some frequently used items out of reach and found myself grabbing a stepladder too many times a day. I met the previous tenants of my place, they're not much taller than I am and it's got me wondering just how gigantic someone before them must have been to put shelves and the bedroom clothes rod so darned high!

I worked up a bit of a sweat lugging and shifting things about and stripped down to a tank top to feel cooler as I worked on the front hall closet where I'm placing my hospital "kits"; various bags that accompany me depending on whether I'm doing a short trip like the radiation appointments this week; the bag that comes when there's a risk of an overnight stay; and the emergency room bag. I know, you're wondering how you can have a life as exciting and adventurous as mine. Sorry to leave you so envious, I get to keep all these thrills to myself.

As I turned to move one of the bags, I caught a glance of myself in the hallway full-length mirror and startled myself. And not in a good way. Who was this bony, gaunt woman looking back at me? Where the heck was the rest of me?

My pacemaker sticks out just below my collarbone (ick alert – you can clearly make out the wires and the ridges on the device. If I looked hard enough I'd not be surprised to make out the serial number), and my size-zero jeans hang off the edges of my hipbones. (I'm really painting quite a sexy image here, aren't I? Hold yourselves back gentlemen!) The frightening thing is that I've gained back about fifteen pounds since hitting my lowest point about four months ago.

When did it happen that I began to look so fragile? And how did I not snap in two, fifteen pounds ago? Incentive enough to not complain again about the high-calorie nutritional shakes I down first thing every morning. On second thought, they remain completely unappealing and I reserve the right to resent needing to drink them.

UNPACKING REVELATIONS – PERHAPS MOVING THIS TIME?
Monday, September 17, 2012

I had to find a home for a great many of my material possessions when we had to leave the house back in June, some of which were really difficult to part with: most of my photography equipment, plenty of books, lots of kitchen items. Much was donated and although I hope items found a home with people who would find value in them; it was still a difficult exercise to whittle a lifetime down to what would fit into a small storage space and later a small apartment. And now I do it again with the realization that all this stuff just isn't going to fit into our new home.

As I unpack, there are moments of regret in thinking of how much I'd like to still have a particular item. It's happened more than once this week that I think of a book I'd like to look at as I'm curled up in bed and realize I've sold it. A print I'd like to hang on the wall and know that it now hangs in someone else's home. What's done is done and I can't hang on to moments of sadness about the tough decisions my daughter and I had to make to lessen our footprint and to find some cash during a time when not a cent was coming our way.

What has become clear to me is that I hung on to some of the "right" things, and darn it these things are going to see the light! The good towels that I'd found on sale a good ten years ago that I'd stored away under the guest bed, taking out only when I indulged in the rare leisurely bath. They now become the everyday towels because darn it, I deserve it.

The bevy of servingware that was gifted by my aunt in Germany at the time of my first marriage. The good silverware, the beautiful platters – they're all getting out for a walk on a regular basis rather than coming out only at Christmas time. Even if it's just me.

Tonight I opened up the boxes of clothing that had gone into storage. (It was only a suitcase-worth that I took to our temporary home, thinking it would only be a couple of weeks.) A rush of sadness in realizing that there are pieces that I feel great in when I wear them, but their season has passed and they need to be put away until the warm weather returns next year. But my favourite sweaters? They're going to get worn this winter until they fall apart! The blankets given to me by dear friends? Pile them on! At the very least I'll not be cold this winter.

YOU CAN ONLY SIT BACK AND LAUGH. A LOT.
Tuesday, September 18, 2012

While a couple of relationships in my life have crashed and burned in the last year (related to the separation), others have delightfully grown into something dear and very special to me.

One level of friendship that must be dealt with concerns my illness. There's no hiding from it – if you're in my life, it has to be understood that it and I are inseparable. Sometimes I have to cancel plans; other times I have a short burst of energy that I'd like to take advantage of with someone whose company I enjoy. Other times there's no need for it to come up in conversation; although it always does because the people in my life care about how I'm feeling and always ask for an update.

An aspect of these relationships is the comfort level with including humour in discussing my health. I've come to realize that the more easily we can joke about my health, the more I know in my heart that the friend is there for the long haul. Not out of obligation or because of curiosity – but because they truly want to be part of my life and know that I want them around too.

Case in point (or two cases actually).

A few weeks ago it was my birthday. Not a big deal, my daughter's birthday follows on the next day and I'd rather concentrate on her celebration. (She was an amazing belated present for me nineteen years ago and nothing could ever top that.) My dear friend Kristee sent me a card and thoughtfully included a scratch lottery ticket, in hopes that I might win big.

I waited until my birthday to open it (I'm superstitious like that, thanks Mom), and emailed Kristee to thank her. What poured forth was a horrified apology from her with the realization that she had enclosed a "Cash for Life" ticket. She'd agonized about it for days, worrying that I'd take offence at the name of the lottery.

We had a good giggle about it (I truly hadn't registered which scratch card I'd been given – I just enjoy the fun of hoping for at least a free ticket). Which I did get, over and over again, until the lucky streak ended yesterday.

An opportunity for a good laugh struck again last night. Kristee had received a call from Costco about having purchased ground beef, which was potentially contaminated. Beef which she'd used to prepare chili for me, which she'd thoughtfully portioned out for the freezer to cover off a bunch of meals if I wasn't feeling up to cooking while I'm going through treatment.

Another worried email, very concerned that although there has been no reported illness, with my compromised immune system it might be a different story. Wouldn't it be something to get this far with battling ECD only to pass of food poisoning? For the record, I'd already eaten a portion last week and was perfectly fine. And perfectly sated – the chili was delicious. Not to make light of the recall, I pray that nobody becomes ill, but this story is of the thread that makes the fabric of my life.

My friends and I can joke about this because if they know me at all, they sense that my demise will have some sort of, "It could only happen to Sandy," component to it. Because that's just the kind of luck I have. And the great luck to have friends who roll with it all.

REMEMBERING WHEN (AND RATHER NOT)
Saturday, September 22, 2012

Since she was little, my daughter and I have played a game that allowed us to check our perspectives on a past event. Sometimes we look back on whatever situation with a similar view (and others not so much).

It goes something like this: "Mom, do you remember the time that I was so sick that I couldn't go out trick or treating at Halloween?" (Plugging in whatever memory, good or bad, that has cropped up).

Memories flood back of the worry of my little girl's fever creeping back over 104 degrees again as it had many times over the last few days that October. Knowing that despite all the preparations of sewing a costume and all the excitement that comes with a five-year-old anxiously awaiting the big day, I was going to have to keep her home with me. She was so ill she didn't even care at that point.

There have to be hundreds of those moments that we'll from time to time call upon to reaffirm our feelings about the event. I remember how disappointed I felt for her and how worried I was, and she recalls how sad she felt to hear the doorbell ringing as her neighbour friends came to the door for their treats and she could hardly lift her head from the couch a few feet away. And that makes me remember that although she couldn't partake, she didn't want me to turn off all the lights and not give out treats that night. Why should the other kids miss out? For the record, her dad went out on her behalf that night with a pillowcase to collect goodies from a few neighbours who would have been awaiting her visit. And when she was better, she was allowed a trip to Sugar Mountain for a good-sized heap of treats of her choosing.

It's those kinds of moments that we look back on to reaffirm our commitment to getting through those challenges together and to see whether we're yet ready to laugh about them in hindsight. Many are now worth a good chuckle; others are reminders that life is sometimes quite tough and painful.

It's been several weeks of evaluating challenges and wondering whether, if given time, I'll be able to laugh about them down the road. I sincerely hope that at least a few of them will give pause and a smile, because they're certainly not right now.

Remember the time when I went through radiation treatment and I was so sore and tired that all I could do was regret that I'd not taken friends up on offers to come stay with me? Radiation 'fatigue' is such a totally off-base description. A semi-coma state is more like it. All I can do is sleep and wish that I had a magic fairy to go make me something to eat. I've just managed my first consecutive two-hour period of being awake in the last two days and the best I can do is drag my laptop a foot over to type this. Up until now, staring at the ceiling was the extent of my exertion.

There are a few dozen challenges over the last few weeks that I wonder to myself if I'll ever laugh about them. If so, it'll be my own private joke and that, in itself, makes me sad. Lost along with this are the opportunities to celebrate the successes when they appear.

At the hospital they make a big deal out of finishing treatment. Everyone who had reason to check my file out yesterday was ready with words of congratulations, a hug, and words of encouragement. Including the volunteer driver who had been notified that this was an important day.

I came home to an empty apartment, exhausted, having to deal with a broken dishwasher, facing once again that really awful carpet that taunts me, listening to the sounds of grating metal from the industrial area just behind me, seeing that my apartment needed a going-over badly with a vacuum and a dust cloth and it wasn't going to clean itself, hungry as could be, and with no energy to make myself anything.

I suppose deep sleep is the kindest gift that can be given to me at this point. I don't want to even think right now if I'll play the "remember when" game about all this in the future. I just want it all to go away for a while and for this apartment to spare me any more unwelcome surprises.

THE TAMPING DOWN OF EXPECTATION
Wednesday, October 03, 2012

When I was pregnant, I was convinced that I was carrying a boy. At the time, I worked in an office represented by many cultures and many of the woman had their own twist on how to tell what gender the baby was. Some would emphatically declare that it must be a boy by the way I walked, others held by time-honoured traditions of the direction in which my wedding band swayed on a string above my belly, or by which foods I craved. (It was tomatoes if you care to know.) Others inquired as to how badly I suffered from morning sickness. (The answer was – to the point of being hospitalized by having changed weight of fifteen pounds in the wrong direction.) Everywhere I went in the building, another woman would have another gender test for me. All indicators pointed to a boy they would say. And I would rub my belly and smile.

I was so sure, and had convinced my husband to the point that when my daughter was born we hadn't even given a girl's name much thought. Sure, we had flown a few names up the flagpole over the months, but we found ourselves so ill-prepared as to what to name this child that we got teased by my nurses that they weren't going to let us take her home until we had a name for the birth certificate.

She did of course get a name, and one that she never had to share with another girl in her class, all the way through school. That wouldn't have been the case for our initial choice of Alexander!

The truth is, I so desperately wanted a girl that I dared not even entertain the thought that I might be blessed with a daughter. I believed that if I set my expectations for a boy, I would have just what I expected; I would be quite content and never look back.

Over the last weeks, I've gone through the same exercise with my radiation treatment. Expect it not to work; therefore I will have nothing to be disappointed about if this is unsuccessful in the reduction of the bone pain in my legs.

I've gotten just what I expected.

There was some initial hope after the first week of treatment. I was walking more easily and definitely experiencing less of the type of pain that I'm infinitely familiar with. As the second week of treatment started, I was having the pain flares I'd been warned about. Intense pain, but unfamiliar at the same time, and hence it was chalked up to flare vs. intensification of my usual pain.

Then the fatigue really kicked in. This was followed by a few more days of less pain, and last week I actually was able to go out for some short shopping trips. I even managed enjoying the treat of a lunch out at a nearby restaurant at the invitation of a friend. Without the company of my wheelchair pad even!

Then everything turned upside down on Friday. Kristee was due to come over and a part of me was telling me that I wasn't up to it and should reschedule. Another part of me was very much looking forward to seeing her and decided to go ahead with our plans.

But I knew something just wasn't right. My heart was rebelling; the pacemaker was in continuous cycling mode, and by bedtime I didn't quite know how to deal with it. My daughter was home for the weekend and I didn't want her to know that I was deeply concerned.

Out for a bit on Saturday morning with my daughter and a friend, and I could sense that trouble had most definitely arrived. Off to bed for the rest of the weekend, and it's where I've been pretty much ever since.

Monday was an especially frightening day. The dishwasher repairman was able to fit me into his schedule, and his ten minutes in my apartment was the only time I've seen another person all week. I have to wonder what the heck he was thinking. His office had called on short notice, leaving me next to no time to take my pain meds and have them kick in before he arrived. (They take about 60-90 minutes.) Why was this woman having such trouble standing up? Drunk perhaps at 10:00 a.m.?

Already that morning I'd started with a bad case of the chills that progressively got worse. And so did the pain. And so did the cardiac problems. I won't give you the play by play, but it came down to being so very weak and dizzy that I had to crawl along the floor to get back to bed. And hours later, I was just strong enough to answer the phone when Sue called to check on me, and she, my good friend, recognized that I was in some serious trouble. I didn't even have it in me to call 911, even though earlier, with a sense that it was going to be a rough day, I'd taken the bag I have ready for hospital trips out of the closet. Sue assured me that she'd take of everything and on my behalf placed calls to the hospital and local friends to get me help. God bless her.

The radiation experiment? Not successful. I'd set my expectations low, and had predicted that in case of failure I'd have no reason to be disappointed. The investment of time (daily visits to the hospital for two weeks and the subsequent fatigue) and the sacrifice of two not-so-bad-looking legs for a forty-eight-year-old (the tattoos are small, but damn it – they seem to leap out at me, and the discolouration from the treatments makes me look like I fell asleep in the sun wearing shorts and socks) seemed a reasonable gamble.

So I shouldn't be feeling sad, right?

Tomorrow, I have my appointment at the local cancer clinic with my pain specialist. This is one of the doctors who cheerfully told me that there was a really good chance that this was going to give me pain relief. I just had no idea that if it happened at all, it would be so short-lived.

A Cancer Society volunteer drives me tomorrow, but I go into that appointment by myself. I've not dreaded anything this much for a long time and I go in with the single goal of not falling apart into a puddle of tears.

The tamping down of expectation didn't work this time. I'm grief-stricken and don't know how to get past this disappointment right now. One more in a long line of significant letdowns.

AT LEAST I'M IMPROVING MY SCRABBLE VOCABULARY
Sunday, October 07, 2012

Yesterday I was bantering with one of my long-distance Words with Friends opponents on the chat feature, and the question of luck arose. I've been on a bit of a winning streak of late with this particular player, and the point was brought up whether it was talent at the game or if I just have great luck in getting good letters. I has said it either one of those, or else I've come to remember an awful lot of almost completely useless words. Having had many years to accumulate them doesn't hurt either!

I love words, and I love expanding my vocabulary. My daughter too has a great love of language; I suspect I've mentioned before here on the blog what a voracious and enthusiastic reader she is. She and I love to engage in word play, and when we really get going the words fly like lightning. Until it was pointed out to both of us recently just how much of it goes on I hadn't realized how easily she and I fall into playful banter when we're together.

In my last post I shared that the radiation treatment had been unsuccessful. I'm trying to deal with that and it's likely going to take a little bit of time to come to terms with my feelings of disappointment. And feelings of failure, however undeserved and inapplicable in this situation.

The side effects however march on. The burns on my legs? Getting more painful with an interesting twist that appeared yesterday. Spots. Many, many spots – an explosion of what look like large, dark birthmarks on the back of both legs. I noticed them when I changed out of my jeans; I'd had enough, for the day, of the irritation of the fabric against my sore skin. Out of the corner of my eye, I noticed something strange against the redness of my legs and quickly called out to my daughter to come see.

I've since learned on-line that hyper pigmentation from radiation treatment is not uncommon and is quite likely permanent. Not only did the radiation not work, now I have a rather obvious reminder.

My daughter and I tried to come up with a description, and the best could do was that my legs looked like those of a sunburned baby giraffe.

Although the spots aren't similar, I learned of an Australian animal called a spotted quoil. How can I not save up that juicy word for a triple play score when I'm blessed with the right combination of letters? At least Chris, you'll know that I haven't invented the word when it shows up on our WWF board!

A GIFT FROM THE HEART WARMS MY SOUL
Tuesday, October 09, 2012

If you've been following this blog, you'll know of my love affair with New York City, a destination I've never visited but had down as my number-one thing to do on my bucket list. You might also know that this is a trip that will never happen for me.

All things NYC are enthusiastically watched and read. I started off the twenty-four hour period that is today watching old episodes of *Rescue Me,* a TV series based on NYFD firefighters post 9-11. I was having trouble sleeping (thank you noisy neighbours and thin walls) and decided to catch up on something deliciously NYC. The opening sequence includes a shot of a city street, with early-morning mist rising off the pavement upwards towards the fire escapes. It's an image that I often bring to mind when I'm virtually walking the streets of the Big Apple.

Early this morning I awoke early as I usually do, and reached for my nearby iPad to check on emails and visit my favourite apps; one being Zite, an online magazine that I check out several times a day. I find fascinating articles there on subjects that interest me. This morning there was an article on NYC's High Line Park, a project that I've been following avidly for the last couple of years. A journalist had been one of a select group who'd been given a preview visit to the last portion of the park, which will be completed next year. It's an old and abandoned elevated railway line running through the city, which through the ideas and commitment of local residents and businesses, has over the last years been converted to a public park.

A couple of hours ago, Kristee texted me to ask if she could stop by for a short visit if I was up to it. Although it's been another bad pain day, what's better for cheering me up than smiles and a hug from a caring friend?

After I greeted her at the door, she handed me a package and made her way off to the bathroom to wash her hands. I noticed that she was obviously holding back a tear, and in the minutes that followed, it quickly made sense.

What she had handed me was a book, a lovely, bound book that had been designed and printed just for me. On my favourite subject. All this had been created for me by a woman whom I've never met (a friend of Kristee's), and she'd obviously gone through a great deal of effort to offer me this tremendous gift. Carolina had come to know about my New York Project, via our Kristee, and had created a book just for me with images and text to help me experience her love of the city.

First chapter? The High Line. Included? Images of those fire escapes that I love. Descriptions of experiences that Carolina has had in my beloved city so that I could share not only in the sights, but in the feeling of being there.

Thank you Carolina. Your gift brought me and your lovely messenger to tears, as she had predicted. Your thoughtfulness is above and beyond, and one day I hope to thank you in person. I'll treasure this gift always, along with the other generous contributions to my New York Project! On any given day, within seconds, I can be there by walking across the room.

THAT WHICH JUST DOESN'T FEEL RIGHT
Thursday, October 11, 2012

I ought to be napping; I do every afternoon for a few hours around this time. Instead I'm keenly aware of my racing heart and how it's keeping me awake. My strategy is keep busy until I'm just tired enough to ignore the odd feeling in my chest.

Today was pacemaker clinic day, an appointment in which the technician downloads the data, tests my device, and then my electro-physiologist reviews the results with me. I'll admit to being nervous today. My last download in April shook me up and set off a chain of numerous diagnostic tests to see what had brought about the unsettling recorded cardiac events.

When I visit my numerous doctors, I usually start off with an answer to the question of "How have you been feeling, Sandy?" with "Not too bad," "Hanging in there," or some variation thereof. Today, blunt honesty: "Awful."

It was decided to adjust the settings on my pacemaker to a higher rate per minute, to try to give me some relief. I was warned that this would mean that I might feel uncomfortable for a while; if it was too much for me to handle, I could easily come back anytime to have it readjusted. It also means that I'll use up the remaining battery on my device that much more quickly as it'll likely be running almost non-stop. As much as I don't want to go through the surgery sooner than I had mentally prepared myself for, I need to feel better and pray that this adjustment helps a small bit.

Yes, it's uncomfortable right now. Not nearly enough to plead for someone to drive me into Toronto first thing in the morning, but enough that my body feels like it doesn't belong to me. That it's going to take some getting used to.

It's a feeling that overwhelms me lately, the feeling of not belonging. Anywhere really, but especially in my apartment. My daughter and I spent over three months without a home, and now I find myself alone (she's back at school) in a place that couldn't feel less like a home to me. Although I've spent almost every hour of the last month in my apartment, it doesn't yet come close to feeling like a place I want to be.

I find myself apologizing to visitors. Please overlook the ratty carpet, don't mind the entrance foyer and the halls. Excuse the boxes, there's just not enough storage room for what we would like to have kept but obviously couldn't. Nothing really matches; it's an accumulation of a small amount of furniture that was spread throughout a much larger house. So please don't assume this is my sense of taste if you've not seen my last home.

My friends know of the numerous challenges that this building keeps throwing at me. I've realized that not only do I dislike being here – I'm coming to hate being trapped between these walls. For the friends and social services workers who help me escape once or twice a week, forgive the over-the-top enthusiasm in giving me a break from being here.

It's especially hard knowing that I came from a house and home I loved; one that I was proud of. Where I'd felt loved for many years, surrounded by my family, and enjoyed being until the life I knew came crashing down around me.

This all sounds to me like a recipe for becoming an old cat lady. We'll have to see how the old part works out...and of course the cat.

Nope, still not sleepy. Just tired of thinking about more things I need to get used to.

AN ABUNDANCE OF BLOG FODDER
Monday, October 15, 2012

A few hours ago, I was prepared to sit down and write a post on a subject that's been on my mind of late. It'll have to wait; a couple of other topics jumped the queue! (This might just be a multi-post evening!)

A few friends know that I've had "neighbour challenges," to put it plainly. I suspect that these neighbours don't even know that they're causing a noise problem, although I have my suspicions that it's one of the reasons that the previous tenant made a move. It's that bad. And almost always during the night when I would rather be sleeping.

This made the knock on the door a while ago especially appreciated. On the other side of me lives a couple. I'd met the husband last week. He's a pleasant British man and he was letting me know that I might want to don earplugs tomorrow. The tiles in the bathroom are to be pulled up and there would be noise and lots of it apparently. His gestures led me to believe he might be bringing in the pavement repair crew from the city with jackhammers and all. Those tiles must have threatened not to go without a fight! A kind thought to let me know what's on tap for tomorrow.

He might have wondered what I was doing in my pyjamas so early in the evening (I hid as best I could behind the door), but the truth is, the alternative would have been less neighbourly of me. It's difficult to tolerate even a slight touch against the radiation burns today; every turn in bed last night resulted in me waking up cursing the sheets against my legs.

Then came more fodder.

A friend emailed to let me know that it appeared that a message, voicing her displeasure, that she'd sent this evening to a political figure showed my email address as the sender instead of her own. I don't disagree with my friend's thoughts on the matter and joked that as long as she visited me in jail after I was arrested for speaking out against the government, all was good.

How did this misaddressed email happen? Months ago when I was left on my own at the old house, I quickly realized that I needed help (and lots of it) to get many household tasks and errands done. I did something that is quite uncharacteristic of me; I asked for the help I needed from friends who'd reached out in the months prior to offer their support and assistance. For me, that was a huge deal. I felt failure in being unable to do what seemed to me were basic tasks. Taking out the garbage, getting groceries, opening up jars whose lids wouldn't budge with the little strength I have left in my hands and arms.

It was likely the most humbling experience I've yet to go through, and not one of those friends I reached out to have ever made me feel anything other than they're glad to help. They know I had to reach deep down to find the courage to ask.

The need for assistance has only grown over time, and now the help of friends is supplemented by social services, the Canadian Cancer Society, and other volunteers who give so generously of their time.

Back to asking for help. One clever friend thought up a solution to help match up the offers of assistance with the need; an on-line calendar. A group of friends gain access with a password, and can check what appointments I have booked any time. (And any of these friends have permission to give me an earful at this moment; I realize that I've not updated the calendar in a number of weeks. Radiation has knocked me on my backside and I've taken a break from most of my regular appointments.)

We surmised that my friend must have been checking my calendar and didn't realize that she was still logged in to my account when she wrote the email.

My friends find the most ingenious ways to entertain me. Intentionally or otherwise!

I SHOULD COUNT TOO
Wednesday, October 17, 2012

I realized a couple of nights ago that I've been in this apartment almost a month and a half and have cooked myself exactly two meals. Yup, just two.

Not that I've been starving at all, friends had very kindly brought by plenty of meals for my freezer and I relished every last one of them. They were truly a blessing when it was hard to even keep my eyes open for more than an hour at a time during and following radiation treatment.

However, my definition of cooking doesn't include heating food up, so in truth I really haven't cooked in this time period. (I should note that we were treated to truly wonderful meals when we were left without a home for the three months. Talk about overstaying an invitation to dinner!) I love to cook, what holds me back?

One very simple reason. I love to cook for people I love and care for. I discovered many years ago that there was a very important difference for me in those extra words. When my daughter was with me, it would be time to break out the fresh ingredients and go to town. On the nights that she was with her father, I'd be eating well if I reheated leftovers but it rarely got to that point. Have you heard of kitchen sink meals? I was the queen of them; eating whatever I felt like grabbing out of the fridge and eating it over the sink so I didn't dirty up a plate. There were some very odd combinations to be had over the years!

Then I remarried and I was in heaven. Trips to the grocery store at least every two days to ensure that I had the freshest ingredients possible, scouring my vast collection of cookbooks and taking great pleasure in knowing that I was putting nutritious and varied meals (in six years there were very few repeats) in front of my beloved family. And as a bonus, they indicated their appreciation for my efforts at every turn.

Some who prepare the family meals may take offence at being given kitchen gadgets for Christmas, but I always looked forward to peeking into my stocking. My husband each year would pay a visit to Williams Sonoma to learn about the hottest new items, and he described the type of meals I'd cook to the salesperson so that they could point him towards an appropriate section with tools to make food preparation easier and more fun.

Nothing made my heart swell more than to see my family well fed and nurtured in the best way I knew how. I felt useful, goodness knows with having to give up the job I loved as well as the ability to do many other tasks, this was one thing I could still do fairly often. And if I may say so myself, I wasn't half-bad at it either.

Sadly, as many of you know, my husband left to find another woman to cook for him. Or if that fell through, he'd rather do take-out for the rest of his days than stay by my side. And I returned to kitchen sink meals.

Sue woke me up to a concept earlier this year that I'm obviously still not clamping on to, but intend to try to move towards. She is often on her own when her husband is travelling abroad for long stretches of time. It would be easy to do the kitchen sink thing, but she, with few exceptions, will every night prepare herself a proper meal. She'll have likely perused her cookbooks, shopped earlier in the day, and set time aside to prepare the recipes without shortcuts. Over the years, I've been lucky to sample many of her creations; it blows me away that she puts similar effort into her meal whether she's surrounded by loved ones or on her own.

Sue values herself and her efforts (and she's been effective at trying to convince me that I should be doing the same for myself). If I care about myself, then I too should be making an effort to feed myself well. It's been a very difficult road to reach even this point. Before leaving me, my husband told me in no uncertain terms how little he thought of me and shared his thoughts with many others, as I'm finding out more often as time goes on. It's challenging to recover from such a bashing and I'm not sure I ever truly will. But I am trying. Knowing the truth helps. (A nod to friends who oft repeated the phrase, "The truth will set you free," to me as I plodded through the fall-out.)

Now, of course, meal preparation comes with heavy restrictions. Almost three weeks had passed before I was in a grocery store this past Sunday. Transportation and the energy to shop are the biggest part of the battle. A very tight budget for groceries is another; many ingredients that I would have used in the past are simply gone from the equation. Then I discovered, as I was making these two meals, the physical strength that I once had has been severely diminished. I have to come to terms with the fact that although I love potatoes – there will be no more meals that require the chopping of raw ones. It was quite a pitiful sight watching myself trying to cut through a couple of Yukon Golds this week.

Stirring for longer periods of time is now out too (or even keeping an eye on the pot). I tried pulling a chair up but the ergonomics just don't work with this stove; a singed forearm is what I have to show for my efforts.

Where does that leave me? With all the best intentions to look after my nutritional needs better, but lacking the tools to consistently follow through. It's now almost 7 p.m., and I'm hungry and tired after a trip to the outside world today, to visit the hospice day program. Time to check out the freezer...

Tomorrow will be better.

HADN'T SEEN THAT BEFORE!
Friday, October 19, 2012

Never a good thing when your doctor tells you that.

This morning, he'd just finished telling me how disappointed he was that the radiation didn't work. That sadly the cancer hospital had no other options to offer me; their research hadn't come up with anything that looked like it was viable for reducing my bone pain. I was being discharged as a patient there and would be sent back to the Toronto Western team for the "balance of my care."

Palliative speak. I've more or less become used to it, but today it hit especially hard. Although I know full well that the radiation didn't work, there was a part of me that was hoping that news would come today that that a different plan of attack might well offer me some relief.

We reviewed the bone scan results one last time. From here on in, it really doesn't matter where the tumours are and where they spread to – the plan of methodically irradiating them one by one, for pain relief, has been shot to hell. I'm not entirely sure if I care to have any more bone scans. I know where the tumours are; it's an all-too-familiar intense burn that feels like hot pokers have replaced my bones. It's getting harder to bear every day, and I'll recognize the feeling when it appears elsewhere.

As we were wrapping up, I was reminded that I was to show him the radiation burns. And that's when the look of astonishment crossed his face. "Sandy, I've not seen that before. It's got to be from the radiation given the location, but that shouldn't have happened." I guess nobody else has the fun of having baby giraffe legs.

The ride home with the Cancer Society volunteer driver and other patients was excruciating. I can say I'm pretty sure that I've never felt lonelier or more alone than I have today. I needed someone to hold me and tell me that it's all going to be okay. Even though we'd both know it isn't. Someone to hold my hand, wipe away my tears as I allow myself to cry out the pain, frustration, and fear.

I'm not afraid of dying, I'm afraid of much more of this ahead of me. Knowing that this only gets worse.

From time to time, it happens that someone will ask me about what symptoms led to my diagnosis. Once in a while, the person will have themselves convinced that they too must have Erdheim-Chester because they have leg pain and/or cardiac issues (and this happened again this week). Or I'm told that that's exactly what their Aunt Sally had, but she's all better now. Sometimes they ask for my doctor's name so they can speak with them to get confirmation that they too have ECD.

I try to be polite and suggest that if they're feeling pain or discomfort they most certainly should have it checked out. But I'm frustrated when others seem to be hoping that they've found the answer in an ECD diagnosis.

On the inside, I feel like screaming that having a very rare illness such as ECD is the very last thing they might want to think about. Pray, hope, wish (whatever works for them) that if it is something serious...that's it's something far more common – an illness that comes with a successful treatment protocol (or a protocol, period), drug funding, answers, and survival rates that are at least a touch more predictable.

I'm not being selfish wanting to have ECD all to myself, or dismissing the pain of others. It's me praying that others don't have to go through something like this where you just don't know what's going to hit next.

Trust me on this. You don't want to be the patient who's been told, "We haven't seen that before." It's not a good place to be.

DECIDING TO NOT DECIDE
Saturday, October 20, 2012

I've spent the last few hours sorting paperwork on my bed. When I had to pack up the house last spring, the contents of the filing cabinet were hastily placed in boxes for future sorting. I anticipated that without being able to work, I'd have plenty of time to get the job done when we had a new place to live.

It hasn't quite worked out that way yet. Six weeks later, I'm still unpacking. It's mostly because I move as slowly as molasses these days, and secondly because I've run out of space to store things. However, tonight I wanted to make a small dent in the piles and boxes of files.

It's been an evening of mixed emotions. I've come across my daughter's old report cards, and cards and letters that she's written to me over the many years. (It made my heart smile to see her earliest attempts at handwriting.) I also found cards that I wish I hadn't come across tonight. (How does someone say that you made him the happiest man alive and is looking forward to many more Valentine's Days together, and then less than three months later say that he can't stand being with me one minute longer and has felt that way for years? That one goes to the top of the heap for a bonfire...)

I also came across old performance evaluations from my tech world days. I'll keep one for my daughter to look at years from now so that she can be reminded that once upon a time I wasn't this shell of my former self. Back then, my nickname at the office was "The Energizer Bunny." (I suppose that's still true to some degree, I am battery-operated after all!)

What struck me was the commentary from various superiors, often noting my ability to stay calm, focused, and decisive in challenging situations.

That's a sharp contrast to what I'm feeling this evening, at least as far as decision-making is concerned. My thoughtful volunteer and friend, Jane, took me out to run two errands today. One was to the post office box, the other was to Sears to get socks. I'd be ashamed to show you the bottoms of my feet the last few months; most of my socks are nearing holes in the bottom if they're not already there. No socks on sale today, but no way that I'm going near the place again on a weekend before Christmas. Sheer madness and very long line-ups. It wouldn't be the first time that I've found what I'm looking for and stood in line, but had to abandon my intended purchase because I just couldn't stand up anymore. Yes I know, suck it up, Sandy and just get the darn wheelchair...

This small amount of walking has had serious repercussions tonight. If you didn't know where my knees belonged on my legs, you'd be hard pressed to locate them with the swelling being so extreme. The weird colouration is spreading to the front of my legs, and the pain is overwhelming. A pain pill that the average adult should take only two of per day, I'm up to one every two hours, day and night. What complicates things is trying to keep them down; they're strong anti-inflammatories that do a number on my stomach and tonight it's a heck of a battle to have them stay put. Note to self: Ask medical team on Tuesday if there's an alternate delivery system. Even if I have to inject like a heroin addict, I'm on board.

For someone who's normally good at making decisions, I can't make up my mind whether to head to the hospital or not. Do I keep pushing through the pain? Or go through the frustration of going to the local hospital only to be sent home again because they've never heard of ECD and don't know what to do with me? Why am I writing a blog post right now instead? (The answer to that is simple. I just don't know what else to do with myself right now, and this is the best distraction I can come up with. And it helps me to feel less alone knowing you're out there reading this.)

Time for another pain pill. Quite simply put, this is wretched.

DECIDING
Tuesday, October 30, 2012

In my last post, I'd mentioned that I had a hospital appointment last Tuesday, back with my care team at Toronto Western. I wasn't quite sure what I was going to tell them about the failure to respond to the radiation. In truth, I had decided some time ago but I had to get my head around it.

Radiation is to be the last experimental treatment I'll be trying. I'm done getting my hopes up, experiencing the side effects, and dealing with the disappointment when the treatments haven't worked. It's time to get off the wild roller coaster. No more bone scans; there is no need to know where tumours have spread to – I recognize the pain and it doesn't help me emotionally or otherwise to get confirmation of location. Diagnostic testing, outside of regular blood work, pretty much disappears. This will result in far fewer trips to the hospitals. To me, in some ways this sounds like a better quality of life. Pain management continues to be a struggle, however, I choose to never again be the first ECD patient to try a new approach to the disease. It doesn't mean I won't sit up and listen if there's a positive new development in research, but I'm not putting myself through this experimental process anymore.

My doctor went through a few scenarios to ensure that I truly understood my decision, along with the repercussions of having signed my "Do Not Resuscitate" order months ago. I felt that we were most definitely on the same page; it's time to let this take its course.

Some readers may disagree with my decision and you may of course do so. What matters to me is that my daughter and I are at peace with this, and we are as best as I think we can be. It's been a surprisingly freeing experience.

My doctor, at that appointment, asked me how I felt about being a palliative patient; a question I'd never been asked before. I told him I'd prefer if it was heading in the other direction, but I can accept that it isn't.

I continued to think about my decision over the coming days quite intently. Not once have I thought I've made the wrong choice; it was an internal thought process about what the journey ahead might look like.

The day after my appointment, I received a rather surprising phone call from the organization that provides my volunteer visitors/helpers.

(Let me add that they're four incredibly giving women, whom I'm grateful to have the chance to get to know better as we go along. All quite different in personality, the coordinator has done a fabulous job of matching me to these new friends.) Might I consider speaking to the group, which is currently undergoing a ten-week course on palliative care, about what a person in my situation might want or need from a volunteer? Quite a coincidence, but then again I really don't believe in those.

I'm immensely honoured. It's a big responsibility to think that a group of people who've made a conscious decision to help and spend time with palliative patients, might be drawn closer to this goal – or perhaps pushed away, by what I would have to say.

There's more than a hint of irony to this. A year ago, it was demanded of me to find a support group to help me be a better caregiver to my caregiver. You might need to read that last sentence twice; I had to make sure I wrote it clearly and accurately. I was marched off to the local cancer support centre to find said support group. I was being told that I had to be a better patient by the person who'd tell anyone, up until shortly before that day, that it was easy was to forget that I was ill because of my optimism and positive attitude.

A huge point was being missed; I didn't want to be defined as a patient. I wanted to be a wife and mother to the two people who mattered most in my life. It was, and still is, me in here – a person who still wants to do what she can despite growing challenges, to love and be loved, and to continue to grow intellectually, spiritually and emotionally. And I suspect many others finding themselves in this position would offer the same sentiment.

And here I am now in a position of participating in the process of teaching volunteers how to support us palliative patients. Irony indeed.

THE MEN WHO RESTORE MY FAITH IN MEN
Wednesday, October 31, 2012

The first part of this post was written last month, just before my laptop died. I was able to retrieve it yesterday.

It's no secret to people who are close to me that there have been men in my life who have treated me less than honourably; some earlier in my life, others more recently. Although there are those who stuck out as princes among men and treat me with great respect, kindness and love, I had over the last year and a half lost some faith in the opposite sex.

Yet there are men who give me reason to rethink this position. Yesterday afternoon, I received a call from the volunteer driver named Bert, who had taken me to my morning radiation appointment. On the drive home with another patient, I'd told the story I'd posted some weeks ago about listening in the oncologist's waiting room to the older ladies discussing tooting on the bus. Bert said that I should write a story like that down, and I replied that I had indeed done so. I then shared details on how to access my blog and we then said our goodbyes when I was dropped off.

This call from Bert was quite emotional. I won't share all the touching details of what he had to say, but he'd told me that he'd spent an hour reading my blog and wanted me to know that I could call upon him if I needed any assistance – beyond his role as volunteer driver for the Cancer Society. Let me clear up something quickly, fearing that any of you are getting the wrong idea. Bert spoke lovingly about his family (including his wife) on the drive to the hospital.

This is nothing other than a decent man wanting to do something to make my difficult situation easier if he could. And I thank the heavens above that this is not an isolated case. More and more, I have men stepping forward with genuine offers of help. And not just offers; actions follow the kind words. Neighbours who helped with household chores before my daughter and I had to leave the old house, men who helped with the yard sale, men who welcomed me and my daughter into their home when we had nowhere else to go, others who accompanied their partners who were visiting me and made themselves useful while they were here.

Men who use their connections to bypass the roadblocks that I run into on a regular basis. Men who call, send emails, and Facebook messages to check on how I'm doing and ask how they can help. Men who tell me that they will never understand how another man could put his wife through what I've experienced, and they apologize on behalf of the gender. That's a concept I don't quite get my head around, I can't imagine a woman apologizing on behalf of all others. But thank you all the same, it's touching and raw at the same time.

Professionals in my life who go well above and beyond the call of duty to let me know that I matter. (Let me specifically note my doctors and lawyers, I know that I've meant more than an OHIP invoice or a billable hour.) Men who didn't blindly believe what they were hearing, but knew that there would be two sides of the story of what led to the end of my marriage. Those men especially earned my respect for acting on their own feelings when the story didn't make sense, based on what they already knew of me.

I'm immensely relieved to know that there are still plenty of good men out there. I trust that the women in their lives know what gems they're blessed to have around to love and be loved by. And a huge thanks to those of you (of both sexes!) who have been checking in on my progress with radiation, now nearing the end of the first week. Today it got a bit rough; it's not easy being here on my own. I wish more than anything that I had a loved one here tonight to warm up some soup for me, rub my head (no pain medication can beat that for soothing me), holding me when an excruciating bout of pain hits.

I don't dare move beyond the bed right now. I wouldn't in a million years wish this experience upon anyone, nobody deserves this. But bless those who want to make things better for me.

And back to now.

Another gentleman drove me to the appointment that I had a few weeks back with the oncologist; the one where we called off any further radiation due to the lack of success of the first round. When I went to find him in the lobby after my appointment, I was visibly upset and he asked if there was anything he could do. At that moment I felt indelibly stained with sadness and loneliness. One of my toughest appointments ever and I'd had to go through it alone.

There were other passengers in the car on the ride home, but for the most part I stared out the side window, tears welling up but not making a sound. I was dropped off in front of the building, and after our goodbyes I made my way to the elevator. All I desired at that moment was to make it upstairs and into my apartment before I fell apart. I didn't quite manage that, but nobody was around to see the sobs seeping their way out of me.

The door locked behind me, I fell into a corner where I must have stayed for the next hour. Sobs that I'd held back for months swept out of me. And then it was time to pull myself together again and muster whatever post-radiation energy I could muster to unpack yet another box.

A few days ago, I received an envelope in the mail, my name and address handwritten. I didn't recognize the last name at first, but as I read the enclosed note, it quickly came to me that this note was from my volunteer who'd driven me to and from that difficult visit with the oncologist. I won't go into details, but I tell you that it was a spiritual gift that lifted my heart. This led to him and me sharing an hour with others this morning, and then I was invited back to his home to meet his wife. It was a lovely visit; they've been married fifty-three years and have lots of stories to tell of their life together. And it sounds like I'll have a chance to hear more in the future; I'm delighted by that prospect. I have a long list to thank for restoring my faith in men. I suspect you gentlemen know who you are.

JUST ACCEPT...
Sunday, November 04, 2012

At astounding speed, old friends are flowing back into my life and new friendships are blossoming. And God bless the friends who just keep hanging in there with me through thick and thin. I don't know why all of this wonderfulness is happening, nor do I dare to question it. Thank you for all the positive energy being sent my way.

The kindnesses, generosity and love lift me in a way I can't begin to explain. 'Tis a brave and courageous thing to join me on this journey. It makes me sad that I can do so little to reciprocate all that my friends and my support network do for me. So many of you are a good distance away and have expressed your frustration at not being closer to help with everyday tasks – please know that I feel your support and good wishes. And without question, this "back office" support helps a great deal too.

I'm learning slowly but surely. Just accept all that is coming my way, it's happening as it's meant to happen. (And I welcome the idea that angels appear around me in human form, nothing could convince me otherwise anymore!) I don't know if I'm here for just one more day or another few years, but for those that are riding this out with me – I'm humbled and so very grateful. And now, I need to go have a really good cry. Because that's just what I do when I'm feeling so overwhelmed with appreciation. Even though I'm mostly by myself in this apartment, my friends are making it impossible to feel alone on this journey.

SHARING THE JOURNEY
Saturday, November 10, 2012

When I'd thought about the conversation I was about to have last Monday evening, I'd envisioned a lonely table in a bar too dimly lit to be able to recognize anyone farther than halfway across the room. Two glasses and a bottle of scotch.

For the record, I don't drink scotch, nor have I ever. Outside of the occasional (as in maybe twice a year) half-glass of wine, I don't drink alcohol; it leaves me feeling outside of myself and it's not a feeling I enjoy. I don't know why I equate solemn conversations with a good stiff drink – too many Hollywood movies I suppose, filling my brain with such ideas.

In a previous post, I mentioned that I'd been asked to speak to a group of volunteers being trained in palliative care. A brave move on their part to participate in this program; the word palliative can scare many a folk away and here were men and women who were embracing the idea of caring for patients with a poor prognosis.

Things happened pretty quickly last weekend, starting with a call on Saturday afternoon from the training coordinator, asking if I would be up to speaking to his students in two days' time. How does one go about preparing to have a conversation like this? To share with complete strangers what it feels like to be facing this journey? To let them know what I need and want from a volunteer?

The safest bet seemed to be to not over-think what might transpire. My first priority would be to establish that I spoke only for myself and my own experiences; I couldn't possibly come near to accurately expressing how other palliative patients might feel about their own unique situations.

I won't go into the long-winded details of the hour and a half that I spent with this large group of caring and generous individuals. I went into it wanting to be of some small help (I feel pretty useless most days), but what I received from them was a far greater gift. I left feeling like I'd had that good stiff drink and had made new friends in the process; the welcome and the goodbye I received from the group lifted me to a place I'd not yet visited along this journey.

My foremost goal had been to not scare these volunteers off the idea of caring for palliative patients; my participation in the evening felt like a great deal of responsibility. Turns out that we shared many fears: The fear of saying the wrong thing, the fear of not being helpful, the fear of offending, the fear of being misunderstood when one's intentions are true.

There was a moment that struck me particularly deeply that evening. We'd been discussing what missteps (and I reiterate that I can speak only for myself here) can happen when strangers say things about my situation that I find difficult to digest. An example might be when I'm chided by a complete stranger for using the elevator when travelling only one level down, instead of taking the stairs like a person my age ought to. In their opinion, I appear to be able-bodied. (Apparently, if I can walk a very short distance into the elevator and stand in it for a few moments, I may as well be running marathons!)

There was a collective sigh of relief in the room when I answered the question of, "Have any of your volunteers made a misstep?" My answer came very quickly, and it was a decisive, "No." Ninety-nine percent of what I need of a volunteer comes from the fact that each of these individuals were in that room on Monday evening; that they wanted to be a part of the journey for patients who have a rough road ahead.

And an important detail, a good deal of the conversation was far from solemn. Champagne would have been a more appropriate accompaniment from my perspective!

Showing up and wanting to be with me on my journey is just about everything I need wrapped in one beautiful package. I thank God and my lucky stars to have so many of these beautiful gifts around me.

WHAT ELSE IS COMING MY WAY?
Monday, November 12, 2012

This is one seriously messed up set of circumstances that I try to maintain some equilibrium within.

One short week ago, I was speaking to a group of volunteers about how palliative patients can be assisted by maintaining some normalcy in life wherever possible, and how much it has meant to me that my team of volunteers has helped me in doing that.

A meeting with my occupational therapist was set up for today, requested by one of my nurses who is keenly aware of my declining health. On the list were the following items; a wedge for my mattress, to hopefully allow me to breathe more easily at night (lying down causes shortness of breath, severe enough that I have to try to sleep sitting up on some nights), and a wheelchair, since it's becoming increasingly difficult to walk or stand for more than a few minutes at a time.

The occupational therapist also recommended some amendments to the bathroom to make bathing easier.

All well and good, yet our regional social services have recently changed their policy so that palliative patients no longer receive any assistive devices. I can have a loan for twenty-eight days, but no longer. So I'd better plan on passing within the month or I'll find myself back at square one.

On top of this, the rubber wheelchair pad that many of you have seen me toting around gets taken away too. This has allowed me to tolerate the drives to hospital appointments in Toronto, to sit on harder surfaces for a short while. I've fought that battle for some months, but solidly lost that one today.

My ex-husband's insurance might possible cover some or all of these assistive items, but the legwork is beyond my current physical and technological capabilities. (Getting around to the various suppliers to get quotes is a challenge, and the computer has died on me once again, so no printer, scanner etc.) On top of that, I need to get a denial letter from the government plan (which I already know I don't qualify for because of a short-sighted decision re: Canada Pension Plan contributions when opening up my photo business ten years ago.)

Is it any wonder that my head is reeling right now, wondering how the heck I'm supposed to manage all of this on my own? I've tried so hard to believe that life continues to throw challenges at me as part of a bigger plan. I'm getting to the point that the longer this goes on, the less I understand how one lifetime can be filled with so many obstacles. It's very difficult to get on with the process of just trying to do some living when one has to spend so much time answering the question of why I'm still kicking around. It's an answer I don't have.

THE DIFFERENCE AN ADVOCATE CAN MAKE
Tuesday, November 13, 2012

I'm bowled over by the volume of support coming my way after yesterday's post. Thank you to all who took time to express outrage and share incredibly kind offers to help improve my situation.

Let me first give you an update. This morning, I received a call from the occupational therapist who had visited yesterday. After leaving here yesterday –visibly upset by the rules that were working against me in trying to be as comfortable and independent as possible – she placed a lengthy call to her supervisors to ask for special consideration for my situation.

Her pleading worked. I'm now permitted to keep my wheelchair pad and I get a wheelchair to go with it. As grateful as I am, I'm disturbed by the inequity in our health care system when it comes to how rare and/or serious illnesses (and the unique situations that come attached to them) are handled.

I'm grateful for the wheelchair that should be arriving soon, but why shouldn't anyone in my situation have the same opportunities for mobility assistance, regardless of which town, city or province they live in? How does it happen that a palliative patient can have fewer (or no) assistive devices available to them than someone who is chronically ill?

Having had far more experience in the health care system than the average citizen, I could write a book on the subject of inequities to be encountered. In my humble opinion, there are lots of wonderful aspects to our health care system in Canada, but there's also plenty of room for improvement for patients with rare illnesses.

And then there's the second point on my mind, regarding what has transpired over the last two days. Over the last years, I've been a traveller through the health care system both with an advocate at my side, and without one. From my experiences, the former leads to better health care. I've come to the conclusion that there is absolutely no doubt about that statement. Someone who sits by as a second set of ears during appointments, someone who makes sure that all questions are adequately answered, someone to think outside of the box when roadblocks are faced.

Someone to spur insurance companies and government agencies to do the right thing. Should it really have taken me being interviewed last year by the CBC to get funding for one of my treatments? And I note that the interview wouldn't have even happened had I not had an advocate tirelessly working on my behalf. Every single step is a battle in itself, and now doing this on my own, I find myself falling between the cracks over and over again.

It's all well and good if one is only remembering what I used to be capable of; I was a person who had perhaps an overdeveloped sense of right and wrong, and would fight for fairness for all parties concerned in a situation. That person just doesn't have much fight left in her; sometimes just getting showered and dressed for the day takes all the energy I have available for the day.

I thank my advocates who've stepped in to make today better: my occupational therapist who pleaded for rules to be bent; the friends who quickly offered to rent/buy the equipment I need to maintain a small amount of independence and better physical comfort.

I'm grateful for the friends (and sometimes near-strangers) who offer this help, knowing how hard it is for me to accept it, and also knowing me to be a person who'll try hard to fix a problem myself before ever letting on that I need assistance. Stubborn old me has to admit it. I just can't get through the rest of this journey without others stepping in to take the reins when I'm too tired to hold them.

MAKING LEMONADE
Wednesday, November 14, 2012

Maybe you're expecting me to offer up the adage, "When life hands you lemons, make lemonade." This is certainly a philosophy I try to follow but really, I'm going to make lemonade.

Despite a lot of challenges happening in my life (when is it not a roller coaster?) I wanted to share some of the lighter moments of the last few weeks. Some of these references might make no sense at all to you; in that case just ignore them – there are thank-you messages in here for friends who I know might be shy about me being any more specific.

Today a new friend, Bert, dropped off a bag of my very favourite fruit, Meyer lemons, never having heard of them but he had read on Facebook how excited I was that they were back in season. Along with that, a jar of Nutella (have I ever mentioned that particular obsession on the blog?) and also very thoughtfully, a new pain cream to try out. Never having tried to make lemonade with Meyer lemons before, it's high time I tried a glassful.

As for the rest of the lemons, they'll be impetus to actually cook something for myself this week. (As terrific as the donated meals have been, I want to break out my pots and pans!)

My friend Deborah's mom wanted to make sure that I was able to get something for myself that falls into the category of, "I would like..." rather than the basics that my very strict budget allows. A very generous gift, which allows me a few treats that I've had to take out of my budget. First on the list? Some new sweaters and a pair of colourful shoes!

My wheelchair arrived this morning, which will be invaluable in hunting down those sweaters and shoes. I'm getting coaching on how to pull off a decent wheelie, something to practice when I can't sleep at night perhaps? Two additional assistive devices have been generously purchased by friends. One, the bed wedge, will be helping me avoid waking up with the "night gasps," which are frightening episodes I could do without, thank you very much. Other friends are helping to ensure I can get more safely into the tub every morning.

Yesterday was quite a therapeutic afternoon, sitting by a campfire with my friend Sandra as we fed the fire. I brought the fuel.

My friends Arlene and Fred enlisted the help of friend of theirs to take me on another delightful virtual New York City excursion. There may be a few too many photos floating around of me as the Statue of Liberty…

There are so many other wonderful moments, but I'll finish with one that will be a long-lasting reminder of what joys can be found in the midst of the messes. In my lap sits the cutest and furriest four pounds of adorableness; my new kitten Scrabble. My conversation with the group of palliative volunteers finally pushed me over the edge to adopt a wee companion. I recognized that I truly need to be needed. I need to care for someone to feel useful, and this little guy needs me.

What has warmed my heart the most is that whenever a loud noise comes from the industrial area situated behind me, Scrabble makes a mad dash for the safety of my lap. Being trusted as a safe place is the best feeling ever. And the tickling I get when he insists on licking under my chin in the middle of the night puts a big smile on my face too.

WANTED - NEW KEYCHAIN
Thursday, November 15, 2012

When the previous tenants of my apartment handed the keys over to me, they were all together on one link. I handed one set over to my daughter, and not having a key chain myself, I kept carrying the new keys over the last few months as they were presented to me.

I misplace my keys a lot, not an easy feat in a small apartment, but my friends who are in the same ballpark in age assure me they're often doing the same. I don't yet have any sort of an entryway table to lay keys and the mail down on, so those items usually travel elsewhere into the apartment. I'm just not yet consistent about the destination. What makes my keys a bit easier to find is the bright purple colour of the keychain.

Last week, one of my volunteers took me to the bank where a trip to my safety deposit box was required. At the customer service representative's desk (I don't think we're to call the staff tellers anymore, are we?) I searched through my purse to find my ID. In doing so (I too have one of those bottomless pit purses in which I'm sure I'd be as likely to find a sink stopper as I would old receipts with the way it looks some days in there), I laid my keys on the counter.

"Ready for the weekend there, are you Sandy?" piped in my volunteer. I looked at her quizzically, and she elaborated. "Always ready for a beer?" with a grin on her face.

All this time I've been going around with a purple beer bottle opener on my key chain, thinking it was a tiny ski.

So for all of you who might have seen my keys, I can only imagine what judgements you might have made. No, I'm not tossing back Heinekens or Coronas to ease my pain; I've never even had a beer in my life. But this keychain confusion has led to some fantastic belly laughs with friends since this happened. If you can't laugh at yourself, there's always someone not too far away to laugh at you. It's far more enjoyable though to beat them to the punch.

Now I just need to find a keychain that won't scream substance abuse issues. For the record, I thought that the raised part of the keychain represented the boot binding. Clearly, I've not skied in my life...but then again, I've not opened a beer bottle either!

NOT DRIVING THE NEIGHBOURS CRAZY
Thursday, November 29, 2012

I have to be cognizant that absence from the blog may lead readers to wonder what's happened to me, I get worried emails asking if all is okay at my end. Thank you for checking in on me.

This blog now averages about 200 hits a day; a good number of those being repeat visitors. I appreciate that so many of you are coming along for the ride on this journey. To know that I'm in the thoughts and prayers of so many means a great deal to me.

The task that's taken the most time is getting back on-line with a computer. Some of you know that my laptop died during the summer (after a slow and painful decline), leaving me without access to much of my data, contacts, a printer, scanner, etc. Quite a challenge when I had pressing legal issues to take care of.

I'm back on line thankfully and working away on getting programs reloaded and data synchronized – but the best part of all has been getting access once again to my libraries of photos.

As the photos moved from my backup hard drives to the computer, images would briefly flash across the screen. It felt like I was greeting old friends. I was explaining to a friend the other day who was asking about some of my older images (and we're talking up to thirty-odd years ago) that I can remember with great clarity what circumstances surrounded the capture of each image. What the weather was like, what sort of mood I was in (and there were generally two modes – joyful or contemplative), who I was with (or had just left or was about to meet up with).

The images form a story of my life. And in the case of the portraiture, the stories of others as well – an opportunity and privilege that I will always hold dear.

THE DIFFERENCE A FOOT MAKES
Sunday, December 02, 2012

The victory of getting a wheelchair was short-lived. In concept, it was wonderful news that social services was making an exemption for me despite my palliative status (which disentitled me to no-cost, loaned assistive equipment), but unfortunately the type of wheelchair isn't suitable for me.

It's just too heavy for any of my volunteers to lift into a vehicle, and has been sitting now for weeks, idle and taking up valuable space in the middle of my apartment. So back it goes. And the red tape with insurance begins once again. (I really thought I had dodged that bullet when I decided to forego any further experimental treatments, but here I go again despite perhaps not having the energy required for the protracted interaction with the insurance company and other parties involved with the application.)

There are some places I've visited over the last few months that make scooters or wheelchairs available to their customers and I have availed myself. This has allowed me to run occasional simple errands with friends and volunteers (or maybe not so simple sometimes – some stores offer better quality equipment than others, not to mention differing widths of aisles for manoeuvrability issues). I'm grateful when I get access to a mobility aid; otherwise the trip has to be either shortened considerably or forfeited altogether.

The most fascinating aspect of the transition to a "less able bodied" individual has not so much been about equipment as it has been about peoples' actions and attitudes.

Shrinking down about a foot in stature when I'm in a wheelchair changes how many strangers treat me. Although there are some very pleasant surprises. (Kudos to two stores that helped me last week, I can't say where or I'll spoil a small Christmas surprise for my daughter. The service was outstanding, no pun intended of course.) But often I'm treated as invisible or seemingly unworthy of the same courtesy as the customer ahead of me in line.

If you've met me in person, you'll know me to be quite friendly to everybody. I enjoy making eye contact and sharing a smile with strangers. If someone appears to be ill-tempered, I try my best to imagine that they've got a tough challenge on their mind and try to be friendly even when they're not.

Sitting in a scooter or wheelchair a foot lower than where I'd normally be has been a learning experience, to say the least. If I thought it was bad when I was walking awkwardly on my own or with crutches, I was in for quite a surprise! Very seldom does anyone make eye contact, even when I'm paying for a purchase. I walk away (wheel away to be more precise) – later asking whomever I was with if it was my imagination. Was I being my usual self? Am I doing anything to make the cashier or salesperson uncomfortable? I'm assured that I'm acting no differently than in other interactions with strangers, but yes – they've also noticed the difference in how I'm treated and relay similar stories coming from others with physical disabilities.

I've point blank asked trusted friends how they feel when interacting with a stranger who's physically challenged, if they find themselves treating the person differently. And in response, I've received some very honest and appreciated feedback. Some of it was difficult to hear, but I wanted to know.

It sounds to me like it comes down to what our families taught us, and what sort of exposure we've had before with the "less able bodied." I hear that some had been taught not to make eye contact for fear that the disabled person might interpret it as staring. Others have been taught to engage as if the mobility aid were invisible.

The latter is a far more enjoyable experience for me, and it just might be for the person who's a foot or so taller than me at that moment too. I'll continue to offer a smile to anyone who'll accept one. Just look down about a foot to find it.

THE "NOTHINGS" THAT ARE TRULY SOMETHING SPECIAL
Tuesday, December 04, 2012

The bag was handed over to me today with, "It's nothing Sandy, really." One of many gifts, favours, kindnesses that are extended to me on a regular basis. Today it was soup and dessert; a dinner I didn't have to rummage for. Frankly the fridge and cupboards are quite empty (for a number of reasons that cause my heart to ache if I allow myself to think about them).

Tomorrow the hospice feeds me lunch, another meal in a week during which it's just been too difficult to stand for any length of time at the stove.

A whole lot of "nothings" that kind people offer to try to make up for the huge, gaping chasm that stands in the wake where I was left to deal with this on my own. So many with tears in their eyes, telling me that they wish they could take all the bad stuff away with the wave of a hand. The hugs that envelop me, trying to hold me away from the edge of what's to come.

There are others around me who understand; who tell me often what I mean to them – leaving loving thoughts for me to hold onto. Knowing that no one wants to leave this life feeling alone. Letting me know that my time here has mattered. Trying to make up for those who have chosen to turn away.

I'm clawing at the distant dream of relief from physical pain, knowing that there's only one way to escape it. That I must steel myself against this pain while trying to deal with the logistical setbacks. Trying to work my way through the minefield of administrative nightmares that seem to pile up higher and higher each week. The phone calls and emails that I'm just too exhausted to tackle most of the time.

The outpouring of "nothings" is everything. I try to go to sleep every night thinking of the day's "nothings," so that I can shut my eyes feeling not quite so alone in this. And I pray that when the end does come, that my heart and my head will be filled with gratitude for those who offered to me what they might have believed to be something quite insignificant, but wasn't at all.

WINNING. AND LOSING
Tuesday, December 18, 2012

A few weeks back, I wrote that when there's a longer stretch between posts, my friends and readers offer their concern for my well-being. This time with reason sadly.

When I started writing this blog, it was a way to share updates on my journey with ECD with friends. Everyone could read the same update, get that out of the way, and then I could then spend my time speaking of more enjoyable matters with them.

I've been told that this blog has been a resource for other patients dealing with this illness who might have been wondering how I've made out with the various experimental treatments I've tried over the last three years as they consider their own treatment options.

Along the way, this blog turned into a story, sharing the medical details of my battle with ECD, telling anecdotes of my family life (funny events have a way of following me around, I'm glad to have added a smile to your faces once in awhile!) sharing quite openly about how I've been dealing with the illness and a rather trying set of personal circumstances.

The truth is that my health has been declining quite rapidly over the last weeks, and although I like to think of myself as the eternal optimist, I need to face some harsh realities. There just aren't that many funny stories to share these days (but they're not completely absent either!)

Some tough discussions have taken place over the last week, including one with my daughter that I wish with all my heart could have had a very different outlook. Sue flew into town on short notice to help me take care of some stupendously difficult tasks that I would otherwise have had to tackle on my own.

So far this sounds like the losing part of the blog title.

When my daughter came home from school this past week, it was blatantly obvious to her that some big changes had occurred in her absence. My heart was breaking as I told her how things appears to be playing out for me, and I told her that I hoped and prayed that she didn't view it as me giving up.

What she said to me was a gift that I'll take with me to the end. Through her tears, she looked me in the eye and told me that as far as she was concerned, I'd won. That I'd been provided with a poor prognosis, and I was still here beyond our expectations.

Perhaps I'll rally again as I have on previous occasions, but sadly things feel very different than when I've gone through other medical crises.

I'm surrounded by people who love me, care for me, and accept me for who I am (quirkiness and all!) and who are making this last part of the story as happy and peaceful as I might possibly hope it to be under the circumstances. But I am very, very tired in every sense of the word.

A CHRISTMAS TO REMEMBER
Tuesday, December 25, 2012

Perhaps I'm not terribly original in my choice, but my favourite movie for as long as I can remember has been, *It's a Wonderful Life*. *Life is Beautiful* runs a close second; such is the life of the almost full-time optimist. A title sincerely tested over the last few years, but I remain an optimist all the same.

Every time I watched *It's a Wonderful Life*, my faith in humankind was lifted just a little bit higher – for at least a little while. It would depend on my circumstances at the time as to how long that feeling would last. There were also a few years in there where the premise of the movie was almost lost on me, including last year. Last December I still had cable and a PVR, and set it to record the movie a few days before Christmas.

For weeks the recorded program sat on the PVR, and eventually I just deleted it – I just couldn't imagine that the movie would do anything other than make me feel even sadder than I was at the time about the situation happening to me and my daughter.

This year has been beset with challenges that I couldn't have even imagined. The circumstances cause everyone to shake their heads in wonder, or more accurately in shock. It seemed impossible to believe that things could get worse, yet over the coming months they did.

Fast forward to a year later.

What's transpired over the last week has been simply magical and breathtaking. The year in whole has been a study in extremes, but right now the good stuff overwhelms.

This year, without cable TV, I haven't been able to catch *It's a Wonderful Life*. And I don't have to. The movie has come right to my front door. And into my mailbox. And over the phone.

Some of it came as financial aid, as it did in George Bailey's case. Friends and strangers put together their own version of a Christmas miracle to help fill our cupboards and fridge again, also ensuring that I am able to get months of the housekeeping assistance I desperately needed in my declining state of health – plus enough to allow me to treat my daughter to a touch more than the pair of slippers which was the only gift she'd asked for. A tremendously generous gift from a large group of people I've never even met, generous in both in dollars and the desire to be of help. The effort led by my friend Kristee, who is one of the most genuinely caring people I've ever had the privilege to know.

I'm able to get a few new clothes; my friends have been very kind in not mentioning the fact that they'd see me in the same wardrobe items over and over again. I'd convinced myself that I was not too old to get away with the look of frayed jeans. I am.

Another lovely surprise this week, a stupendous virtual tour of New York City was hand-delivered. Authentic right down to the samples of the Philosophy shampoo and conditioner that the hotel that I virtually stayed at stocks in their guestrooms. This gift was put together by a friend of my daughter, whom I'd met just once briefly; the assembly of this wonderful gift was months in the making. I just can't put it down; every time I look at it I see something I hadn't noticed before.

Other amazing treats have poured forth. Lots of delicious food (including more than my fair share of chocolate!) a wonderfully relaxing massage, an angel (a reminder of all the here-on-earth Clarences who are watching over me!) and most appreciated – gifts of precious time spent with me in person or on the phone, and through so many lovely emails.

A home visit from my estate lawyer on the afternoon of Christmas Eve (his wife even putting their holiday preparations aside to act as witness) so that I could go into the holidays secure in knowing that my wishes for looking out for my daughter's future would be carried out.

Other professionals and volunteers who've moved heaven and earth over the last weeks to ensure that these weeks that I'm blessed to spend with my daughter over the holidays are as carefree as they possibly could be. And having the sensitivity to step back to leave us to some time alone too. Last night my daughter and I threw tradition out the window and had ourselves a Christmas Eve that we mutually declared to be our best ever, despite that fact that we hardly budged from the comfort of the bed.

Over the years, I'd wondered if anyone could truly feel as special and appreciated as George Bailey did at the end of *It's a Wonderful Life*. The answer for me is most decidedly yes.

Thank you my dear friends, we're so very lucky to have you. It's been a Christmas that couldn't possibly be outdone if we're to measure it by the warmth you've put in our hearts. You've given me the most beautiful gift imaginable by letting me know that you're sticking by my side on this journey.

ALL TIED UP
Wednesday, January 02, 2013

If I thought that my independence was compromised when it was necessary to transition to a wheelchair when leaving my apartment, I was in for a big surprise when something even more limiting was introduced last week – a fifty-foot tether.

With my increased difficulty in breathing, my nurse strongly suggested that it was time to start oxygen therapy. I wrangled with the idea over Christmas Day whether I should proceed or not; having signed a "Do Not Resuscitate" order a few months ago, I didn't know if going on oxygen fell contrary to my wishes to forego life supporting measures as my illness progresses.

A chat with a palliative specialist assured me that even in hospice, oxygen therapy is used to make patients more comfortable, I would not be acting against my DNR. That chat was only part of a longer meeting at my place, during which I finalized all the paperwork for my admittance to hospice for when I, my loved ones, or my doctors decide that I'm ready.

Friday afternoon and evening were a whirlwind. Let me say that getting oxygen set up at the onset of a long weekend leading up to New Year's Eve is no easy feat, but thanks to the persistence and kindness of my nurse, a few friends and my family doctor (who was on vacation but insisted on doing what she could to help me out immediately), I had oxygen within hours. Plus a few new prescriptions to ease my respiration and to take the edge off of the unrelenting pain.

The oxygen is helping somewhat; I can sit up a bit longer than I've been able to in weeks. And conversations are interrupted less by the hacking coughing jags. (My daughter's catch phrase – said with love – since coming home for the holidays, has been, "Lungs. Keep them on the inside please, Mom.")

Over the years, I've been administered oxygen a few times when lying in a hospital bed, but trying to carry on simple tasks around the apartment with a hose up my nose is no easy task.

I learned a tough lesson the second day that one really must sit still for a bit after removing oxygen, to allow the body to readjust. A lesson that I didn't seem to grasp after the first catapult towards the floor, either.

The constant whine of the oxygen concentrator is a rude reminder of my illness. The travel tanks (what kind of trouble can I get into on a three hour outing?) sitting in my living room don't help. (Mind you, the loaner wheelchair resting there doesn't help much either.)

Not to mention all the rules that come with oxygen therapy. No candles, no going near a stove in use. (That's a twist that will be interesting to work around, given that I have a freezer full of meals that need cooking.) A sign on the door stating that on the other side resides a fire hazard. And one cautionary note that surprised me is that I need to check that none of my facial products or lotions contain petroleum. (Out comes the magnifying glass to check out all the labels.) Here I was thinking that the technician told me that they couldn't be used because they could degrade the plastic tubes – it's because they could ignite!

The fun doesn't end there. The government will only supply the equipment for a short time. Here goes another round with the insurance company to get coverage beyond that. I've been warned that given my diagnosis of such a rare disease, this process could be rather problematic. When hasn't it been?

This morning I lost it. Ripped off the oxygen and had a good cry. Which I might add is really not a combination conducive to good respiration. In five short days, I've become so frustrated with nasal prongs that fall out whenever I bend over, tripping over the hose when I tried to get out of bed, and the sharp pain up my nose when the kitten yanks the hose in the opposite direction in a spirit of play.

Tired of having to plan out every move in the apartment, or even just in my bed.

The oxygen went back on after my short-lived cry.

The kicker to all this is that I'm fighting so hard to stay as independent as possible in an apartment that I despise being in. The contradiction can't help but slap me in the face. If you interpret this post as that I'm feeling sorry for myself today, you're absolutely right.

SPECIAL FAVOURS
Wednesday, January 09, 2013

Many wonderful people do very nice things for me. Some I know better than others, but generally, the people helping me out know my situation and go above and beyond to make my days easier.

Most of my interactions these days are over email or over the phone because getting out is getting close to impossible. In the last three weeks, I've stepped out of my apartment just once. (Although it was a challenge to make it happen, I was thrilled to be present for an event that brought a smile to my daughter's face during her visit home from school.)

Although friends and volunteers take care of most of the everyday tasks that I can no longer manage, there are still interactions that require me to pick up the phone – I just have to pick my moments carefully these days and make sure I'm juiced up with oxygen so that I can get out full sentences without a coughing fit.

If I have the choice, the person at the other end of the line need not know I'm ill if it's not relevant to the conversation. It's my chance to feel somewhat normal in a life that is quite far removed from what normal used to look like.

Today I played the "sick card," to get a matter attended to more urgently, and it weighs on my mind. Looking at the situation practically, the matter needed a very quick turnaround – and the only way to make it happen was to very briefly explain why I was not able to appear in person to complete a transaction. That I needed to have an exception made for me because I'm ill, that I needed to be treated differently than the average customer.

Although this challenging health and living situation is with me 24/7, it hits home at these moments just how incapacitated I've become over the last month. Yesterday and today I've learned some particularly tough lessons about my limitations. Trying to do a few tasks on my own because there was no one else to do them, and failing miserably. I can only blame myself for not having had the patience to wait until someone was available to help me, because they always gladly do so.

Things will be changing in a few days after I meet with my case manager. More help is available, and the discussion continues about whether it's time to move me to a care facility. The hope that I'll stabilize lessens as each day passes, despite my determination. My will appears to have little say in matters these days.

This is truly a miserable situation. Especially if I let my mind go back to discussions that were had when I was first diagnosed, about how I hoped things would play out when my health got really bad...and the unconditional support and assurances I received at that time that I would not be going through this alone. It looks less likely as each day passes that I'll be able to end my days in the comfort of my own bed. This thought saddens me greatly.

This week, several people whose opinions matter to me have reminded me that I don't always have to put on the brave face, that I have every right to have the occasional pity party for myself. Today I had to invite a stranger into that party and I don't like it one bit.

SEVENTEEN HOURS
Friday, January 18, 2013

"Nothing fixes a thing so intensely in the memory as the wish to forget it." Michel de Montaigne (1533-1592)

If I'm lucky, I get about four or five hours of sleep a night. To get even that takes a dinger of a sleeping pill to reroute the pain for a short while. Even then, I'm subjected to some pretty horrendous nightmares; one of the possible side effects of this medication. Even unconscious I'm unable to escape this situation.

Being awake at 4 a.m. has always bothered me, there's just something especially unsettling about it. To dodge that hour, I stay up every night until at least 1 a.m., take my sleeping pill, and hope that I make it to at least 5 a.m. before waking. Almost always waking up on the edge of a dream that has upset me, almost always a replay of disturbing events that have happened in real life over the last two years. Very seldom does my illness creep into these dreams; for the most part, I'm able to walk and do pretty normal things. Just under abnormal circumstances.

These days, my level of exhaustion hits new heights. I'm not able to nap due to the pain, so I lie quietly, trying to think of pleasant things. More difficult to do as the weeks wear on. Being more or less confined to bed leaves far too much time to think, despite my best efforts to occupy my mind.

For the sake of argument, let's say I get five hours of sleep. A good night. That leaves nineteen hours. Most days I have a visitor or two (friend, volunteer, nurse, Personal Support Worker). Their visits might add up to a couple of hours.

This still leaves about seventeen hours a day when I'm on my back (or in some contortion that I feel a bit more comfortable in), alone in my room...time that has to be occupied. I don't have cable, so I listen to audio books and on-line courses, watch DVDs that have been loaned to me, try to find something on Netflix that I've not already seen. It's around this time of the month that I have to slow down the online access as I get too close to my monthly bandwidth limit, leaving me even more time to fill in creative ways. Let's not forget the insurance issues I wish I didn't have to deal with on a regular basis; I just don't have the energy for it. And sometimes all I can do is to push away the attempts at distractions and bear down against the pain.

I had a thought-provoking conversation with a spiritual counsellor this week that was of help –the reality is that this really sucks (his words!)

We discussed quality of life. There truly isn't much left. I'm grateful for the visitors, emails, and phone calls. Grateful for the social assistance that's been made available to me in the form of volunteers, nurses and PSWs.

Being hooked up to oxygen, having to limit time on my legs to about ten minutes a day (preferably less if I can get away with it to lessen the aching at night), not being able to escape these four walls, not being able to prepare proper meals for myself. All more frustrating than I could have ever imagined when I years ago thought about what the later stages of this disease might look like. Who would have thought that I'd blister at the top of my ears from the oxygen tubing?

For the next few days I'm able to put this aside. Sue is flying in to be with me, to help me with some lingering loose ends. The apartment will be full a good part of the time with other friends, my daughter will be home too. (An important note for anyone who's had the thought; it's at my insistence that my daughter is away at school. We're in agreement that it's the best way – and our way – to go forward at this time.) We'll laugh, we'll cry. And then laugh again.

Far too much time left over to try to forget things that insist on fixing themselves in my memory. Not a terribly productive use of my time, but it's the reality that is.

Dying alone slowly and painfully is something I wish nobody had to go through. (I know how much the people who care about me hate seeing me like this too. God bless them for their prayers for a more peaceful end to this.) I have to take it hour by hour, seventeen at a time.

WHAT CAN HAPPEN IN 91 HOURS?
Wednesday, January 23, 2013

In my last post, I mentioned that Sue came for a visit from the east coast. She flew out again this morning. Three visits in the last year, but I must admit, this trip we got up to the most trouble – without me ever leaving the apartment!

Sue and I have a friendship that spans just shy of twenty-five years. During that period, we've both been through some difficult times, yet we've never let the many miles between us get in the way of strengthening our relationship. She's been my rock (especially throughout the last two years), unwavering in her support, love, and encouragement.

The last three trips have had their bittersweet moments. In the spring, we met with the funeral planner to make my final arrangements. She helped me pack up my belongings in the house that I had so dearly loved living in and found so hard to leave. In December, she came, knowing that my daughter and I were having a very difficult time facing Christmas, (which in the end we pretty much ignored, it was just too painful to take on this year).

This trip she ran numerous errands for me with the help of other friends, including getting my sweet kitten neutered yesterday. The poor lad is not all impressed by the cone he has to wear for two weeks; he startles himself each time he passes the mirrored closet in the hall. Last night he had two women cooing and cuddling him, perhaps a fantasy for a few other men out there?

There are tough discussions to be made. Sue knows every detail of what has to happen, and what I hope to have happen at the end. Often the tears flow when we have these talks; I know I can trust her to be there for me and make decisions that are best for me and my daughter. There is simply no doubt about that. Given the way the last two years have played out, it's a blessing that never goes unappreciated.

It can't be all sombre though, can it? Saturday, a few friends and my daughter joined us in my "boudoir," to make it a memorable and enjoyable evening. Great food, amazing company, more than a few laughs. With a sly wink it was suggested that it was the best time some of us have had in bed in a long time.

Sue and I were on our own for the last two nights. There just isn't any other way to put it – sheer goofiness set sail on Monday night! No booze, drugs, or other mind-altering substances – just two friends between whom there are no walls. And no judgement thankfully either!

Complete and utter silliness. Exactly what I needed a good dose of.

GRATITUDE–ISSUE #?
Friday, January 25, 2013

I've lost track along the way of how many posts I've entitled Gratitude. I hope that in reading my blog, you understand just how much of it I feel towards the friends and volunteers who've stepped in to ease my journey. It's the little things, it's the big things, and all things in between. It's the things that friends aren't maybe even aware of doing that can help. (Tonight it was a hug that was held just a little tighter and longer than usual when saying goodbye.)

Tonight was my first night as a recipient of a meal prepared by the volunteer organization, Food Train; they'll be providing me with meals twice a week, going forward. Tonight's dinner was actually more like six meals, lots extra for the freezer. The organizer ensured that all my dietary restrictions were covered, and asked detailed questions about what I like and what I don't care so much for. And she also insisted that if a craving for anything struck, I was to be sure to let them know. If tonight's homemade, vegetarian, gluten-free lasagna is any indication, my belly will be very grateful several nights a week!

It's no secret that I really don't like living in this apartment. Nothing I do makes being here any easier. I suspect not having left my apartment in many weeks really hasn't helped matters. (Do I even remember what outdoor air feels like?) However, I made it a mission this week to appreciate some of the things within these four walls. Here goes.

Hot water straight out of the tap. In the old house, it could take a few minutes for the hot water to travel up to the second floor, and it would most certainly run out before the bath was full. Here, in less than a second, beckoned hot water arrives. And it lasts for a good long shower; that's the one activity that I make sure I save energy for every day. These days I have to use a seat in the tub – I'm grateful to have that too.

Delicious smelling soaps, shower gels, hand and body lotions. They make those showers all the better. Almond, chocolate, orange-vanilla, raspberry crème, coconut, and even fortune cookie scent. I've been mightily spoiled over the holidays. If they tasted as good as they smell, you might catch me licking my forearm when I thought you weren't looking. I'll leave that job to the kitten, he's especially fond of raspberry crème; it's hard to get him to leave it where I've applied it.

Turtledoves Gluten Free Bakery treats on my counter and in the freezer. I've never set foot in their shop, but thoughtful friends keep me stocked with their amazing treats. Friday is Cheese Bread day, and along comes Kristee today with a loaf, having heard how much I love it. Toasted, with Nutella. You're welcome to grimace, but until you've tried it, don't knock it! And the lemon squares may or may not survive until breakfast...

Bamboo sheets. If you're going to have to spend most of your time in bed, I highly recommend them. The softest sheets I've ever owned.

Gratitude too for the PSWs and friends who change the sheets for me often so I can have a fresh bed several times a week.

Almond vanilla linen mist. Again, if you have to spend lots of time in bed, sheets with a favourite scent make it a little more pleasant. I go to sleep with my bedding smelling of marzipan. When I wake up from a nightmare, I find it helps to have a scent that I love surrounding me.

Photos of my daughter. She's not thrilled that there's a photo of her on every wall of the bedroom but I'm afraid this is one battle she's not going to win. There's nothing I'd rather look at if I can't have the live version sitting here with me.

Many of the items listed above are here only because of the generosity of friends. Please don't mistake this post as a request for more of anything; the apartment is well stocked at the moment (especially with Nutella!) Just an exercise in appreciating the little things in a challenging environment.

SHAKING THE FOUNDATION
Monday, January 28, 2013

Sometimes I pray that bad things do indeed come in threes. There are times that challenges come at me so fast and furiously that I hope that the after the third one, I get a bit of a break. Sometimes I do, sometimes I don't.

Or there are times like tonight that two challenges have hit close together and I'm braced for the third. And I pray that the saying about bad things coming in threes falters now and again, and I have a better day tomorrow. I need something to go right. It would make a welcome change in the constant onslaught of setbacks. I can't even begin to tell you how badly I need a challenge to have a positive outcome right now. Not just be mediocre, not just be passable, or barely acceptable (which is the current definition of a success around here).

The successes that I have are surrounded in sadness these days. Yay, I found a buyer for my favourite lens! But hey, I just had to sell my favourite lens. Yay, I found a buyer for the dining room table! But hey, I had to sell a custom-made table that my daughter and I loved.

I need something to high-five over, and someone to be there to high-five it with.

Late last night I split a tooth. On something really soft. (Did you know the foods that people most often break a tooth on are soft bread and muffins?) I'd already taken off my oxygen for the night. I wasn't able to move as quickly as I would have liked towards a box of tissues to spit out the contents of my mouth that were suddenly of a texture they ought not to have been. My tongue had already figured out what had happened, it felt a sharp jag along one of my molars that threatened to cut if I veered too close.

Normally, not a big deal. Make an appointment with the dentist, get it taken care of.

Not quite so fast...

I won't bore you with the details but I'll state that I REALLY need a suitable wheelchair. And the friend who took me to my appointment today would gladly beg along with me. The chair I currently have just isn't working out. The saga continues with the insurance company; I've lost track of just how many months this has gone on. And I'll add that I've been made aware that I'll never again be able to have dental work other than a cleaning done in a dentist's office. My cardiac issues do not allow for me to be administered the needle for freezing before work begins, if I need so much as a wee cavity filled I'll need to have the work done in a hospital. I'm one tough cookie, but even I'm not going to have major dental work done without freezing. Though truth be told, at this stage of my illness I wouldn't be bothering with dental work unless something significant happens like part of my tooth snapping off.

An exhausting trek (and that's truly an understatement) resulted in a clean-out of what remained of the tooth and a patch job. A patch job that needs to last...well, just long enough.

As I was waiting out the afternoon in my apartment before the late-day appointment, the fire alarm started alarming. I don't know if there's even an appropriate word for the sound of the fire alarm. Screech? Scream? Shrill? Whatever the name of the sound, it was driving the kitten absolutely insane. Jumping up on me (with nails primed) for comfort, then running around madly. The poor dear, and I wasn't too thrilled about the sound either.

And it kept going, and going. My PSWs have been asked to check in the lobby for notices about fire alarm tests and other building info since I don't get down there, but there had been no forewarning. Then the fire trucks arrived. I couldn't see them (I look out over the back parking lot), but there was no question that they were at the front of the building. The alarms kept ringing. And I heard lots of heavy traipsing (firefighters don't tread lightly in those heavy boots!) Then I could hear my neighbours vacating their apartments to head to the lobby as we're supposed to do in such a case.

The alarms kept on going. And the realization became more unsettling by the minute that in case of a true fire (and I still don't know anything about the circumstances regarding the alarms this afternoon except that my nurse said there was a lot of kerfuffle in the lobby as she passed through shortly after) that I was trapped. On oxygen and unable to walk more than a very short distance and most certainly unable to stand for more than a minute or two at a time, I wasn't going to be able to follow my neighbours. How could I not have considered this possibility as the severity of my disabilities grew? That if there's a fire I'm going to need to be carried down the stairs?

A few phone calls to make tomorrow, to figure out what happens to the disabled when an emergency situation requiring evacuation takes place. I'm not the first person to be in this position, I'm sure there's a perfectly sensible solution. I just don't know what it is yet.

A broken tooth and an emergency in my building have tripped me up. Normally they would have been taken in stride, and I would have done what needed to be done. On the outside, I'm as calm as can be about these two incidents, yet inside I feel a gnawing feeling that I haven't been able to shake. Two more reminders of how isolated I am, and how dependent I've had to become on others.

I could really do without a third reminder this week.

LOVE ME, LOVE MY DNR
Saturday, February 02, 2013

I was chatting with my friend Chris from the UK on Skype this afternoon (I love where playing Words with Friends has led me!) when I mentioned that I was working on a new blog post with controversial subject matter. (With a smile and a hint of sarcasm, Chris quickly piped in, "Sandy, you? Controversial?")

Most days I don't have enough energy for rousing conversation or debate anymore, but there is a subject that creeps more and more into daily life out of necessity. I'm going to shove this one heartily into the arena.

Please offer your loved ones an immense gift (despite this being a very difficult task for most) and share what your wishes for care and final arrangements are should you become seriously ill and/or incapacitated. Most of the people who are aware that I have documented my decisions regarding my care agree that the conversation is an important one to have, yet themselves have not discussed their wishes with the people closest to them. Let me add a request to please get your will sorted out, you'll save your family what might possibly be no end of distress and confusion (and I have a few lawyers to recommend should you not already have one).

Given my current state, many conversations with nurses and other health care professionals start off asking if my "Do Not Resuscitate" order is still in effect, and easily accessible on my fridge and in my purse. Yes. Yes it is. It can be a tiresome question to answer, but one that I'm glad continues to be asked.

I'm grateful that this subject is discussed with compassion and concern; it confirms that my health care team shares my commitment to what my final wishes are (and I'm free to change the plan if I so desire at any point). More so, however, I'm grateful that my daughter won't be faced with difficult decisions should I be incapable of communicating.

There's a plan incorporating emergency access to my apartment, notifying my family doctor instead of calling 911 (to avoid a circus of emergency responders whose assistance won't be required), what measures may be taken if I'm in a bad state – all written and accessible. There's even a government-provided crisis kit in my kitchen, with medications that would ease any extraordinary discomfort, some of which I can self administer or have a nurse deliver to me in my final weeks, days, or hours. There's a fair likelihood that I'll be on my own when these matters need to be addressed; it's entirely possible that I could be relying on a stranger to open up that manila envelope attached to the side of my fridge.

As I reread this, I haven't really even touched upon the controversial part of what I had planned to write. Another day. Today, just a plea to do something very important with, and for your loved ones.

CELEBRATING VICTORIES, HOWEVER HOLLOW THEY MAY SEEM
Wednesday, February 06, 2013

After a long struggle with social services, my ex's insurance company, and suppliers, I received word this morning that I'm finally going to get a wheelchair that fits me, and has the features required to allow me escape from this apartment. Lots of help required, but I'm going to be able to visit the outside world again fairly soon. Wherever shall my first destination be? I'm long overdue for a visit to my Toronto medical team, but that certainly won't be the first place on my wish list.

A victory? I'm celebrating – and my friends are conducting the online equivalent of a riotous stadium cheer for the hometown team's trouncing of the opposition – but put in context, how is this a win? What has this situation come to that we're thrilled to get a piece of equipment that further cements the reality of my declining health? Why months to get to this point?

It seems a hollow victory indeed, as I stand back. It's been a tough lesson in economics, number crunching, and bureaucracy. A fair percentage of the daily challenges I face are. It's often only when a plea for compassion is extended that rules are bent. And they are bent; it's sometimes the only way things get accomplished around here. I detest asking for special favours of others, to be singled out – but I'm learning that it's how the game is played to get what ought to instead be standard issue. Still lots of shortfalls and more mountains to climb. At least now I have wheels to make the physical part of the attempts somewhat easier.

STEPPING INTO THE OTHER PAIR OF SHOES
Thursday, February 07, 2013

At midnight last night, a text message popped up on my iPad. "Are you awake? There's a small problem." I'm always awake at midnight; I quickly replied that I was indeed up.

Although I didn't recognize the telephone number and no name had appeared, the country code was one that was familiar to me. Not because I've ever called it, it's just one of those curious things I look up when I'm bored.

Code 66 is Thailand where Sue and her husband are vacationing, as they do every year for an extended stay. Normally, we communicate over Skype, her cell phone, or now FaceTime, so I'm never left wondering who the caller might be. Except for this time.

A phone call followed a few minutes later, Sue was heading into surgery for an emergency appendectomy. She wanted me to know that she wasn't going to be available for our usual daily call and not to worry.

I was of course concerned for her care and comfort – having surgery far away from home offers added worries. She assured me that the facilities were perfectly acceptable and that she would be out of hospital within a couple of days. And even likely back to the beach soon after that.

Yet of course I worried. I don't sleep much at night in the first place and my unoccupied mind had to be there with her in spirit.

I received a text message from her husband this morning that all went very well, which certainly eased my mind. I'm sure she will indeed be back at the beach very soon; she's a tough cookie, having had her fair share of serious health issues to prove it.

She said something to me last night that many friends have said to me when going through health and personal challenges. "Sandy, it's nothing compared to what you're going through, please don't worry."

The only thing that made the worry for her any less was knowing that her husband was by her side, as he always is, faithfully holding her hand. Even when his work has taken him thousands of miles away, he arranged, as no small undertaking, to come to her when she faced a serious health crisis several years ago. At that time she too said to me, "Sandy – it's nothing compared to what you're going through." In fact she waited until the worst was well past before even telling me, knowing herself how difficult long distance worry can be.

This is never a contest between me and my friends about who is suffering more. I want to support my friends in any way I can when things are tough, I try to never diminish their pain or sadness in comparison to my own. Sadly, I know that often they don't share their own trials because they feel they're not as tough as mine and feel bad about bringing them up.

What this episode did teach me last night was about how utterly helpless it's possible to feel when someone you care about is facing a difficult challenge far away. My friends tell me how they struggle with these feelings, and I always tell them not to worry, that I'll be okay. What I didn't realize until last night was just how much further that worry can be compounded by the thought that they might doing it alone, until I let myself imagine Sue by herself in a Thailand hospital.

But honestly, this episode was a dose of reality for me on a number of fronts. Despite all the preparations, documentation, schedules of Personal Support Workers, visitors, and planning for what happens when the more serious health episodes come along – I'm most often alone when the worst pain comes along. Maybe my friends do indeed have valid reason to worry; I shouldn't be so quick to dismiss their concerns. But that opens the door to worrying about my own welfare and I don't want to let myself go there. It's often easier to dig my head in the sand when it comes to facing my own health challenges. In hindsight, I should have ensured that I had a friend with me for every radiation treatment, every appointment where bad news was anticipated, and every difficult procedure. I made the decisions to not accept offers because I didn't want to be a burden. I'm slowly learning that people who care about me feel better knowing that I'm not on my own; it helps them too.

The discussion comes up quite regularly whether trying to live here on my own is the best option, and as each day passes, I'm not entirely sure that it is.

PATIENCE AND TIMING
Monday, February 11, 2013

The wheelchair rep left a short while ago; we spent about twenty minutes going over all the options available, to ensure that the new chair truly fits. Who knew that it could be customized to the degree that it will be? It's nothing fancy, but at least it will fit me (provided that my outings aren't consistently to the handicapped-accessible Lindt chocolate factory outlet, in which case I should have considered ordering a wider chair).

I had checked out the manufacturer's website over the last few weeks, and I was delighted to hear confirmation today that I could indeed order the chair in a colour of my choosing (at least for the metal bars, the rest will be black). If I must have a wheelchair, I may as well have it match my decor! And so it will – my selection will go nicely with the living room furniture nearby, to where the chair will be stored when not in use.

As for when I'm out in public, there's just no hiding the fact that I'm in a wheelchair. I can have a bit of fun making sure my outfit doesn't clash, but will the combination be attractive enough so that people don't notice that oxygen hose up my nose? Doubtful, but I can hope...

Now the hard part – the manufacturer is running behind with orders and it'll likely be at least two to three weeks before it arrives. Too much time to think about where I'd like to go! Not that getting out will be a frequent event, but it will most definitely be something to look forward to.

Timing these days is an issue. To get out, it has to be one of my good days. Those don't arrive with regularity or the frequency I'd prefer, but once in a while they do happen.

A few things have to come into play to have a better day. First, I'll have had to stay off my feet for at least twenty-four hours prior. Short bathroom trips aside, the key is to stay in bed with no undue pressure on my bones or heart.

Then comes the timing of my medications. At long last, I have access to a pain medication that takes the edge off (most days at least), but it needs careful administering. It's quite hard on the stomach and organs so it can only be taken for a few days at a time. The days in between? I suspect you don't want to know what those days look like.

As effective as the new pain med usually is, it doesn't like to stay down to do its work. Bless my doctor for getting me a supply of an anti-emetic (for nausea) that's normally used in conjunction with chemo – the stuff is magic. Gravol can't hold a candle to it.

Good thing planning and organizing have always have been my forte. Getting out will take much forethought, but I'll have plenty of time over the next few weeks to figure things out.

As for when the nice weather comes along in a few months' time, I'll have quite a different list of desired destinations ready to go. (Unfortunately the wheelchair didn't come with an option for snow tires!)

TAKE FIVE MINUTES
Saturday, February 16, 2013

"People are just as happy as they make up their minds to be."
Abraham Lincoln

A few of my friends and family members are going through a heck of a rough stretch lately. Serious illness, financial troubles; for some it seems that each day brings another unwanted challenge. Yes, I do count myself in all these categories. If you've followed this blog, you know that it's been a really rough go for both me and my daughter. I wish I could tell you that the onslaught has slowed down, but it has not.

The friends and family that I speak of now astound me. Even though we're discussing some deeply troubling issues, they still have a light-hearted lift in their voices, still speak of happy things in their lives, and still laugh with me about the silly and mundane.

I had several lengthy conversations this week with others about happiness. The quote noted above from Abraham Lincoln is one that I remind myself of often, and have shared many times. Just more often than usual this week, as I note how many of the friends surrounding me at this point in my life seem to subscribe to this philosophy.

Yesterday, a large number of people would have seen a middle-aged woman (ouch, it hurt to write that little truth!), bundled up with a grocery basket in her lap as she sat in her wheelchair, oxygen tubes in her nose, oxygen tank fighting with the grocery basket for room. Pushing her was a lovely bundle of energy who always has a genuine and warm graciousness about her.

As others on our journey complained about the cold outside, the bitter wind, and how miserable the week had been – what they might have missed was the sheer bliss I was experiencing at that moment. I was out. Icy or not, it was finally fresh air on my face (even though it was just a few minutes out in the parking lot). After months of anticipation, I was finally in the company of more than a couple of humans at once. They may not have been interacting with me (I refer to an earlier post about how one becomes invisible in a wheelchair), but I was out in public at long last. I pray that nobody looked at me with pity; it's not something I was feeling for myself.

I feel like I share a delicious secret with many of the people who are currently in my life; that true happiness can be found in between all the crap that happens in life. Very few escape challenges and lows in a lifetime. It reminds me of when I've had the flu or a cold, experiencing the relief that comes when I can breathe easily again or my appetite has returned. Sometimes you just need to appreciate the moments that are absent of pain or discomfort.

Of course I complain about tough challenges – I'm unlikely to stop. Nor should anyone. In moderation it sure lightens the load when you can share your burdens.

But if you're not already in the population who can find happiness in the little things, I implore you to set aside five minutes to appreciate the good in your life: the feel of a warm sweater, the taste of a favourite food, the hug from a loved one. And the opportunity to hug the ones you love. I hope you can truly appreciate that last one. (I apologize if I'm coming across as sanctimonious, but on this last point I especially believe that I know of what I preach.)

You can decide that every day will hold a moment to be singled out and appreciated. You might find that there are more of them to be found than you might have believed.

And now, I'm going to hug the person whom I love most of all. Having her home for the next week brings me more happiness than I could possibly express!

GETTING NOSTALGIC
Monday, February 18, 2013

A day of bringing back memories.

A very long chat this afternoon with an old friend whom I've not seen in about thirty years. How sweet it was to pick up where we left off so long ago and have it feel comfortable and warm.

It was to have been a visit in person today, but unfortunately my body wasn't cooperating, with pain levels that have been difficult to get under control over the last few days. I suspect that my Friday grocery trip has something to do with it, but I'm still saying it was worth it. (Though if things haven't calmed down tomorrow, I may look a little less favourably upon the tub of ice cream I purchased on that trip – or just finish it off so the reminder has been removed!)

Cancelling was a difficult choice, but as I told my friend – there are days when I can cover up how much pain I'm in and others not so much. And when it's not so much, I know it makes others uncomfortable to watch and I'd rather not put people who care about me through that discomfort if it can be helped.

I haven't been able to see many friends in person over the last couple of weeks with the pain management dance I'm doing. Getting me to a point of lesser pain, not be nauseated and still awake takes some intricate timing these days. I'm not yet sure if I'm just not getting the hang of it, or the pain is indeed getting worse as the weeks pass. Today I'm going with the latter, and I've needed some pretty intense diversions to occupy my mind.

Tonight I needed interaction with people who exude positive energy, but it's too late to be calling friends. (I know a few of you will be wagging a finger at me to remind me that you've offered an ear 24/7, but in reality I just can't see myself calling at this hour.)

Instead I did something that I've been putting off because I thought it might make me too sad, but in reality it was just what I needed.

I played a YouTube video that I'd compiled several years ago as a marketing tool for my portrait business. What gorgeous smiles, and seeing them put a big one on my face.

ANOTHER ONE PASSES WITHOUT CHANGE
Wednesday, February 27, 2013

Today is International Rare Disease Day, the fifth observance since I was diagnosed in 2009 with Erdheim-Chester Disease.

I'm sad to say not a lot has changed in Canada regarding the availability and funding of treatment of rare illnesses.

Several years later and I still find myself embroiled on a regular basis in arduous applications (along with a fair amount of begging and pleading) for funding. The battles for me are no longer about experimental treatments in hopes of slowing down the progression of this disease, but instead are pleas for pain relief, mobility aids, and oxygen; items to make a poor quality of life just a smidgen more tolerable.

Might things have turned out differently if access to treatments and medications had been more readily available? Would I have given up on treatments as I did after the high dose radiation sessions in the fall? I just didn't (and don't) have the strength anymore to keep on fighting. Perhaps I'll be judged as giving up, as weak – but truly, until you've walked in these shoes... (And I pray that you never need to.)

I thought about listening to the radio segment on rare illness I did for CBC almost two years ago, but decided against it. I'm afraid to hear the hope that I had in my voice at that time, for myself, the fellow ECD patient interviewed (who sadly passed not long after, his family remains in my thoughts and prayers) and other rare illness patients in this country.

The system has exhausted me. Fighting this illness and all the challenges surrounding it has annihilated me. I've raised my white flag, and it's awfully hard to keep waving it.

THE INBOX
Tuesday, March 05, 2013

Thank you for the huge wave of support sent my and my daughter's way after my most recent post. Although I'd mentioned it in last year's Rare Disease Day post, I had decided that I wasn't this year going to mention the petition asking our government for help addressing rare illness. What point? After almost two years, it sat only around 1200 signatures.

Thanks to my daughter and Kristee, who shared a request on their Facebook pages to sign the petition, it now sits a little higher. It's certainly not representative of the hundreds of thousands of Canadians who suffer from rare illness. But it's a start. And the lovely notes and words sent our way were heart-warming, especially for my daughter who was for the first time widely acknowledging to her circle of friends what we're up against. I'm so proud of her bravery. As she stated, "People are so kind if you let them be." I concur – most of the time.

With my body not cooperating much at all, I truly have no choice but to be confined to bed very close to 100% of the time. I've written about my various diversions – learning continues to be a preoccupation with me.

One subject that I've tentatively broached over the last few years is the subject of how to die. I'm learning through the wisdom of others about different ways on how one can go about it when death is known to be on its way.

I'm often given the opportunity to speak freely with my palliative team, friends, and volunteers about their own experiences and about how I'm doing on my journey. When I was first diagnosed it was reasonable to speak in increments of years, but realistically, that no longer applies.

This week I've been reading a book called *Final Journeys* by Maggie Callanan. It's meant for caregivers of the terminally ill, but I found it helpful nonetheless.

One simple paragraph from the book lifted a huge weight off my shoulders today. "We are never done. The inbox is never empty. The desk is never cleared. The dreams are never all realized, nor the projects all completed."

This past week, I've been able to tick a few major items off my to-do list. It lifted weight off my shoulders, yet it nags at me what I still feel I need to accomplish before I leave.

Being the uber-organizer that I am (a few of you who know me all too well can stop laughing anytime now...I'm not blind to how annoying that trait can be at times!) I need to give myself permission to accept that I won't get everything done. And to believe that those I love will see what I was able to do, and not what was left undone on my list.

LOOKING INSIDE THE DOOR
Wednesday, March 06, 2013

My uncle's 90th birthday today has brought me some luck and good news.

I need to preface the balance of this post by saying that by marrying my aunt and joining our family around seventy years ago, he fixed himself in position to be one of the most important people in my life. Unwavering in his love and support for me, he has throughout my life been my role model for what I've come to believe unconditional love to look like.

The new wheelchair arrived today. It's an interesting perspective to realize just how excited I was about it getting here; you'd think I'd just been handed the keys to a Porsche.

It's been a long and very challenging trek to get to this day; it was back in October when I conceded to the urgings of my support team that it was time to give in and use a wheelchair. It felt like a failure on my part to do as much for myself as I could. I've since been able to look at things a little differently, for now it's my ticket to being able to get out into the world once in awhile. And to stay in my apartment perhaps a bit longer than I could without it.

I've had loaner and rental chairs in the meantime, but none of them fit me properly. Or they were much too heavy for my friends and volunteers to lift into the trunk of their vehicle.

This one is light, comes apart for transport, and it fits. The delivery person laughed when he saw the rental and the newly purchased chair beside each other this afternoon, the difference in size was remarkable.

More good news was to come. The phone rang a short while ago and I saw that it was my contact at the insurance company. I thought she might be calling me back to acknowledge the message I'd sent to thank her for all her efforts to get me the chair.

Instead, she was calling to let me know that my oxygen treatment funding had been approved. Within 24 hours. You could have knocked me over with a feather. Maybe not the best way of putting it; you could knock me over with the lightest of drafts these days!

I had steeled myself for yet another long insurance battle. More letters from doctors, more pleading, more of everything that I really didn't need on my plate.

My government funding runs out March 28th, and the insurance coverage kicks in that day. The thought of having to do without the oxygen that has eased my breathing considerably might have paralyzed me if I had let myself consider that scenario.

I won't lie; it's a royal pain in the behind to live with the nose prongs and tubing. I trip over the hose, it gets caught on corners, and trying to propel a wheelchair and keep the hose out of the way (and not run over the kitten who insists on lying down in front of the wheels) is a talent I'll have to work on developing. But gasping for air and coughing so hard I choke and gag is a far less attractive option, so I'm learning to deal.

I celebrate both successes tonight. I'm by myself in my apartment this evening, but feel far from alone. And Happy Birthday to my uncle, who unknowingly (but most characteristically) shared his good tidings with me today.

LOVE IS IN THE DETAILS
Friday, March 08, 2013

People around me may believe that their words and actions are small and insignificant, but perhaps don't realize how powerful an impact they so often have for me.

Today, remembering kindnesses has been what's gotten me through the day. There's no need to go into the details of what today looked like; it's like yesterday but harder. And yesterday was more challenging than the day before that. The trajectory of this illness is undeniable, unrelenting, and some days – like today – almost too difficult to stare in the eyes.

I'm paraphrasing what someone else who is seriously ill posted recently on Twitter. I need a vacation, but unfortunately I'd have to take me along.

Time for gratitude is set aside every day, but it also floats in throughout my day unexpectedly. Those moments are as far away as I'm able to get from the challenges I'm facing, and I savour them. Just a few recent gestures that I'm appreciating tonight. There are so many more, enough to fill a book or two (but likely even more) if I were to list them all.

A call from a volunteer who'd delivered a beautifully prepared meal days earlier, thanking me for the thank you message I'd left on her voicemail. Apologizing that she might have appeared awkward when she entered my apartment, admitting that she felt uncomfortable with my health situation and hadn't known what to say. Her children are lucky to have a mother so giving, honest, and courageous.

An email today from a newer friend who has come to know me well enough to feel comfortable in sending me a short essay. It was written by a young woman and was guaranteed to rip my heart open, and know that it would be a launching pad for something positive for me to leave behind when I go.

A call from Jane letting me know that even though we may not be in touch every week, I'm in her thoughts every day.

A note from my daughter letting me know that she's feeling happy today. I so desperately want her to have as many of those days as possible, knowing what a feat that is right now, with the worries that weigh upon her.

The smile from a bank employee who saw past the wheelchair and oxygen tubes. Not understanding the gravity of the reason why I had to access my safety deposit box, she couldn't have understood how much I needed the kindness at the moment,

The offer of a kind friend to sell what's left of my photographic art prints in her shop, and a promise that my daughter would continue to receive the proceeds after I'm no longer here.

Kristee's desire that I meet her beloved mom. I'll see for myself where such a big heart has come from.

So many kindnesses have gone unmentioned. For all of you who think that the little something that you said or did for me was small, know that they're all significant pieces in letting me finish off my journey knowing that the world can be a very kind place indeed – something I might not believed many times along the path.

NOT DOING MYSELF ANY FAVOURS
Monday, March 11, 2013

It was two years ago today that I was interviewed by CBC Radio on the subject of rare illness in Canada. How difficult it is to recall that day; hope that a new treatment would offer relief from the pain (which it did to some degree for about six months), and my husband cheering me on teary-eyed from the green room – telling me how very proud he was to be at my side throughout this battle. And he spent the next few days emailing just about everyone he knew to tell them about the interview, letting them know how much he appreciated that I continued to keep a smile on my face, that as best I could, I was trying to keep life "normal." It seems a very cruel joke that the particulars of that day stand out so clearly in my memory as I soldier on by myself.

What is normal? My days look very different than they did two years ago. If you visit me at home in my bedroom, besides the oxygen hose you might be hard pressed to know that I'm ill. I'm constantly told how well I look. But if I try to stand, it quickly becomes apparent that something is very wrong. Going without the oxygen means that I'll have difficulty speaking. So in bed, hooked up to oxygen is how I must stay most of the time.

What is a terminally ill patient supposed to look like?

Growing up, in my ignorance, I believed terminally ill meant a patient confined to a hospital bed; machines clicking and whirring above the laboured breathing of the patient.

Not until I met other terminally ill patients over the last two years did it hit me that one could know that death was on its way within a somewhat predictable time frame; yet the patient might still look quite healthy and still be active with family and friends, perhaps even continuing to work.

I've come a long way in understanding what "living while dying," could look like. Sadly I'm now much closer to the scenario imagined in my youth; however, I continue to engage in however many ways I can with friends and family.

I have no idea how to respond to others telling me, "But you don't look sick!" when they visit. It's well-intentioned and caring, and I don't dismiss that.

There's a firestorm on the inside; pain, discomfort, conflicting feelings about what is happening inside me and around me. A clear understanding that this battle is nearing the end. I refuse to say that I'll have lost the battle when I pass, that would suggest I haven't tried hard enough. You may interpret my decisions along the way as you wish; my definition of "trying hard enough," is my own personal business. I'm at peace with my treatment choices (or choices to forego treatment) and that's all that should matter.

My gift to myself every day is to save whatever energy I have to take a shower (with quite a creative set up to accomplish this on my own), to dress, and to put on a face. Not a lot of make-up, but just enough to add healthy-looking colour to the sallow pallor that presents itself on my freshly scrubbed face. Then a rest of some length, to recover from that process.

This daily ritual makes me feel better. If it's all that I'm able to accomplish in a day, so be it. But being clean, dressed, and made-up isn't doing me any favours in helping others understand how the inside of me is being eaten away by this disease. Although as Sue and I laughed about last night, is it any easier to be told that I look terrible?

"FATIGUED"
Thursday, March 14, 2013

I've just finished a phone call with Sue, who has been vacationing with her husband in Thailand for the last six weeks. It's an annual trip to the other side of the world, yet she doesn't let distance get in the way of checking in with me every day.

She's just heading off to bed, and I'm somewhat into my day. "Day" is a loose definition these days for me; last night was pretty typical for the way things play out. I was up until after 4 a.m., then up again at 7 a.m. It's noon and I've not yet felt strong enough to haul myself out of bed. (That treat of my daily shower still lies ahead!) Quite simply, it's pain that keeps me awake. Nothing seems to knock it down enough these days for me to be able to get decent rest.

Sue and I chatted about some difficult matters that require discussing, regarding my declining health, and ended our call with recalling my last blog post. "Soldier on by myself," was the term I used, and we began to imagine what that might look like if we were to be literal about it.

It started out with army boots. Getting my socks on these days requires great effort, are army slippers an option? The wheelchair would need to be repainted with camouflage shades (which I wouldn't mind so much anyway, there's no way I'd describe its colour as the copper I ordered, it's Halloween-ready with that shade of orange).

Next, the enemy line would need to be very close. No farther away than the length of my apartment, that's about all the steam I have in my arms to propel the chair (it's also the length of my oxygen hose). And do they make army fatigue yoga pants?

Pretty useless as a soldier, wouldn't you say? Yet the fight continues whether I'm up for the challenge or not.

Sue and I ended our call as we often do – recalling some funny event from our day, laughing so hard that it's hard to finish our sentences, yet knowing each other as well as we do we usually know the words that didn't get out. As I hung up the phone, I wiped away tears of laughter, wondering which wins out more often these days – the tears from laughing, or tears of sadness and pain. I don't think I want to acknowledge my honest answer to that.

ANTITHESIS
Monday, March 18, 2013

Polarity, opposition, extremes – my life is full of contradiction.

The physical challenges continue to mount. My nurses visit daily now, and the need for assistance from friends and volunteers has again increased. I often sit on the edge of very tough decisions. An illusion perhaps; it would seem most are out of my control.

It seems that that the more I require assistance with my daily routine, the more I miss my independence. If I let myself think about it that is. I'd rather not go there, and I invest significant effort to direct my attention elsewhere.

Donna, our family doctor from our Toronto days – and now dear friend, reminded me last week that there is a huge difference between giving up and surrendering to reality, I struggle to keep that delineation clear. If I'm able to do something myself, I will. If I can't, I'm learning a difficult lesson of acceptance that the goal is beyond my capabilities.

I liken the experience of my declining physical health to that of going through labour when I gave birth to my daughter. My body is going to do what it needs to do, and I have little say in the process.

I've mentioned before that I have vivid dreams when I sleep (which is now more of a precious commodity than ever). Asleep, I can run, jump, drive, cook. Asleep, I live the opposite of my waking hours. Circumstances that gnaw at me while awake have a way of creeping into my dreams.

A life of extremes. A body suffering, yet a spirit richly nourished.

Knowing that when I need help, I need at least all my fingers to count out the number of friends who would in a heartbeat drop whatever they're doing to come to me, with their gentleness in understanding that asking for help sits well outside my comfort zone.

Learning more life lessons in this lifetime than I thought possible. Finding out that despite a very bumpy road dealing with plenty of difficult situations, there is far more love and kindness to be found than I ever imagined. Some of the most challenging periods of my life have not been shared on this blog – believe me when I tell you that I've firsthand experienced the opposite of love, however you might define that. Hate? Indifference? Fear? (Which reminds me of a quote I shared with some friends last week. "I don't have time to hate the people who hate me, I'm too busy loving the people who love me.")

Finding out that while there are some people who don't seem to care a shred beyond meeting their own needs, there are far more with so much good in them that they have not only enough to share with their own friends and family, they have an ample supply in their hearts to spread around to strangers.

Great pain endured, and love sent to me in abundance at this time. To me, it seems the universe has me going in two very different directions. In the bigger plan, maybe they have to go hand in hand for me to better understand each.

INTENTIONS. WE PREFER TO ASSUME THEY'RE GOOD
Saturday, March 23, 2013

A few weeks ago, a fellow blogger who is living with terminal illness put up a post about things that people sometimes say to the dying (and their loved ones) that can come across as hurtful or upsetting. I'm not using the exact phrasing, for reasons that might be become clear in few moments.

Dozens of examples were provided, and her readers added plenty more over the following days.

Although I could relate to many of the comments that patients had found upsetting, I felt that perhaps the author might have embarrassed people who would recognize their own words. Recognizing some phrases that had come out of my own mouth over my lifetime when speaking with ill friends and their families, I discussed the blog post with a few friends.

I at no time ever meant to be insensitive; I just didn't know what to say. Sometimes when I don't know what to say, the wrong words come out. My friends shared that they'd had similar experiences over the years. I'm generalizing, but I'd say that in North America we're not as comfortable addressing death and dying as some other cultures around the world.

Yes, in rare moments I do bite my tongue at something someone's said. And when it happens, it's almost always someone I don't know well to whose words I took offence. I remind myself that the speaker was most certainly well intentioned and caring and I have no wish to let them know that the comment might have hurt a bit, or that it reminded me of something I don't wish to be reminded of.

A few days ago, however, something was written to my daughter that floored me. Someone from our past sent her an email with a request for her to do something to benefit the sender. No offer of help, no recognition of the struggles she's going through. The request was prefaced with a phrase that deeply offended both of us. No, life is not treating her well. The sender should have a pretty good idea of how tough her life is right now in trying to balance getting an education, with having a mother who is dying without a caregiver. Not to mention all the other usual stuff than can crop up in a nineteen-year-old's life.

Despite our best efforts to keep my daughter at school and me at home, something had to give. And it did over the last weeks. For the moment, that's a private matter until we have more details sorted out.

The mother bear in me reared up. I told my daughter to forget the request, forget the email – just concentrate on the exam that she was stressing over. That I would look after the issue, and I did.

Let me just say that despite the fact that she and I both try to put on a brave face with a smile as much as we can, everyone may safely assume that our situation is pretty lousy at the best of times these days. This is really hard on so many fronts.

We appreciate the smiles, hugs, and kind words. A lot. We appreciate the offers of help; we appreciate when we can share how we're feeling. And also appreciate that sometimes it's understood that we'd rather not talk about what's going on and just want a pleasant diversion.

The next while will be even tougher as we face some difficult decisions, realities, and consequences. I won't always be around to stand up for her, and frankly that truth hit me pretty darned hard across the face this week.

TOUCHING DOWN
Tuesday, March 26, 2013

Overall, I think I do pretty well with not dwelling on what I've lost. I do have my moments, but considering how many things in my life that I loved have disappeared over the last two years, I believe I'm entitled to feel sadness over the losses once in awhile.

This evening is one of those times. For the first time in ages, I put on music to entertain myself, instead using other diversions to keep my mind busy.

Going through my playlist of most often-played songs, I'm saddened to realize that in the past it was hard to keep myself from singing along. My natural impulse is to join in, regardless of how awful my singing voice is.

I miss my voice. It's become hoarse, creaky, and sometimes entirely missing in action. A symptom of the mess in my chest. Some days I'm grateful just to get out full sentences.

Singing is entirely out of the question. So is dancing to the music. These things have to take place in my imagination now. They still do, sometimes as fleeting daytime thoughts, but more often in my night-time dreams.

I have to wonder if my body knew all along that I'd lose so many of my physical abilities. It seems that I've gone through my life taking note of how good it felt to walk, run, sing, dance, jump, spin, and so much more when I could.

A memory floods back of teaching my daughter how to jump rope at our old house in Toronto. We'd tied one end to the fence, while she and I took turns making the rope turn circles. I didn't care that the neighbours were watching a woman edging into her late thirties skipping rope like a schoolyard girl. I so clearly remember my feet hitting the ground beat after beat, appreciating the connection to the ground, and then feeling glee over the weightlessness at the height of the jump. And praying that my daughter might also learn to appreciate these small moments of bliss that can enter at unexpected moments.

Another memory of being at a dance theatre when I was married to my daughter's father: After a performance, the dance company to which he belonged as a performer and its guests had moved to the foyer. The stage was mine alone. I leapt up from the seating area onto the stage and ever so quietly led myself through a ballet routine that I vaguely remembered from the dance classes I taken when I was very small. I'd performed with my class at the since-long-gone Eaton Auditorium in downtown Toronto. I believe I was only five or six years old. I can still remember the feel of the sequins of my purple butterfly costume wings between my tiny fingers. (And I was tiny, until about the seventh grade I was always the shortest in my class. Always at the end when the teacher lined us up by height.) On that stage I felt strong, tall, beautiful, and capable of executing a complicated dance routine. In reality of course, it was a few strides, spins, and waves of the arms that might have caused any of the professional dancers to giggle. The delicious part is that that they would have been laughing with me, not at me.

I can think back to so many of these moments of awareness of feeling happy. I wonder if I was given this gift to help me through the challenging times. I cling to this belief; it seems to make sense to me. The ability to bring forth a happy memory whenever I need one.

Tonight I need these memories. Thunderstorms, the softness of my daughter's cheek when I kiss her, the frenzied enthusiasm of a puppy let loose, finding the daisy among the tulips, a squeeze of my hand when I'm scared.

I'm still trying to make more of these happy memories. I'm grateful that my mind is still sharp and my memory is still good. (Though at rare times I wish it weren't so much so.) That I can still feel, be it good or bad.

I pray that for as long as I'm here, I can still see the beauty in the faces of the people who surround me, hear their loving voices, and feel their touch when they hug me.

Tonight however, I'm allowing myself to grieve a little. Yet still trying to find space in the pain to be grateful that I can hear the music, even if I can't sing along.

SACRIFICE
Saturday, March 30, 2013

As parents, we make sacrifices to help our children reach toward the goal of being productive (and hopefully happy) members of society.

Many years of teaching them, trying to set good examples, doling out gentle discipline and above all, offering love, in hopes that our children will become adults who feel good about who they are and the choices they make.

As parents, we sometimes sacrifice opportunities for personal or financial gain, and give our time (and in the early years, many hours of precious sleep!) with the intent to do what is best for our children. If we expect nothing in return, we may truly delight in whatever joys come to us through our children.

Not every child grows up this way. I speak from personal experience. I don't care to have a go at my parents in this post; it's no secret that my upbringing was less than idyllic.

I wanted my daughter's upbringing to be different than my own. My parenting choices at times have fallen under criticism, but my goal was and always will be to be a parent that can be counted on through thick and thin. My daughter went through tough times after her dad and I divorced; and then again when her stepfather left. I didn't care how much ribbing I endured about running to her side when she said she needed me – nothing could stop me. Whether it was dropping whatever I was doing, or taking her 2 a.m. phone calls when she was in first year university, I was going to do whatever it took for her to know that I would be there for her. That I could always be trusted.

My daughter has many times told me how grateful she is that I never failed to be there when she needed me. Not to say I didn't make many mistakes along the way in raising her; absolutely there are things I might have done differently, given another chance. As my own mother told me, the first child is the "try baby." You try to do your best, but hopefully learn from what does and doesn't work and refine your technique with subsequent children.

My daughter was my one and only shot at parenting. One could argue until blue in the face how much of a child's behaviour and personality come from nature vs. nurture, but I'm going to allow myself a small amount of credit that trying to do right by her led in small part to her being the wonderful young woman she is today.

In an ideal world, I envision myself easing her mind when she has jitters about entering the work force, listening to her as she stresses about wedding planning, reassuring her that she's doing her best when the toilet training of her little one isn't going as smoothly as she hoped. Reminding her that along with the tough challenges in life come moments that can bring such joy they can seem surreal. It's unlikely that I will be around to support her as her life plays out. If we allowed ourselves to wallow in this reality, we wouldn't have room to continue to make new happy memories together while I'm still here.

Sometimes she tells me she's fearful that she'll make poor choices if I'm not around to offer guidance. If I allow myself that I did the best I could as her mother, I tell her that I have every confidence that she already knows the answers that are right for her.

I'm lucky to have had a child to make sacrifices for. Although in my younger days I was convinced that I didn't want children, by the time my daughter came along, there wasn't anything I had ever wanted more.

My daughter is now making tremendous sacrifices for me. It's the last thing I would have ever wanted; my goal was always to do the best I could in my role as her mother and send her off into the world to find her own life. I knew that I would always be included as an important part of her future, but she was free to make her own choices – my job was more or less over.

She's putting her future on hold to help me. Come September, she's not returning to university.

It's been a tremendously hard school year for her. As much as I tried to keep the details of my declining health from her (with that you may correctly assume that I've also not shared many details with the readers of this blog), it was impossible to shield her from the visible evidence when she would visit home.

Coming home became more and more of a challenge for her; the guilt of leaving me at the end of a weekend visit became more agonizing for her. It became more difficult to concentrate on her studies, and it wasn't made any easier by others suggesting that she ought to be at home with her ailing mother instead of at school.

If it were my choice, I'd ask her to go back to school. The thought that she might not go back later scares me. She has passion, potential, intellect, and an unwavering curiosity. Good things lie ahead for her, of this I am sure.

It's time to sit back and trust that if I have done the best job I could do as her mother over the last nineteen years, she's now making the best choices for herself. Even if it means shelving immediate educational goals to be by my side.

How blessed I am that my daughter would make such an immense sacrifice to ensure that I'm not alone on the next part of my journey. It's a gift I didn't expect, and didn't ask for, but will appreciate with every last breath. And I will pray that karma ensures that the remaining decades of her life bring less heartache to her than the first two.

SCORE!
Monday, April 01, 2013

One very rocky night for pain tonight. I gave in to the lure of the Zofran/Toradol cocktail. The first pill to keep the second one down, the latter following fifteen minutes later, in hopes that within an hour I'll have been given a slight bit of pain relief.

Each time I take this cocktail, it's a game of pro vs. con. Pro? A bit of pain relief – it even comes with a boost to my appetite for a couple of hours. The con – Toradol is simply wicked on the stomach. Although the Zofran helps with the nausea that hits soon after ingestion, the day afterwards I have to be prepared for moderate to severe stomach pain.

Every day I weigh the trade-off, and I'm usually on the losing end. In most cases, I regret having taken a chance on pain relief and therefore, most days go without. Tonight, I went for it – the alternative wasn't looking so pretty.

Pain management has been a challenge to say the least. With my allergy to opiates, it leaves nothing very effective on the table for me to try.

I've been blessed with a high tolerance for pain; even after bone surgery, I requested nothing stronger than a regular Tylenol. However this is no regular pain that I deal with day in and day out. Tonight the cat snuggled in as the pain got worse; I feared I might drown him with the tears streaming uncontrollably down my face if I didn't down my cocktail. My friends, we had a solid 8.5 on the pain scale of 1-10.

I'm smiling as I type this (and with this you may gather that tonight the cocktail helped). Undoubtedly, one or two you might wonder if an alternative pain reliever might be effective. If we're on the same page, the answer to the question you might ask is yes. I have indeed tried marijuana for pain relief. It's surprising to me how many people have helpfully (and sometimes in the most humorous of ways) let me know that they could help connect me to a trial dose.

The first try was about eighteen months ago. Imagine the scenario – in my late forties trying weed for the very first time. Not that it wasn't around me when I was younger; there was ample opportunity to smoke up. I just chose not to; it wasn't for me. One bout of alcohol intoxication at sixteen taught me that I didn't care for the feeling of losing control of what I was doing.

My first high was quite the experience. I was at one end of a Skype call with my daughter, she wanted to make sure that I wasn't on my own and could call for assistance if I had a bad reaction.

I kept my daughter amply amused. I was convinced that the back of my head had turned to mud, and that I'd developed a magical talent for saying words before I'd actually thought them. I think you had to be there, but for my daughter it was raucous entertainment.

The second time didn't go well. I became so very sad over something I couldn't even pinpoint. I imagined that perhaps it might be what depression feels like, and it felt simply awful. It was a feeling I didn't want to repeat. And neither experiment provided any pain relief anyway.

As the pain increased, I was talked into trying marijuana one more time this past summer – this time, legal, medical-grade supply. I was told that the high might feel different than the last time and it might, in turn, provide better results for pain relief.

We (I had two accomplices who were taking great delight in bearing witness, in hopes that I might break out in goofiness) snuck outside on a beautiful summer evening. By then I'd already developed difficulty in sitting up for more than a few minutes, and they arranged me on a lounge chair so I could recline. I'm rethinking the "snuck" part of that sentence, it's been impossible for me to sneak anywhere unnoticed for quite some time. Lumbered outside? How dainty!

I did not disappoint them. I announced I was having "thoughtful thoughts" interrupted by periods of having no thought in my head whatsoever. For anyone who knows me, that's quite an absurd concept! Ask me anytime what I'm thinking and I will never, ever say "nothing." Except, it would seem, when I'm high. Unfortunately however, it provided no respite from the pain.

The helpful offers to "score some pain relief," continue to pour in. Thank you, it's kind that so many would like to be of service in easing my pain. I'm sincerely grateful. And so many offers to share the experience with me! Thank you for such thoughtfulness <grin>

ANTICIPATION
Wednesday, April 03, 2013

Many years ago when I was employed in the corporate world, it seemed that the weeks leading up to a scheduled vacation would feel longer and more hectic than usual. The closer the vacation date came, the more I felt that I needed the break and would count down the days. The final days at the office could feel endless, knowing that a reward was so close. Rarely would the break be anything more than a "staycation" at home, but the idea of spending uninterrupted time with my daughter had tremendous appeal.

Although it's only two and half weeks until my daughter comes home from university (and it's only been four days since she was home for Easter) I feel as if I've never missed her as much as I do right now. It's not necessarily a negative feeling; I'm glad that she's focused on completing her final exams. Despite her delaying her third year of university, she's still committed to doing her best in finishing off this semester. I'm so proud of her determination to stick to a plan, regardless of how drastically it has been revised due to my illness.

Back in those corporate days, I was unfortunately never very good at completely leaving the office behind. Like many of my colleagues, I would keep my pager on, and let my supervisors know that I'd be checking my email and voicemail should a work emergency arise. The ties were never severed for more than a couple of days. Where did that get me?

A similar sense of unease comes to me now, in anticipation of my daughter's homecoming. Wouldn't it be wonderful to be able to leave my health issues (which seem like a fulltime job) completely behind and enjoy our time without reminders? Wouldn't it be absolutely fantastic to be able to forget that I was sick for at least a few days?

Years ago I had the choice to sever ties with work for a week or two. In hindsight I should have, but didn't.

This time around we can't escape.

This wish isn't for me; it's for her. Deep down, I know that we'll be able to continue making wonderful memories, but I wish that oxygen tubing wasn't in the way. She and I (perhaps unfortunately for her!) share a similar sense of warped humour, and I can't see a wheelchair getting in the way of that. In fact, it's often the source of a good laugh these days.

We'll make the most of our time together, we always do. No matter what disagreements have come up between us over the years (and they will continue to, sharing a one-bedroom apartment won't be easy!) never for a moment have I ever not wanted to see her beautiful face. No matter how angry we might be with each other at the time.

It would, however, be lovely to kick my illness to the curb for a break now and again. Don't think we won't try.

THE PIGGY BANK
Thursday, April 04, 2013

I was always good with money. Starting from an early age, I had paper routes, babysitting jobs, and even a lemonade stand or two. Bless my neighbours who would fork over a nickel on a hot summer day for a glass of refreshment; with it being a quiet crescent that led to nowhere else, my friends and I were unlikely to have had anyone besides those who lived on the street pass by our table.

There was a summer job every year. The one at age sixteen, cleaning guest rooms at a downtown Toronto hotel taught me tough lessons about respect and dignity (or lack thereof). I had been hired in another capacity, however – when the housekeeping staff went on strike I had to, along with everyone else, quickly learn what "all hands on deck" meant. I could go into the gruesome details, but I learned how little respect some people have for others with evidence of the messes they leave behind. Sometimes from people you'd least expect. This is a lesson the universe has tried to teach me over and over again in my adulthood, am I finally learning to steer clear?

Leaving home at a very young age, I had to find gainful employment while still attending high school. To get by, I had one job at Sears, in the bedding department, (a source of endless amusement for my schoolmates) and I also waited tables at Pizza Hut.

The budget was extremely tight. Like many students, I subsisted on a diet of instant soup and ramen noodles. A car was necessary to get back and forth to school and jobs; thank goodness I'd saved and invested my earnings from earlier years to buy that old rust bucket of gold Hondamatic. Even with the tight budget, I understood the value of looking out for my future and opened up my first RRSP (retirement savings plan) at sixteen.

I even managed to go to university on my savings, but my money ran out mid-way through second year and I had no choice but to quit and work full-time. This may help you to understand why, although it's for different reasons, it's so difficult for me to watch my daughter leave school at this time.

My habit of watching out for the pennies never wavered. Before getting married seven years ago, I was so very close to retiring my mortgage on a house in Toronto and had a healthy retirement fund. Some of you know that didn't turn out so well in the end for me financially. I'm left with deep regret about making decisions during my marriage that I believed were for the overall financial health of our family, if looked at it as a long-term objective, but ended up being very poor choices indeed when my marriage ended suddenly. Hindsight...

Today, I'm back to that student budget. It is what it is. I had a reminder yesterday of just how embarrassed I am to be in this situation when a health care worker asked me if I'd moved in to my apartment in the last few weeks. The furnishings are sparse, and as in my student days, boxes double as furniture. When friends or my nurses visit in my bedroom, they either jump on the bed or sit on outdoor chairs loaned to me.

Besides living with a very strict financial budget, a budget of another sort needs adhering to; that of my energy. Of the two, this is the one that I find more of a struggle these days.

After another recent downturn in my health, I've realized that it wasn't just a bad patch. It's just bad. To be simplistic, let's say that in one twenty-four hour period, my reserves will allow for:

One hundred steps. Five minutes of standing. Five hundred spoken syllables. Fifteen minutes of sitting upright. Ten minutes of reading.

Out of that reserve come trips to the bathroom, maybe about seven steps each way. A visit to the kitchen for a glass of water might be thirty-five steps, round trip. Answering the apartment door? Probably fifteen steps each way.

Standing is the really tough one. Part of that allotment is already shot with walking in the apartment.

Where does the wheelchair fit in? It's reserved for the rare trips outside of the apartment door. It's impossible to wheel the chair within the apartment while trying to keep the oxygen hose out of the way, and the carpeting (I detest that carpet!) makes it difficult to manoeuvre the chair with my limited arm strength.

As for the syllables, I dearly miss my long conversations with friends. I waste my words in discussions that I'd rather not be having as I try to wade my way through endless red tape.

Where do I fall into debt? Laundry, meal preparation (heating up food is the extent of my cooking repertoire now), opening and closing the window in the apartment for temperature control. Part of that debt is recouped by taking strong pain meds, and I've written about the consequences of taking those. It's a loan that carries an exorbitantly high interest rate.

It's taken me a long post to get to the point that I started out with in my head. I only have so much energy and I'm pushing the boundaries every day. If I don't reply to an email or phone call promptly, I truly apologize. If I ask to cut a visit short or cancel altogether, I know you understand – but also know that I'd rather I'd had the energy for a proper catch up.

Being with the ones I love and enjoy spending time with is my top priority. I hate that other chores as basic as taking my daily shower chip away at that small reserve of energy.

As for writing the blog, it's therapeutic for me and keeps me busy in the hours in which I'm awake but it's too late to have visitors or chat on the phone. I have a system worked out now, with a bed table to hold my laptop, my phone, remotes, iPad, and notebook and pen within easy reach. Meal replacement drinks are within steps, and I'll admit that a supply of chocolate is usually not too far away either.

Adhering to a strict budget of any sort can be challenging. The cutbacks I have to make on my expenditure of energy are by far the ones that hurt the most. They cost what is dearest to me, and put me in a position of feeling more isolated than ever.

OPENING DOORS
Friday, April 05, 2013

At the end of a very long day (although at 10 p.m. I likely still have at least four hours of wakefulness ahead of me to fill), I'm physically exhausted but feel spiritually fuelled up.

A busy day in my world includes a visit from a Personal Support Worker, one of my nurses, three deliveries (if you're keeping track of my "step allotment" from yesterday's post, I'm already well past my one hundred in just answering the door). And then, added bonuses – two visits from friends to round out my day. I love when visits from friends overlap and they have a chance to meet each other, it makes my world feel a bit bigger and warmer when these connections are made.

Even the people delivering somehow find a way into my circle. The Canada Post delivery person knows that I'm not able to leave my apartment and will personally bring up items to me that don't fit in my mailbox rather than leave them in the lobby as he does for other tenants. I hope that I don't come across as grumpy when I come to the door; he often rings the buzzer at 8 a.m. – a jolt when I've only gotten to sleep a few short hours earlier. At the very least I'm always dishevelled and I wonder if he thinks I spend the whole day in my pyjamas. The oxygen tube might suggest that, and it somehow bothers me that anyone might believe that I don't clean myself up every day. He remembers that I have to pick up the cat before opening the door, a bit of an effort for me but it prevents Scrabble from making a mad dash down the hallway. I can't imagine what excitement he believes lies beyond our front door; the young lad has a pretty good life on this side. What is it with this quest for greener pastures?

The gentleman who several times a month delivers my medications from the pharmacy always has a smile on offer and a few words to say about what's happening in the outside world. My apartment is far off his route (a favour extended by my wonderful pharmacist) but you'd never hear him complain about it. Another funny (or not so much) twist to being palliative, the insurance company only doles out a thirty-day supply of each med at a time. Heaven forbid that they give me more and they go to waste should I pass in between! And I've given up on getting them all coordinated to be delivered once a month.

The volunteer who delivered a hot meal to me (tonight, spicy curry with fish and shrimp, so delicious!) is among a group who initially signed up for preparing a meal one or more times a month (a rotating roster that provides shut-ins like me – is there a more appropriate term? – with fresh meals twice a week). The volunteers have each extended themselves in offering to do more than cook and deliver a meal; all have reached out to allow me to get to know a bit about who they are, to introduce me to their children, and to offer to do things to help, on top of cooking a meal for me. People who are essentially strangers are offering to come clean my apartment, run errands, do whatever they can to make my life easier.

And so it goes. Day in, day out. Tough battles buffered by so much kindness around me.

My original intent tonight was to write on another subject, one that addresses bridging the extremes. I have two full days ahead of me this weekend without any visitors. (I wish I could bank steps and syllables but it doesn't work like that, unfortunately.) You might hear more from me over the next few days, or I might have fallen into a sugar coma thanks to the treats that Kristee brought for me today. It could go either way...

HOW TO MAKE THE BAD STUFF GO AWAY
Sunday, April 07, 2013

A very young lady by the name of Emma just made my day. Years from now, it's unlikely that she'll remember our conversation, but it's one that I'll not soon forget.

A week or so back, her mom brought me a hot meal as part of the Food Train program for which she (being Mom), and about a dozen or so other volunteers donate their time, ingredients, and cooking talents to make sure people like me in our area get a chance at regular, hot, nutritious food. Without meals (and yummy snacks!) being brought to me by these volunteers and my friends, my diet would mainly consist of meal replacement drinks (not a terribly attractive option at the hungriest of times) and Babybel cheese (but even unwrapping those on some days is more than my fingers can handle).

It was her mom's first visit to me, and I was looking forward to meeting her. That day was not a good one physically, and I was confined to bed. As luck would allow that Monday afternoon, a friend was visiting who could take care of door duties. I had let my friend know that if Mom felt comfortable, she could come down the hall to the bedroom so that we could meet.

When my friend opened the door, I could hear additional voices – voices of little people. Before I knew it, I had Mom at the bedroom door holding her toddler, and young Emma (kindergarten-age) was standing at my bedside, close enough to put her hands on the covers.

She was very engaging young lady, and we spoke of school, red ponies, and various other topics, which she covered with enthused expression and gesture.

It was one of those moments that filled me with great delight (as a former family photographer, this sort of interaction would have been the absolute highlight of a photo session), but it also made me miss my photography days so deeply.

On Friday, I received an envelope in the mail. It's the day that my mail is usually fetched for me from downstairs; typically it's bills, flyers, and nothing that's likely to put a smile on my face. This envelope however had Emma's name in the top left corner. I waited until after my PSW left before opening it. Inside was a letter, a picture Emma had drawn, a sticker, and a tattoo.

What she wrote is between her and me, but I will tell you it let forth a torrent of happy tears sliding down my face.

I wanted to thank Emma for her thoughtfulness, but wanted to wait until I had a bit of a voice to speak with – it went AWOL again Friday night and had returned this afternoon. Well, now it's gone again – but I take my opportunities when they come.

Just a short while ago, we finished a lovely chat, she on speakerphone so I could hear her parents' contributions to the conversation as well. We've made a plan for her to come back to help me apply the tattoo – of Cinderella. Emma has selected my elbow as the perfect spot. I'll wear it proudly. And I'll be careful not to scrub it off in the bath so it lasts as long as possible.

Emma told me about soccer practice this afternoon, and then said that she has something very important to tell me. "I love you." At that moment I was so grateful that she was on the phone and couldn't see my face. I tried to keep a steady tone to my voice, but inside I was melting.

It made me realize how much I miss having children in my life. The photo sessions always lifted me to a place of remembering how much I enjoyed the different stages my own daughter went through. When asked if I missed a particular age/stage, my answer was always the same – it only gets better as each day goes along.

And it has. I enjoy my daughter's company more than ever. The nice thing about memories is that they can be recalled and lived over again, so I've never truly lost those moments when she used to crawl up into my lap and snuggle into the crook of my neck, animatedly tell me about her school day, and proudly show me her latest creations. In the late hours of last night, when neither of us could sleep, she sent me a link to crazy science discoveries that she knew that I'd enjoy as much as she had.

This morning started out with heaviness in my heart as I was reminded of just how warm the day is becoming, and that I can't go out to enjoy it. I was thinking about my short and quite reasonable bucket list, and how not one of the goals came to fruition. (I should qualify it with an acknowledgement of how many generous souls tried to give me the New York City experience – top on my list - in other ways). That in trying to help someone else who was in my life at the time realize the most important item on their bucket list, I had forfeited my own.

Sometimes you need to ask for what you need, and sometimes what you need just gets handed to you. Thank you Emma, I love you too. Blessings appear everywhere when I keep an open heart.

ACCOMPLISHING LITTLE
Monday, April 08, 2013

A few days ago, I wrote that I had forty-eight hours on my own lying ahead of me, and I had hopes to accomplish something of merit.

I shouldn't do this to myself. I continue to set lofty goals, and am then disappointed in myself when I accomplish little to none of what I set out to do. It's not laziness, lack of willpower, or distraction.

It's trying to do something, and not being able to follow through due to exhaustion, pain, and plain and simple physical inability. Limbs don't bend and move the way I would like them to anymore, and staring at something heavy won't lift it off the floor. It stays there until someone comes along to move it for me.

I concern myself too often with trying to accomplish what I believe others expect of me. I'm embarrassed that I can't be productive, useful, and helpful in so many of the ways I used to be.

What do others expect of me? Now there's a question.

Lately, I've been reading several blogs, books, and listening to audio books written by others who face/had been facing death. Most recently the audio book, *Mortality* by Christopher Hitchens.

It's reassuring to find that I'm not the only one who feels like she is letting others down when serious illness strikes. That willing oneself to accomplish more just isn't enough. Limitations are what they are; wanting things to be otherwise is of no use and only leads to feelings of failure. The one thing I did accomplish this weekend was a load of laundry; a load of fine washables that had been piling up in the hamper. Maybe that doesn't sound like a difficult task to most of you, but to me it's quite an undertaking.

It was after midnight last night when my daughter emailed me to ask if she could come home from university for the afternoon; that she needed to see me. She's in the middle of studying for final exams and we have just two weeks to go before she comes home for an extended stay. My answer of course was yes; nothing could make me happier.

When she arrived late this morning, she immediately noticed that I was wearing a blouse that she had given me at Christmas time. One that I had washed yesterday before I knew she was coming home today. A broader grin on her face wouldn't have been possible, and she snuggled up beside me for a hug. It's a very soft blouse and I like to believe that it gets me extra long cuddles.

I had needed that moment; an ever-so-small sense of accomplishment that the effort to do a load of laundry yesterday meant something to my daughter. She wouldn't have expected it, and likely would have insisted that the laundry wait until she was here this afternoon, if she had known of my plans. It was my luck that the one load of laundry I felt up to tackling included the sweater she'd given me. It felt good that in a rare instance, I could exceed expectation. The feeling of letting others down is simply exhausting and I needed a short break from that.

IT'S NICE TO BE MISSED
Saturday, April 13, 2013

Still here.

To my faithful blog readers, I didn't mean to alarm you. I've received dozens of notes over the last few days, asking if I was okay after having taken a few days' break from writing the blog.

What I was doing was racking up more subjects to write about – whether I'll get to them all is another matter entirely. Quite a bevy of topics to select from!

Sue flew in from Halifax again to visit for a few days.

We (and I use the "royal we," it is she who did all the work) spent time clearing out some closet space for my daughter who arrives home next weekend. In our one-bedroom apartment there's one tiny clothes closet, which was inconveniently divided by the previous occupant into two levels that allow nothing longer than a shirt to be hung. My wardrobe has become very small, yet it easily fills up the available closet space, leaving no room for my daughter's clothes.

Items that used valuable space in the front hall had to go find new homes. In particular, my corporate work wardrobe. Try not to laugh when I tell you that I left the corporate world about eleven years ago and saved my good suits and shoes. For all these years, I believed that I might have occasion to don them again.

Clothing-wise, nothing really has compared to how a well fitting, classically styled suit would make me feel. My work clothes were an investment, and each suit was nipped and tucked by a seamstress immediately after purchase, to fit me like a glove. The suit, a pair of pumps and a fresh haircut – I'd feel like I could take on whatever the day could throw me.

It was time to let them go. Seven months ago when I moved here I couldn't do it, there was still hope left. As silly as that may sound.

This week, it didn't hurt at all. Okay, maybe a wee bit. Likely far less because I knew where they were going. At the suggestion of, and with the assistance of a friend, those suits (and those beautiful leather pumps!) were delivered to a women's shelter. They'll be made available to women who could likely use clothing that helps them feel like they can take on whatever the day could throw at them when they face their abusive partner in court.

To the women who might wear these clothes under challenging circumstances, I send wishes for strength and courage to get through those difficult days. I'm sure from time to time I'll think back on how wearing those suits made me feel and I'll be thinking of the battles these women face. May they believe in themselves and trust what they know to be the best path for themselves and their children. If I may speak from experience, this might well be the most important part of the battle.

THE REVISED BUCKET LIST, PART 1
Sunday, April 14, 2013

A few years back, I wrote about my bucket list; as of earlier this week, unfulfilled.

As you might know from my last post, Sue spent the better part of this week with me. Before she arrived, we spent time discussing how she might be able to help see items on my bucket list come to fruition while she was here.

When I was first diagnosed, I would repeatedly tell my family how grateful I was that my appetite wasn't affected by ECD – this girl loved her food! I had hoped to keep cooking meals, or at the very least to eat pretty much whatever I had a penchant for.

Little by little, this wish crept away. First, it was the inability to drive; I could no longer fetch groceries. In the beginning, my ex would happily fetch whatever ingredients I needed and I kept cooking for my family. Like many family cooks, I prepared what my family wanted and rarely made anything that suited my tastes if it didn't match theirs.

Then bone pain, fatigue, and weakness became more of a hindrance. My ex had never cooked a meal during our marriage, so prepared food was the only choice. For a short time, I had more of a selection in what I ate. With individual portions available in the prepared-food section of the market, I could ask him to get me items that I particularly enjoyed without worry about what didn't appeal to him.

I had to make major adjustments last year when my ex moved out and I was left on my own. I couldn't fetch my own groceries, nor could I have cooked for myself anyway. I found myself eating a lot of Babybel cheese that Janet would buy in bulk at Costco for me. (Calcium for my brittle bones!) The medications were really starting to take a toll on my insides. A combination of intense stress and stomach troubles had led to a weight loss of over twenty-five pounds, in a few short months. My clothes took over me; even size 00 jeans required a belt to stay up.

As grateful as my daughter and I were to have the Miele family give us a roof over our heads for over three months last summer, I was in no shape to cook, despite Janet's offer to use the kitchen whenever I wished. We were made to feel part of the family and were invited to join in with all meals, but I just couldn't eat much, despite how wonderful the food always was.

Expectations had to be radically adjusted when I moved into this apartment in September. Lack of appetite, loss of strength to make meals, and a shortfall in financial resources to allow the purchase of prepared food led to a general disinterest in eating at all. With revised expectations, I went from "living to eat," to "eating to live," as a philosophy.

From previous posts, you might already know that a wonderful group of volunteers stepped in a few months ago to deliver delicious hot meals several times a week. And friends often bring treats that they know I enjoy. One can only stand so many of the meal replacement drinks each day before finding them abhorrent, the gifts of food were/are welcomed and appreciated.

This group of friends and volunteers has urged me to let them know if I have any cravings, and said that they would do their best to fulfill any special requests. But you know how it is, when you crave something – the sooner the better! So I try to not let myself think of cravings, and instead enjoy whatever has found its way into my fridge and cupboards.

One craving however has stuck with me for months. It shouted out to me as something I wanted to have just once more; a nod to my bucket list wish to eat foods I really enjoy. It wasn't something that the volunteers could prepare – and until I sold some jewellery a few weeks back, it wasn't in the budget.

A part of that small windfall was going towards my bucket list, no question. Just a few hundred dollars, but it was going to be spent on something that put a smile on my face. And Sue was going to be my accomplice and partner in crime.

Wednesday night, with help of Kathy and her husband Tony from the Food Train taking care of the transport (each and every one of the volunteers has offered to help in some way beyond making meals); I had in front of me the object of my desire.

One damned fine Keg steak (for non-Canadian readers, The Keg is a restaurant chain that has built their reputation as a carnivore's heaven), with a side of crab legs. Garlic mashed potatoes and melted butter on the side. Although I tried to apply some grace in how I ate that meal on the tray while propped up in bed, anyone watching might have believed that it was the first meal I'd had in days.

I wasn't being a complete piggy, the small windfall also allowed my Sue to enjoy her own steak dinner beside me (and after all her considerable generosity over the last year, it was such a small gesture in return). She however, went about things far more elegantly than I. And there was more than enough to enjoy leftovers the next night.

If that's the last Keg steak I ever have, I'm okay with that. It was even better than I'd remembered, and I'd shared the experience with Sue – and very importantly, my stomach didn't rebel against it (a small miracle).

And for my Canadian readers, The Keg doesn't do take-out. I have Sue's perseverance to thank for getting that fantastic meal in front of me.

We weren't yet done for the week...

THE REVISED BUCKET LIST, PART 2
Tuesday, April 16, 2013

If you've been following this blog over the years, you might remember that the item on the top of my bucket list was a trip to New York City, family by my side, camera around my neck.

That didn't happen, and won't happen.

Over the last year, friends, acquaintances, and strangers have participated in, "The New York Project," and have in many ways given me NYC through their own eyes. There are photographic diaries, scrapbooks, printed books, souvenirs, and postcards, and especially precious to me are the written accounts of their own travels (and some hilarious adventures!) to the city.

Not that I'm hinting or anything <grin> ... but the New York Project remains a going concern. Stories of favourite places, adventures, amazing meals (food always sneaks in there!) are much appreciated.

I mentioned in the last post that Sue wanted to help me realize some bucket list wishes while she was here last week.

New York was out, but perhaps my second favourite city was not. It's been four months since I was well enough to travel to my Toronto medical team. Not that I don't want to see them again, but our goal on this adventure was to hit a favourite spot of mine in the city...and it wasn't the hospital.

We were going to do this right.

A few days prior, a friend who is a make-up artist came by to give me some tips on looking less gruesome. (Those are my words; she quickly and kindly disagreed. We'd simply try to make me look like I'd had a good night's sleep – something that hasn't happened in a very long time.)

A limo was booked, courtesy of the leftover funds in my small bucket list fund. Perhaps an extravagance, but truly the only way that it seemed that I could be somewhat comfortable for the minimum hour-long drive each way. We'd pad the seats with blankets and pillows and I could recline on the way there and back, saving my sitting "allowance" for time in the wheelchair at the destination.

After visiting my favourite spot, the plan was (energy permitting) to stop by three places that offer some favourite food items. If I was looking to satisfy cravings last week, we weren't going to stop at the steak dinner. I could rest in the limo while Sue jumped into each location – none of the three were wheelchair accessible anyway.

For days, we watched the weather. It wasn't looking good; rain and cold winds – but I really didn't care. After being trapped indoors all winter I'm not sure that I would have even noticed the cold.

The morning of the trip, it became apparent that Mother Nature really wasn't going to cooperate. Freezing rain was forecast, not a day that anyone should be on the road if avoidable – bucket list or not.

Having gotten myself ready with help from my friend, (blow-drying my own hair isn't something I can do anymore), putting my face on, and getting dressed, I realized that the trip would have to be cancelled regardless of the weather. I'd exhausted myself with the preparations to such a degree that the trip was no longer viable anyway.

For the last months, if I had a short trip outside of the apartment planned (I can count all my outings since October on one hand), or had visitors coming, I kept myself to strict bed rest the day prior, to save up my energy and reduce the strain on my bones and heart.

This formula no longer works. I get what I get when I get it. Without question, moving about at all will exacerbate the pain, but resting beforehand is no longer a guarantee that the pain and exhaustion will be lessened.

As disappointing as it was to give up my revised bucket list trip, it wasn't devastating.

If I look at it pessimistically, I can say it didn't hurt that much because I've become numb to being let down. By my body, by people who I had thought would stick by me through this ordeal, by the constant barrage of challenges on which I often find myself on the losing end. What was one more letdown?

The optimist in me can revel in the joys of the planning of our adventure, appreciate the fact that despite not getting out the door I still had my best friend with me, and that instead of getting out, I had the pleasure of spending time with a few new friends who came by for a visit.

Not to say that I won't attempt the trip again in the future, but often, the thought of something enjoyable has to take the place of actually doing or having what I'd like. And often, that's enough.

Still more to come on bucket list week...

THE REVISED BUCKET LIST, PART 3
Wednesday, April 17, 2013

The next bucket list item that was to be tackled last week is not so much a wish to be fulfilled, as it is a philosophy to be maintained.

On my bucket list of several years ago was a desire to keep laughing with people I enjoy being with, to maintain the ability to see the humour in situations, and to be able to laugh at myself. I was a "glass half-full" woman, and I intended to go out the same way.

Goodness knows that this philosophy has been challenged in the last two years, in ways I never thought possible. There were moments that I thought that our situation couldn't get any worse, and then my daughter and I would get blindsided again.

Although there were many months that I believed I'd never be able to pull off a sincere smile again, smiles did come back to my face. And along with that, laughter.

One might have thought that it came because others tried to cheer me up, but it surprised me to realize that it came from within. My friends were in shock as they watched what was happening. They grieved along with me and tried to do what they could to help. Laughing wasn't a priority – getting a roof over our heads was.

I don't remember when exactly I found myself smiling again; I'd suggest that it accompanied the gratitude I felt as the groundswell of support grew around me. A safety net that allowed me respite from the unthinkable circumstances.

Sue's last evening of her visit here last week had its sombre moments. We've parted now a few times over the last year not knowing if it was the last time we'd be hugging each other goodbye.

Yet without fail, our visits include lots of laughter.

It started out on Friday night innocently enough. My cat was stretched out with all limbs extended. This reminded me of Sue's last visit in January when she brought back to mind the name of a toy I'd had as a child but couldn't remember the name of. A cheap rectangle of suede with fur on it, when stroked it would rise up and down like a caterpillar. For years it had bugged me that I couldn't remember, and in one quick second she delivered to me the answer, "Squirmin' Herman."

We then began to look up retro '70s toy commercials on the iPad, one favourite of mine being for, "Super Slider Snow Skates." I used to love saying those syllables over and over again when the commercial came on, to the point of seriously annoying my mother as I begged for a pair for Christmas.

Sue hadn't remembered ever seeing that commercial when she was young, and asked me if I got the skates for Christmas as I had hoped. I answered that I hadn't. Watching the commercial, I saw now that my mother had wisdom and insight that at that time I didn't possess – they would have been a recipe for a cracked limb, given my lack of athletic prowess. A klutz like me might have done herself in hurtling down a snowy hillside wearing those contraptions.

More laughter ensued about the '70s styles, products, and fads. Suddenly my Sue piped up, "Do you remember the Man They Call Ravine?"

What was I not catching on to here? Why call a man a ravine? I looked at her quizzically.

In a deep voice, she started singing, "The Ma-HAN They Call RAVINE!!!!" holding long and strong on the last word.

It was explained to me that Raveen, not ravine, had been a popular performer/illusionist years back, who had passed away a few days earlier. I didn't remember him, or the commercials. But the song in the background of the commercials for his shows that we viewed on YouTube? Sue was not going to head to bed until I could sing the words with the right intonation and tone. A few tries and I received her okay to stop trying. She says I got it right, I say she couldn't stand one more round of my singing and was tired – it was well past midnight.

She headed off to the bedroom "nook" (if you've seen my apartment you know what I'm talking about) and had turned off the light by the time I headed to the bathroom to brush my teeth.

Wouldn't you know it; I just couldn't get that tune out of my head. Something about the way the words boomed out, the expression on my Sue's face as she tried to imitate the baritone singer, and my misinterpretation of what was being said in the ad had grabbed my funny bone and wouldn't let it go...to the point that I was laughing so hard that I thought I would choke on my toothbrush. I assumed that Sue might already be asleep, so I was trying to do so soundlessly.

I thought I was doing a bang-up job of keeping pretty quiet until I opened the bathroom door. By that time I was laughing so hard I could barely stand, and certainly couldn't take another step. Trying to stifle it was making it so much worse. I leaned against the wall certain that I was going to fall over or collapse to the ground if I didn't steady myself.

Sue, it turned out, was still awake. And alarmed. She interpreted the muffled giggles as sobbing and called out to ask if I was okay.

All I could get out was..."The Ma-HAN they..." "The Ma-HAN..." After what seemed liked minutes I was finally able to slow down the chortling and snorting and shuffle off to bed, my shoulders still heaving and a huge smile on my face, I turned off the light and thought about how lucky I am to still laugh like that, and how grateful I was to have my best friend with me to share the giggle with that night.

Sue called a short while ago from her home in Halifax. A quick glance at the call display assured me that I was safe in answering the phone with, "The Ma-HAN they called..." I didn't make it to the last word this time either.

FORGETTING PAIN
Friday, April 19, 2013

Muscle memory. Sometimes I'm glad for it, other times not so much.

Although at no point any more am I free of physical pain entirely, the intensity of it varies according to a few factors.

Time of day can make a big difference. Pain grows as the day wears on after having been on my feet or sitting up. At this time, I'm still able to get to the bathroom on my own so at least a couple of times a day I travel a short distance within the apartment. At night, I'm hoping that my bladder is less demanding. A reminder of needing to get up one last time to go to the bathroom before bed is one I dread.

By the same token, mornings are sometimes a beast. Especially when I've done something completely idiotic the night before (as in last night) in trying to retrieve an item that the cat swiped under the fridge. Never, never again will I get down onto the kitchen floor. Doing it while alone was even more asinine. Allow yourself to imagine the visuals, it causes me pain just to think about it much less describe it. I made it even worse by trying to sit on the balcony for a few short minutes last night, to enjoy the mild temperatures. Both were well intentioned but stupid actions, given my current state of disability.

Pain medication alleviates the discomfort to a small degree, for a few short hours at a time. It's however often not worth the side effects that kick in afterwards.

Distraction can play an important role, but there's not nearly enough of the right kind of it around here. This situation changes in two days when my daughter arrives home from school – there's nobody I'd rather have helping to keep my mind off of the pain. And such a lovely distraction she is on top of it. I've got lots of her adventures to catch up on from the last few months.

At times, like this morning, due to last night's antics, the pain went to epic levels. I had to leave my bed to allow the PSW to change the sheets and for several hours I had not a clue as to how I was going to get myself back to the bedroom from the couch.

At times when the pain is not at epic levels, I quite simply forget how bad it can get. I chide myself for having put my body under of the strain of the pain meds, certain that I could have done without. I truly forget how unbearable it can often be.

As Sue says, if women were unable to forget the pain of childbirth, the world would be full of only children.

I might have mentioned that I've been taking on-line courses, of late in the area of neuroscience. I'm fascinated by how the brain works; especially intrigued by the admission of neuroscientists that there is so much not yet known or confirmed about the workings of the human brain.

It's quite a blessing to able to forget severe physical pain. One I'm grateful for every time another round hits me, otherwise I suspect that I'd live in deep fear of the next onset. I don't.

Emotional pain I find to be quite a different story. I don't live in a world of sadness, but if I choose to think about a painful emotional event, the memory can still feel raw and searing. Over time, the pain has diminished somewhat, but can be brought back if I allow it.

I happen to think that as much as the emotional pain hurts when I think back to it; it helps me in my drive to better myself as a person. Perhaps we can be more sensitive to others' emotional pain if we've experienced, and remember, similar emotions ourselves. I can sharply remember feelings of sadness, humiliation, embarrassment, shame, and disappointment, among others. They can all come back if I call upon them.

But on the flipside, I can also remember joy with similar clarity when recollecting. It's happened numerous times over my lifetime that I've been doing some lone, mindless task thinking a pleasant thought, and someone has asked me what was on my mind. I'd had a silly grin on my face and the other person wished to be let in on the secret.

It's still somewhat easy to do. I'd like to think it's a wonderful gift I've been given, to be able to bring forth a joyful memory when I need it the most. The contrast to unpleasant memories make the joyful ones all that more precious.

THE ORDER OF THINGS
Saturday, April 20, 2013

This has been a challenging week, primarily due to my diminishing physical abilities. Something as simple as trying to budge a bar of soap that had adhered itself firmly to the shower shelf when it dried had me upset with myself.

The hand that was free to attempt the soap's removal caused additional frustrations. A couple of weeks ago I banged it pretty hard on the grab bar, in trying to break an impending fall in the bathroom. (Isn't that irony?) It would appear that I might have broken a bone or two in the process. Thank goodness for voice dictation software, otherwise nobody would have had emails returned by me this week. My one-handed typing technique is coming along nicely too.

A day of mishaps led me to feeling frustrated and a little beaten down tonight. When Sue called this evening I was ready to answer the phone with a shriek, holding a fistful of hair. But with a hurt hand, I couldn't even get that right.

We speak every day, but tonight was a longer call of over two hours. The first part of the call, she listened as I whined. I don't do that often, but there was a long and torturous (for her) whine stuck inside of me that needed to escape. There are a handful of people in this world upon whom I can inflict a rare pity party for myself. She's always the first volunteer in line and she gently urged to me to get it out of my system this evening.

That complaining being mostly emptied out of me (I still have a good cry deep down inside that needs to get out sometime) we could get on to the cheering up part of the call.

We traded stories of misadventure that had happened when we were small. Bangs, scrapes, cuts, split lips. We were laughing uproariously – the injuries hadn't seemed nearly as hilarious at the time.

A couple of incidents that I shared after our exchange of war stories correlate quite well to my frustrations of this week.

My mother has many times told me the story of how when I used to fall into puddles, instead of using my hands to lift myself up I'd cry for someone to come get me. The idea that getting a bit dirtier meant I'd be saving myself sooner was beyond my comprehension.

When I was in kindergarten, one afternoon I came home and broke into tears as soon as I saw my mother. It took a great deal of convincing on her part to get me to share why I didn't want to go school the next day. For the record, I LOVED school. As far as I'm concerned, I'm still in school and always will be. I never tire of learning.

The look of alarm on my mother's face suggested that she wondered if something quite sinister might have happened that day. In reality, my teacher had gleefully announced at the end of class that the next day we'd be doing finger painting. The mere thought of dipping my hands into the coloured slime was fodder for nightmares. I'm sure that I was excused from doing it, but remember being pretty ticked off with myself as an adult when my daughter and I fingerpainted together. How could I have wanted to avoid such a wondrous mess?

This week's frustrations have mostly been about my inability to keep up with the high standards of tidiness that I set for myself. If there's a mess, getting it cleaned up these days is usually a task not completed according to my exacting standards, due to my mobility and weakness issues or it doesn't get done at all until somebody arrives to do it for me. More than a handful of friends and family would recognize an unattended mess as being something that could drive me around the bend. And it has this week.

When all else was crashing around me growing up, at least I could control the state of physical space around me. It's been one of my coping mechanisms since I can remember. When I moved out, at a very young age, I was teased mercilessly by my friends about how my wardrobe was sorted by colour. White at one end, black at the other with a carefully coordinated rainbow in between. The spices in the kitchen were sorted alphabetically; every receipt and slip of paper had its place.

I can assure you that as I got older I loosened up a lot; having a child left me no alternative than to be less precise about the order of things so that I could enjoy quality time with her.

But I'm still a neat freak to some degree, and disorder will often grind my gears. Not so much because of the mess itself these days, but more so due to the fact that I can't return things to order on my own any more.

It's a process of letting go of what I could once do but can no longer, and grasping as firmly as I can onto what is still possible. What a mess.

There was one pleasant connection for me. For all the times I was quite a sissy about getting dirty, I must have been equally adventurous, in order to have accumulated so many childhood injuries. (We'll ignore the part about being a complete klutz.) There were bikes to be ridden with abandon, hills to be tumbled down, horses' backs to fall from, jump ropes to trip over, and eyes to be blackened after trying to turn a guest bed into a trampoline.

In life, you don't get dirtied and you don't get hurt if you just sit on the sidelines. Although physically I'm not on the field, in spirit I'm still in the game. An albeit messier one.

THERE WILL BE DAYS LIKE THIS
Monday, April 22, 2013

It's often happened that soon after I've written a blog post, something will happen to hit the point home in some sort of ironic twist.

Yesterday was a case in point. In a, "One day I might find this funny, but it could take awhile," kind of way.

You might remember from previous posts that my daughter was due to arrive home this weekend from university. She's not returning in September so that she can instead take care of me.

My gratitude towards her is overwhelming. I could go on, but I'll save that for another post. I'm not missing any opportunities to tell her directly.

My wish was to make her feel as welcome as possible, for her to feel that this is truly her home. Until now, she's been at this apartment for the occasional holiday but hasn't yet lived here without the expectation of being on her way again.

To make the apartment feel welcoming, my wish was to make space for her clothes and personal items, find a way to give her a small amount of privacy in sharing a one-bedroom place, and to have her not feel the true weight of what caring for me entails right off the bat. Part of that was to have a clean apartment waiting, and as of Friday afternoon that was the case, thanks to the lovely woman who cleans it for me every ten days.

Within hours, the plan started crumbling. Anything that could drop, break, spill, get tipped over, overflow, or clog did exactly that. I didn't have any visitors coming, and for the most part I wasn't able to rectify much of it myself.

By yesterday midday, after the cat had a fight with his litter box (and won, it would seem), I had spilled a bag of kitty litter on the carpet (used, of course, quite fitting with the way my weekend was proceeding). The bathtub had clogged, there was a sticky flood on the bathroom floor with shards of glass mixed in, (let's not even go there with as to how that came about), dishes were piled up on the kitchen counter, and the cat had tipped over his food and it was strewn across the kitchen floor.

There was very little cleaning up that I could do. Imagine trying to keep the oxygen tubing out of the way, as well as attempting to not use my injured right hand. Not to mention that I can't get down to floor level on my own, and the pain that is brought on by any moving about.

A phone call went out to my daughter who was packing up her apartment at school, with my sincerest apologies for welcoming her in a few hours with a disaster zone. I was beside myself; this was quite far from how I'd envisioned welcoming her. The truth is that if she hadn't been coming home to stay this weekend, it would now be time to have a serious chat with my support team about how to move forward.

The crushing reality is that I can't be on my own for extended times any more, as I have been for sometimes days on end since moving into this apartment. By way of physical weakness and disability, I can't always get myself fed, dressed, or stay hydrated. Fetching a glass of water is at times impossible, opening up a sealed bottle of water usually a task beyond my capabilities too.

The forethought that went into each day became exhausting. Had I asked the last person that was here to fetch me enough drinking water (or pre-open bottles for me)? Move wet laundry to the dryer? Fill the humidifier? (A necessity on oxygen therapy) Take out the garbage so that it didn't start to reek in the passing of a few days with no visitors?

Asking is already hard enough in the first place for me, realizing after they'd left that I'd left out an important request...worse.

With her return, my daughter has given me gifts that I can never repay. Above all, time with my favourite person. Next, more time in my own home before facing the possible necessity to go elsewhere. Next, fewer physical challenges/more time resting (and accordingly, possibly less pain).

I sense that I was being delivered a lesson yesterday, that despite my objections to my daughter leaving school, it has to be this way for now and I need to accept her assistance graciously. In many ways, it's harder to accept help from her than it is from friends and volunteers. She's supposed to be off making a life for herself. It should be me looking after her, instead of the other way around.

On the other hand, if I could have only one person by my side as I each day become more vulnerable, it is her. I trust her with my life. With the end of my life.

A NEW VOCABULARY
Thursday, April 25, 2013

My daughter arrived home on Sunday and we've had a wonderful time catching up. It's amazing how quickly we've fallen back in pace with each other.

But boy, she sure brought a lot of stuff from school! Finding a place for everything is an exercise in planning, motivation, and execution. We could use a touch more of the motivation part, but for now we're trying to balance enjoying our time together with the chores. Well, her chores. I'm not a lot of help; a backseat unpacker shall we say?

Looking at this as a long-term arrangement requires far more than just the desire to spend this time together. We need to be flexible, understanding, compassionate (towards each other as well as to ourselves) and patient.

In addition to looking after me, my daughter will need to take care of herself and what's important to her. It will be at my insistence that she gets out (beyond the part-time job she returns to tomorrow) to visit her friends, go on outings, or maybe just sit on a park bench to give herself time alone with her thoughts.

We need to take cues from each other, both verbal and non-verbal.

Did you ever play the game of drawing something on a piece of paper, guided only by the physical description of the item coming from someone who isn't allowed to use gestures or say the name of what it is or what it's used for? We've had this sort of comical exchange several times already over the last few days. The most common scenario; she in one room, me in the other as I try to explain where an item is stored as best as I can remember its location in the apartment.

Although we're very close and communicate quite well, it's amazing how four semesters at school for her, and a steep decline in independence for me has brought about the need for some new vocabulary between us.

What thankfully hasn't changed is what a hand stretched out towards me across the bed means. Mom, I need a hand hug. And my darling, a hand hug is what you shall have as we do our best to get through this together.

IN GOOD COMPANY
Friday, May 03, 2013

I may or may not have a wee infatuation.

Kristee and I have a running joke about our TV boyfriends. Neither of us watch much TV at all, but in chatting last year, we discovered that we are in agreement that actor Peter Krause would be welcome to drop by anytime for coffee. (No disrespect intended towards my Kristee's fiancé, he's quite a catch himself and my Kristee and her man know how lucky they are to have found each other.)

That discussion led to her lending me the entire series of *Six Feet Under* DVDs last fall, and me making sure that I caught every on-line episode that I could of the show, *Parenthood*. In keeping with the manner of dark humour that creeps into this household, I'm still allowed to look at and appreciate a good-looking man. I'm not dead yet!

There are other men that I find quite attractive for various reasons. A great conversationalist is at the top of my list, and if he's got a good sense of humour and is physically attractive it certainly doesn't hurt either.

For many, many years I was a diehard *Coronation Street* fan. When my daughter and I were without TV and bandwidth this past summer, it went by the wayside and I lost track of the plotlines.

After I settled into this apartment, the only option that was within my budget was hooking up to the apartment building's antenna. On a good day, I get a decent image on three or four channels. The one dependable station is CBC, Canada's national network.

After the flurry of moving-in activities died down, I made an attempt to catch up again on my beloved *Corrie*. Not having a DVR/PVR, I had to make sure I had the TV on in time, so as not to miss it. It became habit to tune in while eating my dinner and catch up on the nightly news while I was at it.

After over thirty years of hardly missing an episode of *Corrie*, I found that I just wasn't that interested anymore after my long break from the show. However, the programme that falls in the time slot just before it comes on caught my attention.

George Stroumboulopoulos Tonight. Affectionately nicknamed "Strombo," (a moniker that gives the rest of us a break from consistently misspelling his surname), George interviews his guests with an ease and humour that I find very enjoyable to watch. And his rotating trio of sidekicks can always make me laugh. (More of comedienne Jenn Robertson please; I've been a fan of hers for years!) And...George is not hard to look at.

You can imagine my delight when a bobblehead George was delivered to me yesterday afternoon by a mutual acquaintance. Last night, my daughter and I had a blast deferring to George throughout the evening. "Yes, it is time for a piece of chocolate, don't you agree, George?" "George agrees with me, Mom – time for you to rest," as she tapped on his forehead to make him nod.

Now, George – isn't it time for another piece of chocolate?

ON THE BEACH
Tuesday, May 07, 2013

A Royal Navy term meaning, "Retired from the Service."

Also the name of my favourite novel, written by Nevil Shute. I was what you might call a precocious reader when I was young; my Grade Six teacher Mr. Bone would score me the brochure for the Scholastic Book Club that was reserved for the senior elementary (Grade Seven and Eight) students, not normally available to the lower elementary grades. It was our little secret, and it was with great excitement that I awaited the monthly delivery of my new books. (That's about the only thing I would spend my allowance on; the apple hasn't fallen far from the tree with my daughter either.)

On The Beach isn't what I would classify as great literature, it's generally not deemed Shute's finest work. The story is that of several characters living in post-apocalyptic Australia, aware that certain death is to follow after nuclear bombs are presumed to have wiped out the rest of Earth's population after the eruption of World War III.

I was watching a bit of TV last week; a show in which a young cancer patient is asked by her therapist what her favourite book is. To my shock she cited *On the Beach*. My jaw could have dropped.

It's not that it's an unknown entity; the book was made into a movie in 1959, and again as a TV movie in 2000. Many of you may know the story.

It's that this book, read over and over again throughout my teen years, had been my guidebook from an early age as to how I would hope to cope with adversity.

What struck me at the first reading was how the characters each face imminent death in their own way. Two characters, Lieutenant Peter Holmes and Commander Dwight Towers, became my heroes. Despite knowing with certainty that in just a few short months, they will die of radiation poisoning, they go about their daily lives with as much normalcy as they can muster and circumstances will allow.

Gardens are planted, dinner parties are thrown, and new friendships are forged. They continue with the mundane tasks of life as if nothing has changed, yet acknowledge at the same time that everything has indeed turned upside down.

My heroes. Facing the end of their lives not with anger, but with acceptance of what is to come. There is no hope, yet grace and gentility reign.

I'm sure that I'm not alone in having thought out in my younger days how I might handle a diagnosis of a life-limiting illness. If and when those thoughts ever crossed my mind, my mind would go to this book.

The game plan I had imagined for how I would deal with serious illness is pretty much on par with how things have actually gone. I knew that I would investigate and try treatments, but would have a sense of when enough was enough. I reached that point last year when I decided that I'd no longer put my body through experimental treatments, nor would I have any more diagnostic tests done. I don't need to know any more details of the ravages to my body; the knowledge offers neither comfort nor advantage.

Despite the overwhelming challenges to keeping some sort of normalcy, we do what we can to shelve my illness for at least a part of each day. I may not leave this apartment, but as a dear friend recently noted – it appeared to her that I seem to do more "living" between these four walls than some others on the outside world do.

It was not without a sardonic twist when I named this blog *Without a Manual*. To be certain, I'd had very little experience with serious illness and death in my lifetime, but I'd had plenty of adversity thrown my way. I'd like to believe that all the challenges along my path were practice for the biggest and most difficult of them all. I don't presume to know the answers; I can only acknowledge what I believe to be the right path for me. I can only walk in my own shoes.

I'm on the beach, looking out to the sea's horizon. It's there waiting for me and it's my prerogative to choose whether I let the current carry me out or I swim towards it.

I am not afraid.

FEAR NOT
Saturday, May 11, 2013

"I am not afraid." I ended a post last week with that sentence, but perhaps it could bear elaboration.

I am not afraid of death. Not so thrilled about the suffering that has to be endured before that happens, especially if it's the painful death that seems to be in the cards for me. But I'm not afraid of no longer being alive.

I can't tell you if the lack of fear comes from a spiritual, intellectual, or emotional place inside of me, but it just never occurred to me to be afraid of death. I realize that may sound strange to some, I've been told so up front many times. I don't wish to diminish the fears that others may have about facing the end of life, it's just truly never been an issue with me for whatever reason.

Not that I've lived without fear. A friend gently asked me a few days ago if I could write about how fear has been addressed in my life, and it's taken me a few days of consideration to frame my thoughts.

I can't leave any of you thinking that I'm some sort of kick-ass storm trooper who can face anything without trepidation. Far from it. But I'll admit that at times I'd prefer it to look that way.

Admittedly, I don't think I'm afraid of very many things. Now. I suspect that any courage that I've been able to muster in facing the challenges of recent years has come from having gone through some pretty harrowing ordeals in my lifetime. You couldn't make this stuff up if you tried; it's quite unbelievable that these challenges happened to one person in just one lifetime.

There have been obstacles that at times I simply believed could not be overcome. I can't even begin to offer a formula for managing to get past them, for some I don't know how I even did so. But generally, we do what needs to be done, dust ourselves off, and hope that tomorrow will be a better day.

One significant fear that I've struggled with is the fear of letting others down. Throughout my life, pleasing others (or more so, not upsetting them) was an overriding concern. To the point that I often allowed myself to be diminished so that others could feel better about themselves, or permitted those others to do whatever pleased them, to my own detriment −sometimes subjecting myself to abject cruelty as not to rock the boat.

Learning to assert my value as an equal to all others has been what I consider to be my last big lesson for this lifetime. Not that I'm terribly good at it yet, but making progress toward it has lessened the fear that my tolerance of past disrespectful behaviour towards me has set a poor example for my daughter.

Not surprising to me, she's been my greatest teacher for this lesson. Another fear that I can let go of before I leave...she's on the right track and I'm grateful that I've been here long enough to learn from her. Perhaps her modus operandi will sometimes require her to do the opposite of what I would have done when facing difficult situations in her future; whatever gets the job done with her dignity and sense of self-worth intact.

ACCEPTING PAIN
Monday, May 13, 2013

Shortly before my nurse arrived today, I came across an online article about the abuse of pain medications. Although that's not a concern of mine, there was a quote that caught my attention.

"Learning how to cope with pain can be more empowering for patients than trying to find a pill to completely eliminate it." This coming from Dr. Mitchell Katz, director of the Los Angeles County health department.

During her visit today, my nurse asked if I'd like her to once again raise the issue of my pain management with my doctors, in hopes of finding something more effective.

I shared the gist of the article with my nurse, and explained how the quote I'd found quite nicely summarized how I felt about my pain management strategy. It's highly unlikely that we'll find anything to eradicate my pain completely, but it's comforting to know that I can relieve it to some degree when it becomes too much for me to bear. Which happens more frequently as the weeks go on; you might accurately surmise that I have a very unhappy stomach to match.

Not having an expectation of complete pain relief is what gets me through my days and nights; I just didn't see it as clearly as that until today, when I read the article. I think I'd be struggling far more emotionally with this illness if I didn't accept that there will be zero days in my future without pain. I just hope to have some days with less severe pain than others.

This philosophy is one that has been in the background throughout my life. I don't know anyone that gets through a lifetime without hardship. It makes the good times all that much sweeter. I suspect that's been my secret to finding happiness in the spaces between the challenges; accepting that no life is without battles and tears.

When my husband first blindsided me with the news that he was leaving me, he said that 95% of our life together was great – but the 5% of unhappiness he was experiencing was more than he was willing to go forward with. He expressed that he deserved to be unabashedly happy all of the time with a partner, and was going to leave me, in order to find someone who could provide him that desired state of absolute and utter happiness. Over the coming weeks and months, the ratios changed – in his version of our history, he apparently had very rarely experienced happiness and that became his truth. I disagreed, but it really didn't matter what I had thought in the matter. A decision had been reached without me.

What I do accept as my truth now is that a certain percentage of my week is spent in moderate physical pain, some at higher levels. There are discussions with my medical and support teams as to how we will proceed as the pain ratios change for the worse. We're together creating a plan with open and honest communication.

I leave you with another quote that I came upon today.

"A lot of people end up unhappy because they made permanent decisions on temporary emotions." There will be no rash major decisions in my future, only ones that have been given lengthy consideration and debate, of that I can assure you.

INDEBTEDNESS
Tuesday, May 14, 2013

Like many others, I've always felt that I had a duty to return kindnesses with something that was of at least equal value or effort. When it wasn't possible, despite best efforts, to give back to the person who did something generous for me, it made me uncomfortable. Isn't that the way the world is supposed to work, so that everyone both gives and gets to meet needs (and as a bonus, experiences the joy of feeling like an active participant in the game of life)?

Even my cat seems to agree. Scrabble finds it impossible to just accept cuddling and being petted without at least a good part of that time returning the favour with attentive licking. With his rough tongue, he might well lift off a layer of skin if we allowed him to persist. If only he didn't like to go after that ticklish part of my throat just above my collarbone!

Delivery of prepared meals (and favourite treats), help around the apartment, errands run, visits from near and far, time spent checking in on me, offers to take me outdoors (it's been six weeks, I pray that it'll soon work out. My body hasn't been cooperating in the least!), loans of movies and audio books to keep my mind busy, numerous gifts, and help from friends and strangers. I fear I've left out mention of a particular kindness, there are just that many of them that come our way.

Today, a call from friends offering to come over for a slumber party so that my daughter could have a night away from the stresses of looking after me. These friends, among others, recognize that my daughter needs a break now and again to be able to keep herself healthy both physically and emotionally. Since she's mature for her age, it can be easy to forget that she's only nineteen, and carrying this huge weight on her shoulders.

I've come to the point of realization that there's no possible way that I can ever repay the wonderful things that so many have done for us. It's been an issue that I've raised a few times on this blog; I have to get better at accepting generosity with a simple, "Thank you," without feeling as if I'm not holding up my end. Quite a difficult task.

This feeling of indebtedness that can't be rectified during the balance of my life makes me pray ever harder each day that I will have opportunities on the other side of this lifetime to offer something meaningful to those who have been so kind to me.

A quote I came across today: "Be thankful for the difficult people in your life, for they have shown you who you do not want to be." This may hold true and is a concept I've taken into consideration when I reflect on my experiences. What I like even more is to paraphrase it to, "Be thankful for the beautiful souls in your life, for they have shown you what is within each of us to be."

Thank you to so many of you for reminding me on a daily basis of what selflessness looks and sounds like. I am forever in your debt.

AN INTRODUCTION
Saturday, May 18, 2013

I've likely made reference to my daughter in just about every post over the last few years. As you might have gathered over the last four years my of writing this blog – I think she's pretty darned amazing. And it's time that I introduced you to my Suzanna.

Why now? Suzanna will be doing me the honour of taking the steering wheel on this blog now and again. She insists that she isn't, but I happen to think she's quite a talented writer and I'm sure that you'll enjoy reading whatever she has to say.

She's welcome to post anytime she wishes, and I'm pleased to say that's she quite excited about participating! Suzanna has also committed to letting you know of any significant updates should I be unable to write. This story needs an ending, and as many of you have very gently and respectfully requested over the last while – you will have it.

Here is Suzanna's first post; I look forward to sharing more of her contributions!

> As my mum has previously mentioned in an earlier blog post, I've made the decision to take the next year off from my education at university to care for her during the end of her journey. It's not that I want to take a break from school, and it's not because it seems easier. In fact, it's an exponentially (here's my science nerd side coming out!) harder experience. So why am I doing this?

I am taking time off to see her through to the end because it is the right thing to do.

I've got to admit, it's really hard being home. For one, I am not free to go and do as I please anymore. I can't take off on a whim, wait six weeks to finally do my laundry, or eat pickles for dinner three nights in a row without it affecting someone else. In my two years away at school, I became accustomed to being totally independent and enjoyed that. Moving home has definitely changed my level of freedom. Secondly, while away at school I didn't have to face how hard my mom's declining health really was. When I was away, I could take my mind off of her for short periods while I concentrated on lectures, labs, and work. Living at home, I see the daily struggles she faces, and how much work goes into making a day go smoothly for her. Physically seeing my mother get sicker before my eyes is – not to be dramatic – heart wrenching. This is the woman who cared for me for years, and now she needs my help caring for her. There is no one else who can do what I do, which brings me back to the point of doing the right thing.

It would be easy to go back to another year of school and try to forget about what is happening at home. I don't believe that I could think highly of myself, however, knowing that I neglected my mom when she needed me most. Doing the right thing is a great source of pride for me. I am proud that I am running a household of myself, my mom, and two cats that cause so much trouble and mess that I liken them to toddler twins in their terrible twos. It has been hard to have to grow up faster than others my age, causing a disconnect between myself and my peers, but I know that it will be beneficial in the long run when I don't have a mother to teach me all of these things later in life when I actually need these skills. This experience has taught me a lot more than just skills in how to run a household, and I feel I have grown as a person because of what I have been through and continue to go through.

This journey has been as hard as I have expected it to be. I am a person who expects the worst, and hopes for the best. In this case, it was closer to the worst, but at least I came prepared. As difficult as this is, it is rewarding too. Knowing that my mom appreciates what I'm doing (and she thanks me a lot, at times excessively!) makes me feel like I am making a positive difference in her life, and that I am needed. My mother is my best friend, and knowing that she won't be enduring the end alone is a bigger reward than I could ever have next year at school.

SHE'S LEFT THE BUILDING (BUT COMING BACK!)
Sunday, May 19, 2013

What's the phrase? I'm so proud I could bust a gut?

My heartfelt thanks to my daughter Suzanna for writing the last post. When she expressed an interest in contributing to the blog, I assured her that she could write about anything she wanted to. There would be no editing on my part, with one exception. I would only review content to catch any details that she might have inadvertently shared that we've mutually agreed are not (or not yet) for public consumption. As I expected, there was nothing at all in her words that needed revision. I'm sure I'll have to give in to her sharing the occasional embarrassing tale; I do seem to have a knack for providing fodder!

The notes of support have flooded in, giving Suzanna confidence in visiting here again sometime soon. Thank you for the kindness and encouragement sent her way; I've shared with her all the comments that came to my inbox.

She's away for a night visiting a friend from university; I'm pleased and grateful that we've been able to make it work. Things were quite rough here for the last few days with my health, thankfully I rallied a bit this morning – enough for her to feel less nervous about being an hour's drive away.

What preparation is required for her to be away for more than a couple of hours?

Lots of water bedside. Suzanna had the excellent idea to bring the full Brita pitcher to the bedroom as a back-up for the three tall glasses she'd already filled for me. And as an extra precaution bottled water with the cap already unscrewed. I hope she's not disappointed if I don't finish it all!

Food at hand. I'll sheepishly admit that part of the supply includes Kernels SuperKid flavoured popcorn. (Thanks to Kristee. She'll know I must really be off my game for it to have lasted this long!) I may be forty-eight, but sometimes I have the cravings of a seven-year-old. Luckily, I have friends who indulge me instead of making fun. Okay, they make fun too but that's all right. The forty-eight-year-old in me can take it.

The side of the bed that Suzanna usually occupies is strewn with my laptop, iPad, land line and cell phones, chargers, TV remote, lip balm, hand lotion (I've jumped up another level in the oxygen airflow, it's desiccating me from the inside out), notebook/pen, tissues, and a cat. You'd think that the cat would be a transient visitor, but somehow Scrabble knows when I'm on my own and rarely leaves my side.

The litter box is clean, cat food and water bowls amply filled. The door is locked; Suzanna will arrive home in time to let the PSW in the door tomorrow at noon.

Laundry is all caught up, garbage has been taken out, and lights other than in the bedroom and bathroom have been turned off. The bedroom window is opened wide. (Who would have guessed that this apartment would get so hot? I haven't managed to get it to a comfortable temperature since I moved in.) If only we could turn off the volume from outside. Visitors who park out back likely have no idea that we're subjected to every word they speak when the factory noise from just beyond the wall doesn't drown them out. Today? "Grandpa smells so old, why did you hafta promise that we'd come back next week, Mom?"

There's a long checklist to go through every time Suzanna steps out. She shared with me a few nights ago that it's now all become second nature after four weeks of trying to settle into a routine.

Her taking care of all these chores is the reason that I'm not in a nursing home now. Whether leaving school was the right thing to do I can't answer, but if she tells me it was the right thing for her I will trust her. And I'll continue to be very, very grateful.

Something she always makes sure to do before she leaves? A hug, a kiss on the cheek or forehead, and telling me that she loves me. And with that, even if I should pass while she's physically away from the apartment, I'll not feel that I died alone. We're in each other's hearts always.

PERKS OF THE JOB
Tuesday, May 21, 2013

My daughter is a voracious reader; typically the only item that would be on her wish list come birthdays or Christmas would be a gift certificate to Chapters bookstore.

She knows that if I read at all these days (eye strain has become an issue) my tastes lean towards non-fiction lately. There was one book, however, that she had suggested I read, *The Fault in Our Stars*, by John Green. She warned me that it was sad, and that it was undoubtedly going to make me cry. She rarely sheds tears for the characters in her books, so I knew I'd best have a box of tissues at hand when it was my turn to tackle the story.

I won't spoil it for anyone who has plans to read *The Fault in Our Stars*, but I will share one thing from the book. Cancer perks.

Erdheim-Chester Disease is at this time still not officially classified as a cancer, but recent studies have it leaning that way. The research community has been making significant strides, thanks to several teams around the world focused on learning more about ECD. Even better is the news that the various researchers have been sharing findings and coordinating efforts. An excellent example they're setting for politicians!

Cancer perks. Things that come your way only as a result of being seriously ill; offered with kindness and compassion. I've often written about my challenges in learning to accept graciously what is offered to me.

Asking for special favours is another thing altogether. Suzanna and I loathe playing the "sick card." Just about everyone has some sort of burden upon them and neither of us feels that we should get special consideration because of my illness.

As you might have already read here, Suzanna has left university to take care of me. The last months of classes were particularly difficult for her to get through as she grappled with making a decision for herself.

More than a few of my support team members suggested that Suzanna let her student advisor know what was going on at home. I learned that sometimes adjustments to grades can be made to compensate for the strain that a student may be under from circumstances beyond their control.

Suzanna wouldn't hear of it. Whether it was good or bad, she felt it imperative to earn every mark on her own without, in her words, pity.

I applaud her for this decision. She passed all of her classes, some grades better than others – but she carries with her the knowledge that she earned every mark on her own.

The apple doesn't fall far from the tree on this one, I'm afraid. Unless it's essential to the conversation, I just don't see any reason to mention to others on the phone or in emails that I'm ill. Before needing mobility devices (crutches, the special cushion and then the wheelchair) and oxygen, getting away with being perceived as "healthy" had given me a bit of a thrill. A chance to fade into a crowd.

I played the sick card last night, and it burns me today thinking about how hard I had to slam that card down.

We've had intermittent, yet continuous problems with our Internet and phone connections since moving in here. Techs have come and gone, yet the problems weren't resolved.

We nearly had emergency services here a few days ago when a PSW was trying to call from the lobby downstairs. The only reason I even have a landline is to be able to buzz visitors in, and when it's not working, I can't get anyone inside the door. Protocol with my palliative team dictates that if I don't answer the phone, help is to be summoned.

That particular situation turned out all right when another tenant opened the door for her more than twenty minutes later, but I'm sure you understand the importance of having a phone that works. Unfortunately my service provider didn't see it the same way.

A call to the technical support line last night landed me a Thursday appointment for the repair; four days away. It was suggested that I have visitors call my cell phone, and I could go downstairs to unlock myself the door in the meantime. I respectfully explained to the agent that due to disability I'm not able to leave the apartment. That still didn't get me anywhere.

I explained that not answering my phone would be setting off alarm bells with my support team. Still no luck.

So I did it, I played the sick card. Apparently, the situation I'd already laid out still wasn't enough to warrant sending out a tech the next day, but telling the whole truth finally got things moving. Being disabled wasn't enough of a reason, but being palliative is.

Cancer perks? Not this time. Just the provider stepping up to do the right thing, as I see it. Sometimes the bar needs to be raised for those who need special consideration. I'm not thrilled to be stuck on this boat, but I am getting braver about asking for the rules to be bent on behalf of myself and others who sit in the boat with me.

DWINDLING PIGGY BANK
Thursday, May 23, 2013

Last month, I wrote a post that detailed how I needed to reserve my energy, taking it down to the number of steps I estimated I could take each day without pushing myself too far.

It seemed to be about one hundred steps, and no more than five minutes of standing each day. Today those numbers feel very far away. How dramatically things have changed.

That allotment needs now to be spread over several days if I'm to lessen the excruciating pain that accompanies having used my legs too much. If not the pain, it's the accompanying respiratory issues that have me returning to bed as soon as possible.

There's a dilemma in choosing how much to share with my daughter about the pain levels; it usually flares up at night when we're trying to enjoy some quality time. This time usually consists of light-hearted banter and "punnery" whipping back and forth; the breadth of topics we can cover in an hour is a source of amusement to us. She has to take care in not saying anything too outrageously funny for fear of getting me gasping for air. (She's nicknamed me the Coughy Monster and she's not far off base.) Not an easy task, she has a terrific and wry sense of humour.

By end of day, my part of any conversation is usually held at a whisper, but between hand gestures and Suzanna knowing me well enough to know which words would have come out of me next, we've made it work.

We're getting creative on how to keep my "leg time" and talking to a minimum. During the day, if Suzanna is away, the apartment door is left open for friends and palliative team members to let themselves in. (No worries, there's absolutely nothing of any value here left to steal – least of all me!)

When the pain escalates, I get quiet. I worry about offending her, that she'll think I'm not appreciating her attempts at keeping me entertained. I worry that she'll think that I'm in more pain than usual that evening because she didn't do enough for me during the day to keep my allotment of leg time to a minimum. When I do tell Suzanna that the pain levels are difficult to manage, it's so that she can understand why I'm not reacting as quickly, or at all, to her comments or questions.

This concern in not wanting to offend others by not participating fully in conversation has me withdrawing, at least to some degree, from my circle of friends and support team. The truth is, phone calls and visits do place additional strain upon me. There's no question that there's a price to be paid for doing anything other than just lying quietly in bed. I know that my friends also feel badly when they realize that interaction has been taxing for me.

I realize that I'm likely to hurt some feelings in saying this, but some relationships going forward may need to be maintained more often over email and short phone calls. I do hope that friends who are wondering if they can visit will ask me or Suz, and understand if she or I tell them that it's not something I'm up to.

Although I may be talented at budgeting when it comes to money, I have to apply the same principles to my energy reserves. The piggy bank is dwindling. It used to be that I had a balance that went up and down from day to day, finding a way to save up energy for an upcoming visit. Now, there are only withdrawals.

I know how I want to invest the balance. The biggest gift I'm getting now is having my daughter is here, and that she approves of the spending plan.

REMEMBERING PENELOPE
Saturday, May 25, 2013

Back in 1969, the year I turned five, Hanna-Barbera Productions aired a cartoon entitled *Penelope Pitstop*. It was just for one season, but I found the show and the lead character memorable. Race car driver brave (most of the time!) and extraordinaire, for a time in my childhood she was my role model and idol. So much so that for many years afterwards when asked what my favourite TV show had been as a child, I would mention Penelope.

Except for maybe once or twice, my answer would be greeted with a lack of recognition. Very few remembered the show, and at times I would be asked if perhaps I was confusing a character, or it was suggested that maybe Penelope was instead from a printed comic. I'd shake my head, insisting that she had been on TV.

I'm not entirely sure at times whether an excellent memory is a blessing or a curse, but I knew what I knew. (The Internet has since proven that I had remembered Penelope accurately.)

Having grown up as generally quite a shy person, I had assumed that I blended into the background and was easily missed or quickly forgotten, as it seemed Penelope had been. It didn't help that I had poor self-esteem and didn't believe that anyone would have reason to remember me.

Things did change a bit over time; career successes brought with them more confidence. However, I maintained the belief that once out of someone's life, I would also have fallen out of their memory and thoughts.

Through my writing this blog and my CBC radio interview, a few people from my past have been in touch to say hello. To my surprise, the emails and phone calls have often started out with the phrase, "You probably don't remember me, but..." I remembered everyone who has reached out, and with great delight had the opportunity to recount memorable highlights of time spent together.

It amazes me that others sometimes also feel that they've not had a significant enough presence to be remembered; that it's not just me who can feel invisible. And I certainly would say for the majority that reached out that I hadn't thought of them as lacking in self-confidence as I had/have been.

Last night, I unexpectedly received a letter from the mother of one of Suzanna's friends from elementary school. We hadn't been in touch since Suzanna and I moved away to another city, eight years ago. This mother and I hadn't known each other very well, but I have memories of some lovely conversations when we and our girls were together at school events, birthday parties, and play dates. (My bookish daughter did indeed have somewhat of a social life despite being the homebody that she is!)

The letter was beautiful, and brought tears of joy, in reading that Suzanna and I had held a special place in their memories, as they had in ours.

Reminders come along frequently that despite thinking that I haven't had any significant impact during my time on this earth, I have made footprints. Perhaps sometimes there are ones that I regret having laid down, or wish I had taken in a different direction, but all the same, I was here.

I'm often feeling like I haven't accomplished even a small part of what I was supposed to in this lifetime. How can one at forty-eight? A harsh realization came to me this week when my uncle, at ninety, was hospitalized once again. I was fondly remembering a few of his many adventures since I was born; when he was just a few years younger than I am today. What difference could I make if I were to be around for another forty or more years? It's only quite recently that I began to accept the idea that my actions and presence have at times made a positive impression in the lives of others.

I have no idea if the creator of the character of Penelope is still around (I'm feeling very old when I realize it's well over forty years ago), but I wish that he or she could have known that despite not being well known, Penelope made a difference in the life of a five-year-old girl a very long time ago.

A PICTURE'S WORTH
Tuesday, May 28, 2013

Infrequently, I have days when the ache inside my heart (the one that I use to love with, not the one that runs on a pacemaker battery) exceeds that of the physical pain in my body. Sunday was one of those days.

A few months ago, my daughter asked me how I would feel if she were to book a photo session with a pro photographer for herself and James, to mark their three-year anniversary of being a couple.

Suzanna brought the request to me ever so gently, knowing that with me having been a family photographer for the years before my "retirement," I was going to be very sad about not being able to photograph the two of them myself as I had done several times before.

And I am. Terribly sad about not being able to do the session myself, but at the same time very happy that she's come to value photos as a wonderful way to mark special occasions and the passing of time.

I of course gave her my blessing to go ahead, and she gave me the opportunity to contribute with discussions about her outfit, hair, and make-up for Sunday. It sounds like she and James had a wonderful time and I can't wait to see the proofs.

Part of getting ready, for lack of a better term, for my death has been the exercise of determining what to do with all the photographs I've taken over the course of almost forty-five years. (I still have my first camera, a Diana that I received at age five.) In my estimation, I've likely topped well over a hundred thousand images that need sorting. (It's running about 50/50, landscapes to portraits.) Now there's a job nobody is offering to take off of my hands!

Although I've always preferred to be behind the lens, it makes me sad that there are so few photographs of me for Suzanna to show her own children years from now. Most of my childhood photos were destroyed. (You can't imagine how much I'd value having some of my yearly school photos, as horrid as they may have been.)

I have a few photos that my high school boyfriend took (bikini photos, not exactly how I'd like my grandchildren see me solely represented in my school years!) but other than that just a handful of images. As designated photographer at just about every occasion it was rare that anyone took the camera from me.

I know that I've smiled for the occasional photo over the years, but unfortunately have very few images to pass on to Suzanna. Hopefully, in time, a photo or two will make their way to her.

Sunday was indeed tough to get through. It was also the two-year anniversary of my husband telling me that he no longer wanted to be married to me. With all that has happened, I honestly can't say if it's been the longest two years of my life, or that it's flown by; the answer changes on regular basis.

Incidentally, just weeks before that, knowing that I wasn't well, a photographer friend offered us the gift of a family portrait session, with the generous thought that my daughter and husband would appreciate having images of us together. I had put it off waiting for warmer weather (and for my face to deflate a touch more, a sorry side effect of the prednisone). But in hindsight, any photos would be too painful to look at now. I suppose the universe was doing me a huge favour at the time.

You might wish to suggest to me that it's not too late to have photos taken, and you're right – it isn't. My daughter and I regularly goof around with the camera phone. But it's just not a look that I'm rocking right now though.

What I'd like to suggest in return, dear readers, is that you make an effort to capture your loved ones (and don't shy away from a camera yourself either!) at every milestone, at every special occasion – but mostly in the moments in between. While life is being lived.

As for Suzanna, I know that when she shows her children the many pictures of her childhood self, she'll tell them that someone who would have loved them very much was standing close by on the other side of the lens. I'd like to think that I'll still be taking in the scene at those moments too.

PERSPECTIVES ON PAIN
Wednesday, May 29, 2013

Sadly, I have a number of friends who are at this time experiencing various ailments causing considerable physical pain and discomfort. Invariably, a few times a week I'm asked how I manage to keep a smile on my face, given the considerable bone and cardiac pain.

I'm often told by visitors that I'm good at covering it up. Mind you, they're usually not around when the pain is at its worst in the wee hours of the night. It's at those times I'm found as curled up as my stiffened body will allow, and permitting myself occasionally to let the tears silently stream down my face. Not terribly desirable – I'm then stuck with a wet pillow.

A few weeks ago, I had a conversation with Donna, who used to be my family doctor in Toronto, and who since moving away, I've been blessed to call my friend. She was my physician back in 1996 when a mysterious virus hit me.

It wasn't so much pain as severe discomfort. Endless months of intense nausea, vertigo, and retching made daily life unbearable. It was next to impossible to keep anything down (although the Ovaltine biscuits that my father-in-law would bring me seemed to often magically do the trick when a touch of appetite would finally arrive around 3 a.m. each night).

I was beyond miserable. I couldn't work; I couldn't care for my daughter properly. Even turning over in bed seemed an ominous proposition. There were too many trips to emergency as my body repeatedly went into severe dehydration.

My doctor had given me her home phone number; I remember calling her one Saturday afternoon as I reached my breaking point, after over six months of this torment.

She gently assured me that despite numerous tests not having yet determined a cause, this would end – she would keep trying to find an answer. It would be okay. Admitting how much I was struggling had brought me to my low point, hearing her caring words brought me back up again.

In case you're wondering, it's impossible to know if that rough patch was a precursor to my diagnosis of Erdheim- Chester Disease. It was, however, yet another of many prolonged spells of ill health, with the most serious yet still to come. I sometimes wonder what surprises the pathologist will come upon when it's time to take a look inside. Wish I could be around to hear the results, they might explain quite a lot!

When Donna and I had our conversation a few weeks ago, I reflected upon how I had handled my illness at that time, compared to how I was dealing with my current situation. Mentally, I've dealt with each quite differently.

When I've been seriously ill in the past, attached to it was always desperation to get better. The discomfort had to eventually let up, right? Something had to work, and eventually something would.

This time, it's completely different. With no expectation of getting better (and a reasonable assumption that with each day, week and month I'll be feeling worse) at the risk of sounding cliché, I can embrace the pain. It's part of me now, and there will only be one way to escape it. There's a comfort in knowing that eventually this will be over, just not in the way I'd hoped with previous health challenges.

I don't have to fear that tomorrow the pain might be worse, I already know that there's a fair chance that it will be. I don't have to worry that this illness will kill me; I already know that it will.

To my friends who are going through illness and injury, please don't shy away from telling me how bad you're feeling, in concern that it pales in comparison to what I'm going through. Neither of us can know that, but be assured that I can understand how overwhelming it can be.

If what you need is for me to just listen, I will. If what you need is to hear that it'll all be okay, I can say that to you. Sometimes, even though that might be straying from the truth or from what can be known for certain, those words can be golden in their intention alone.

STANDING UP FOR CHOICE
Thursday, June 06, 2013

I'm prepared to learn that perhaps two or three out of every ten readers of this blog might decide to not come back after I share my thoughts today on a topic that is quite relevant to my situation.

That would be in line with the stats that tell us that 70-80% of Canadians support an issue that's been hotly debated for some time, but it would seem especially so in the last few weeks.

This issue is one that falls under many names. Dying with dignity, end of life options, gentle death, physician-assisted suicide, the right to choose. You might be aware that Vermont recently became the third US state to allow physician-assisted death for patients falling within a stringent set of parameters. It likely won't be long before more states pass similar legislation, to allow a dignified, peaceful death for individuals dealing with terminal illness.

The reason I'm coming forward with more detail about my personal situation is because I strongly believe that Canadians should be given the opportunity to make a decision that is right for them. As a person with a life-limiting illness, I deserve a voice in the matter.

Dying with dignity is an option that I would like to be available to me legally. I'm not saying that I'm certain that assisted suicide is the right thing for me, or if it is, what I would want the timing to be.

What I do know is that as my health continues to decline and my independence diminishes day by day, I'd like to have some control in how my last weeks or days play out. It's my life, my body.

Issues surrounding my wish to have a more peaceful death have been under discussion for quite some time with my family, my doctor, my palliative team, and the local hospice. By no means has this been an easy road, but it has been for the most part been addressed with respect and compassion.

Well over a year ago, I made two important decisions. The first was to sign my "Do Not Resuscitate" order. Under no circumstance do I wish to have heroic measures used to save my life if my body has decided otherwise.

The second was a decision to not have my pacemaker replaced when the battery runs out. For anyone wishing to do the math, it was implanted in 2003. The time I've been using it is a whole lot longer than the time that is left on the battery.

This issue is not nearly as simplistic as perhaps I'm making it to be; I'll share more in the coming weeks. For now, I will leave you with a passage that my daughter shared last night with me from the book, *Life of Pi*, written by Yann Martel. After reading it, she asked me if this is what dying slowly felt like to me.

"Oncoming death is terrible enough, but worse still is oncoming death with time to spare, time in which all the happiness that was yours and all the happiness that might have become yours becomes clear to you.

You see with utter lucidity all that you are losing. The sight brings on an oppressive sadness that no car about to hit you or water about to drown you can match. The feeling is truly unbearable."

I told her that perhaps I didn't see it as unbearable – yet – I try very hard to not allow myself to go there. The passage did strike me as particularly poignant, looking at it from the perspective of a younger person who will not have the opportunity to live to a ripe old age.

The fact is that the end in many ways looks like it could be quite ugly. Yet there are measures that can be taken to ensure that the end is not as awful as it might be. That to me is something worth speaking up about.

A GOOD DAY, BUT...
Friday, June 07, 2013

Back in April, I wrote about a failed attempt at a revised bucket list trip to Toronto, instead of my original wish of going to New York City.

Almost two months later, it still hadn't happened. Both my health and the weather were working against me. And I was suffering from some serious cabin fever.

As the weeks went by it became very clear that I wasn't well enough to travel to and from Toronto. However, could we perhaps manage a destination that was closer?

With the help of Suzanna and our friend Sandra, I finally escaped these apartment walls for the first time in almost three months. (Previous trips were no treat; one to the dentist and the other to a Hamilton hospital.)

I picked a spot that is special to me, a spot in which I've spent many hours photographing and walking. A spot that was perfect for when I had needed quiet contemplation. Seemingly a perfect spot for my great escape.

Poor Suzanna. Let me say that we're learning the hard way to not take the words "wheelchair accessible," (starting with our apartment unit and building) at face value, and Tuesday was one of those days. What a trouper she was in pushing my chair along deeply rutted gravel paths, despite my urgings to turn back so that she didn't hurt herself. And thanks to Sandra, who hauled the heavy spare oxygen tanks. It turns out that we needed all three; I'm sucking up the stuff big time these days.

I was thrilled to be out in the fresh air. The sun was on my face, and when we had a short clearing of smoother path, Suz gave me a fast enough ride to have the wind blow through my hair. Not something I had anticipating feeling again, and it was simply blissful to have those moments with her.

As wonderful as it was to be out, it was a mistake to set it up for myself as fulfillment of the top item on a drastically revised bucket list.

A beautiful spot, but a substitute for New York City it isn't. There are the rare times that trying to see the glass as half full just doesn't work that well, and Tuesday was one of them. It didn't help that it was a spot that I had gotten to know so well as an able-bodied person, and that the grand majority of the property was now off limits to me. I think going forward it's healthier for me if I don't get such a close look at what's out of reach.

LAYING IT ON THE TABLE
Monday, June 10, 2013

Some (I think especially my female readers) might relate to one of my small pleasures in life. Getting my hair washed when preparing to get my hair cut.

Always the highlight of a salon visit, especially when head massages began to be incorporated a few decades ago. I practically purr when someone is playing with my hair!

I'm not able to get to the salon anymore, yet my hair still annoyingly continues to grow. A friend connected me to a stylist who was willing to come to my apartment to cut my hair – and also make allowances for my difficulty in sitting up and needing oxygen. My friend also happens to be an aesthetician, who takes care of my pedicures for me now. (I can't reach my feet anymore.) Today I lucked out in having both aesthetician friend and stylist friend come over at the same time.

To make things easier, I suggested that Suzanna could wash my hair before their arrival. Normally I'd have washed it seated in the shower, but my daily shower had already taken place hours before. Certainly my daughter and I could figure out a way to get the job done in the bathroom that wouldn't be too uncomfortable for me.

Think back to your own visits to the salon, leaning back into those big comfy chairs with your head titled back over the sink. Imagine if you then found when you tried to get out of the chair that you couldn't. Your muscles (or lack thereof) just wouldn't put out the strength that was needed.

It wasn't just hesitation; it was flat out lack of cooperation on my body's part. The most frightening part was the lack of strength in my neck. Then it hit me that my stomach muscles weren't up to the task of getting myself upright again. I'm already used to not being able to get out of chair by myself without a grab bar, but I couldn't even reach out for anything to pull myself up on.

Suzanna of course was there to help me up, but I can't ever remember feeling such helplessness in realizing how badly my body is failing me. The sobs poured out of me.

It's not just the lack of strength. Over the last week, I've had to go off my pain meds due to stomach bleeding and we have nothing to replace them with. I won't even try to describe what going without has been like.

Swallowing has become a lot more difficult; it'll soon be time to switch over to a liquid/soft food diet. For anyone who knows how much I love good food, you might understand how much this reality is kicking my behind.

Then there's the ongoing discussion about when it's an appropriate time to have a catheter put in. It probably won't be long and I'm dreading the arrival of that day.

Sleeping is another interesting proposition. No position is the least bit comfortable; the only way I can get three or four uninterrupted hours of sleep in a row is to knock myself out with a strong sleeping pill. Even then, more often than not these days, pain prevents the pill from working for several hours (I'm almost always still up at 3 a.m.), or pain wakes me up again far too early.

I'm done with sugar-coating how I'm really doing. If we're to have open discussions about dying with dignity, I'm going to lay it out on the table what it's like to be living in this body. The realities are harsh.

Even so, I'm still trying to greet each day with smile. When my daughter awakens beside me each morning, I tell her that I'm happy to see her beautiful face.

The measurement of quality of life? Ultimately, that should be mine to define.

WHY JUNE 12TH IS SPECIAL
Wednesday, June 12, 2013

I pay little attention to the calendar anymore, there's little need to. All upcoming visits and phone calls are logged on to my iPad, and it keeps me notified of what needs to be prepared for the following day. Most days that consists of little more than asking Suzanna to wash the spare set of sheets so that the PSW can freshen the bed the next day.

There are days that I don't wish to remember. Days that I used to count down to celebrate, but have no reason to anymore. Today was one of those days. I probably wouldn't have registered the date in my brain had it not been that I needed to figure out that I have only a few days left for the insurance company to reimburse me for the monthly oxygen charge before my credit card balance is due.

06/12 had been a very special day for me for many years, and for that reason I used those numbers as my cell phone voicemail password, for the combo lock that stored the spare house key, and my debit card password. (Don't worry, they've all been changed. I wouldn't be announcing them to the world at large!)

Instead, June 12th will be remembered for the following reasons:

Today I saw for myself that a friend was on the mend from a recent and very serious health crisis.

Today we welcomed a new volunteer to the team, and both Suz and I very much enjoyed her warmth and positive spirit. Angels everywhere I tell you.

Today I received an enquiry from my work website for a quotation and information on my wedding photography services. For a very short instant a punch to the gut, but when I learned that the referral came from a guest that had been photographed at an event I shot five years ago, my heart filled with joy. When I looked up the young woman who had done the referring on the Internet, I immediately recognized her beautiful face although I had never come to know her name. What an honour to be remembered in the way that she had remembered both me and my photographs.

An added joy was hearing that the venue for next year's wedding was a spot that my friends and I, while in high school, had a few times snuck into for midnight tobogganing on the snowy and pristine hills. I wasn't always such a goody two shoes! Needless to say, I had to decline the opportunity to provide a quotation, but it was a thrill to have been asked.

Today was a day when a dear friend came to visit; she sat on my bed and so lovingly listened as I lamented about the further decline of my health.

Today was a day when my daughter surprised me by coming home early because she wanted to be here instead of elsewhere.

Although each day holds its own challenges, each also holds its own joys. Today was special for many reasons, just as I'll find tomorrow special for different ones.

SHE WAS IN THERE ALL ALONG
Thursday, June 13, 2013

Darn it, I am brave. I'm finally going to take ownership of that.

Whenever anyone has ever told me that they thought me brave, I would dismiss it in saying that I was only doing what anyone else would do in whatever situation I was up against.

What brought this acceptance to me today was the gift of more than a dozen photographs from my childhood. Photos I'd never seen. In reality I had little concept of what I had looked like as a child and teenager because I had only my memories to go on. That in itself was quite a surprise. I wasn't the ugly and awkward duckling I'd believed myself to be. I was actually a fairly cute kid if I may say so myself!

Several pictures took me by surprise. I believed that I'd only ever been brave when there was a need to make a bad situation better, but that I hadn't been one to push my limitations for reasons other than survival.

One photo of a young girl doing a back flip into a pool from a diving board struck me. When it was sent today, it was a "guess who," and neither Suz or I could be sure of who the subject was. It's me, and although I do remember the time it was taken – I've never quite been sure whether I had just wanted to pull this off, or had actually done it.

I don't know how to swim. Am I allowed to say that I'm totally impressed with almost thirteen-year-old me?

Other photos followed today, all taken when I was between the ages of five and thirteen. Horseback riding (not a trail ride, me alone across fields at my uncle's and aunt's farm), driving a horse-drawn sleigh on snowy back roads by myself, and travelling unaccompanied to Germany when I was five.

These photos brought back a flood of other memories. Sticking my arm into a goat's insides in the wee hours of the night, to turn her kid around when the birth became complicated and going off to sleepover camp for two weeks when I was ten without knowing neither any other campers, or anyone who'd ever been to that camp.

Although most who knew me as a child would say that I was timid and hardly spoke, inside, the beginnings of a warrior princess were emerging. Albeit, a rather quiet one. She's served me well.

ZERO MINUTES OF FAME
Saturday, June 15, 2013

While sorting through my photographs on a hard drive, I came across one of my favourite images – and it has a good story to go with it.

The photo was taken in Caledon, Ontario at dawn, after having left home at around 4 a.m. to reach my destination in time. Although I had a digital camera at the time, I often preferred to shoot film for my landscape work for both colour and black & white.

For several years, my photographs had been represented by a Toronto gallery, which rented images to set designers for TV and movies. Imagine my thrill when I received a letter from Twentieth Century Fox asking permission to use this image on set for the movie *The Sentinel*. Of course I said yes!

We went to go see the movie in the first few days of its theatrical release. Could I have missed it in the background of one of the scenes whilst I was concentrating on the plot? (Which I thought might have been hard to do given my level of excitement?)

When the movie came out as a rental months later, I gave the search another try. Still no luck. If actors could deal with ending up on the cutting room floor, certainly I could handle a bit of disappointment.

What made it less disappointing was hearing that the framed image had indeed been used in the movie, and that one of the actors liked it enough to personally purchase it. My gallery wasn't at liberty to tell me who the purchaser was, but given the secrecy I'd like to believe that the image now resides in the collection of Michael Douglas, Kiefer Sutherland, or Eva Longoria.

I may not have had my moment of glory, but it's always nice to be invited to the party.

THE SLOW BURN
Sunday, June 16, 2013

A topic that comes up with others: Am I grateful that I have had my chance to say goodbye, or would I rather that my death would have come without warning?

I don't know that I could answer that one consistently; there are many days that I believe that it would have been much easier on myself and my daughter had I had a quick and fatal heart attack. Goodness knows that my heart keeps unsuccessfully testing out that game strategy.

There are days that the suffering for us both can be unbearable. We're trying to make the most of our days together, yet me being so limited in my energy and mobility makes it all that more difficult to forget that which always hangs over our heads.

Knowing that my time is limited, this is not how I would choose to spend this time with her. I'd have taken her travelling, to all the places I promised I would when she was small. We'd be zipping around the city together, visiting whatever restaurants caught our fancy. We'd go to the movies and we'd entertain our friends. On summer nights, we'd drive into the country far away from the city lights to watch the meteor showers, lying on our backs, anxiously waiting for a chance to wish upon a falling star. We'd chase the Northern Lights. How could I have lived in Winnipeg for two years and not noticed them? It was a time long ago when I didn't yet appreciate the wonders around me.

What I wouldn't have chosen is for her to be here day in, day out looking after my every need. My heart breaks for her. Every morning I wake up it starts to hurt all over again.

This morning we had quite a fright. There was a small electrical fire here in bed that could have had dire consequences had we not been awake at the time.

Had I been on my own this morning, things may not have turned out as they did. Suzanna's quick thinking and ability to move much faster than I can saved the day.

As much as I'm overwhelmingly relieved that Suzanna was unharmed and our neighbours were spared danger today, the experience awakened in me a deep sadness in being reminded that more suffering still lies ahead for both of us.

When Suzanna comes home tonight from a visit with her father, she'll snuggle and as always tell me how much she loves me. A big part of me will be wishing that my body would just let go and allow her to get on with the rest of her life. I'd think it far from selfish if she were wishing for the same, a chance to bring this chapter to a close and no longer live on this tightrope.

LEARNING TO TRUST
Monday, June 17, 2013

I'll trust you until you give me a reason not to.

This wasn't an easy philosophy to embrace; it took me almost thirty years to get there. I'd been provided with ample opportunity in my early life to learn that sometimes people had hidden agendas; that their actions could be highly destructive to others. That some could act with utter disregard for the welfare of others, leaving a trail of misery behind them. And I've been reminded a few times since.

I wanted my daughter's world to be different. It's not that I wanted to do the impossible and shield her from all that was difficult or painful, but I did want to teach her to give others the benefit of the doubt.

It started at home. To this day, I've never searched her personal belongings. Never peeked in her diary, never opened up her phone (and she can attest to the fact that I can't even figure out how to turn the alarm off when it trills while she's in the shower, much less look up any info).

The deal was and is, unless she gives me reason to worry about her safety and wellbeing, her privacy is respected. And she respects mine. It's brought us to a place where we can feel safe to speak to each other about anything on our minds, and it's an amazing place to be with her.

When it came to others, I asked her to assume the best of intentions. When someone cuts you off in your driving lane, they might be trying to reach a loved one who's taken ill. When someone is rude to a store clerk, maybe they've just learned that their job is in jeopardy.

We all have bad days, and we all at times take it out on others. And yes, sometimes people are complete and utter jerks. My suggestion to Suzanna, however, was to give them more than one chance to prove it.

I'm not entirely sure at this moment if this is indeed the healthiest way to look at the world. I've found myself too many times over the years excusing inappropriate behaviour, thinking that surely the person who was being hurtful was just having a bad day and tomorrow would be better. Surely nobody could be that indifferent to the feelings of others. Indeed, sometimes they can.

Our faith in the world outside of this apartment has been tested again over the last weeks. A casual acquaintance of my daughter's was found murdered recently. Disturbingly, Suzanna had been a stone's throw from the young man's body before it was discovered. Due to the actions of a person who drove into our old clunker and left without leaving a note a few days earlier, she was at the neighbouring car repair shop. Our car (nearly as old as Suzanna) had been literally held together with a bungee cord on the drive there, to prevent her from being pulled over by the police.

A racist comment from a customer at her place of work…and not the first one. Me tripping across the "hate map" online, a deeply disturbing mapping of tweets sent from across the U.S. containing phrases indicative of racism, homophobia, and intolerance for the disabled. Would a Canadian "hate map" prove just as unsettling?

A theft from our apartment – ill intent has also crept in here. Really? We have next to nothing as it is, yet someone helped themselves to a little bit of the little we have left.

I still have numerous examples held up to me daily about what is good in the people around me, and I won't let go of the faith that there's far more good than bad out there.

However world, please show my daughter a sign that despite the risks, trusting in others is ultimately more rewarding. A few jerks are blocking the grander view right now.

STILL HANGING IN
Thursday, June 20, 2013

Sue will be paying us a visit tomorrow; a quick stopover in Toronto in the midst of a heavy work schedule that has her crisscrossing Canada for three seasons each year.

I'm always very happy to see her. However rare our opportunities have been to get together in person over the years, distance has never been an obstacle in our friendship. Granted, we've likely seen more of each other in the last eighteen months than in all the years leading up to them combined.

We'll greet each other with a big hug and enjoy our hours together. The goodbyes however, get more difficult each time we part. We both know that it might be the last time we see each other. Yet we continue to end our visits saying that we'll see other soon again.

There are friends whom I see more frequently, others less so when distance and busy schedules get in the way. There are also the friends (and family) for whom I know seeing me is overwhelmingly difficult.

I try to understand.

The hard part for me is not knowing if the last time I visited with a friend will be the last time I'll have seen them. I suspect for some, their perspective is that they've already said their goodbyes to me. Sometimes I wonder if I missed it. Were they saying farewell and I didn't recognize it for what it was?

Looking from the outside in, this situation is ugly. I'm hooked up to oxygen tubing, confined to bed, and I know it's hard to watch me try to shift about in bed, or hobble to the bathroom, or see me wincing when I'm not doing a good job of covering up the physical pain.

From the inside out, however, I'm still me. I still want to converse about everyday subjects, joke around and share in the ups and downs of the lives of my family and friends.

Inside, I'm still very much alive. My body may be wasting away, but my mind is sharp and wanting to keep engaged with life outside of this bedroom. It just has to come to me now.

My hope was, and is, that I'm not going to need to say goodbye to anyone. I'll hopefully just slip away in the night, and would be happy at the prospect of friends saying, "I just spoke with Sandy the other day, discussing the kids, our vacation plans. Who would have imagined that she'd be gone just like that?"

Of course it's not "just like that"; the way out the door has been agonizingly prolonged. Even so, I'm not yet ready for goodbyes. In fact, I'm still making new friends along the way. (A brave lot, wouldn't you say?)

DROPPING THE BALL
Sunday, June 23, 2013

Not a ball exactly. A little pill less than a quarter of the size of a pea. But what an important little pill it is.

It was 2:30 a.m. when I was getting to bed, and as usual, I reached for my night-time dosage of my medications. My hands are often quite shaky, and one of the pills slipped between my fingers. I noticed before I had put them to my mouth; usually I do a quick inventory with my tongue to make sure no pill went astray between hand and lips. You can't be too careful when your hands aren't steady.

In the dimness of the nightlight, I couldn't tell which of my pills was missing somewhere in the carpet. My first thought was concern that the cat would get to it first. He's quick, and I'm not able to reach the floor. My second thought was the hope that it wasn't one of the expensive meds for which the dosage is closely monitored by the insurance company. The carpeting in this apartment is pretty grungy and the thought of putting the dropped pill in my mouth was completely unappealing. There's one medication in particular that I can't get refilled until I only have just two pills left, the insurance company will only cover thirty days-worth at a time of any of my meds. And no automatic refills so my doctor has be bothered each time. There is no end to the additional red tape that comes with being of palliative status, I really didn't need a replacement pill being one more headache for me to address this week.

I needed Suzanna's help, and called over to her side of the bed to give me a hand. She quickly got up, found the pill, and got me a replacement. It had been my beta blocker, a cardiac medication used to help regulate my very irregular heart rate. Not taking it would have been problematic, as would accidentally taking a double dose, if in the dark I had guessed the wrong medication to be missing from my hand. Thankfully it wasn't a pill which would require a call to the pharmacy, it's the one for which I need to adjust the dosage based on how my heart is behaving so I'm provided with a bit of wiggle room in my supply.

Prior to the last six months or so, dropping something wouldn't have been such a big deal. Not being able to pick anything up off the floor has been very frustrating for me. Adding to the frustration was the fact that I had taken off my oxygen a few minutes earlier to wash my face and brush my teeth, I was unable to get enough air to speak to Suzanna. I had to communicate with her through gestures and whispers.

Ever so gently she placed the replacement pill in my hand, and after I put them in my mouth she handed me a glass of water. These days I have to hold a glass with two hands to drink, and my teeth clink annoyingly against the glass as my hands shake.

She then replaced my day bed wedge (steeper to allow me to lie at a higher angle in bed) with the night wedge. (My head and chest need to be raised while I sleep to help avoid the dreaded night coughing and gasping).

Suzanna takes wonderful care of me, but I can't help but dread what else my failing body will cause me to drop the ball on. With that, comes the responsibility for her to pick those balls up for me. I detest the reminders of how the scale is tipping more every day.

YOUR CHANCE TO STRIKE IT RICH
Wednesday, June 26, 2013

Aside from some truly enjoyable visits with friends, this week has been a quite the downer. I'll eventually get around to writing about the events of the last few days and the coming ones, but I'd rather end today on a higher note.

I'm the queen of thinking of creative solutions for predicaments, but then saying, "Someone should invent a device that does..." without realizing that I'm the one who just then might have invented something quite useful. Many ideas I'm sure would have been complete duds, but had I invested a bit of time on research and development, I imagine that it's entirely possible that I'd have a patent or two under my belt.

When I was in the corporate world, for years I worked with a woman who then and in the years since, has been a close and trusted friend.

Deb and I have never been at a loss for topics to discuss, and can't imagine a subject that we've not chatted about at least once over the years. Many times she'd hear my ideas for a new product (oftentimes we'd quickly agree that it was one for the trashcan), but occasionally she'd tell me that I really ought to act on the notion.

One idea particularly sticks in my head. I detest feeling cold. I'm not that thrilled about feeling overly hot either; the Canadian spring and fall seasons are by far my favourites. I prefer temperate, rainy, foggy days and my photography archives certainly reflect that.

Wouldn't it be a great idea to invent a vest that's battery operated for warmth, just like an electric blanket? Deb jumped all over that idea, and every time I mentioned it she urged me to pursue the concept further.

Jump ahead fifteen years, and I'm going through one of my experimental ECD treatments. And I'm cold. Not just chilled, but iced down to the bone. Walking around the house wearing a blanket tightly wound around me even though it's on the cusp-of-officially-being-summer kind of cold.

I was already in pretty dire financial straits by this time, about to be without a home, and with absolutely no income other than the proceeds of a garage sale (a whopping $263) to get me and Suz through who knew how many months ahead.

Time to kick that electric vest idea into gear!

That high lasted all of the two minutes I needed to search the Internet to see if someone else had the same idea.

They had, about three years earlier. Had I acted on my creation way back when, I might have had a good ten years or more of raking in the big bucks.

Of course, chances are that would never have come about, but it gives me pause sometimes to think about the ideas that got away from me.

Now I'm going to pass the baton over. Something needs inventing, and it needs inventing badly. Somebody please invent it, and make a gazillion dollars in the process. Put a little aside for charities, I have some names of wonderful organizations to offer up.

Wireless oxygen delivery. I know, I know, a crazy idea. But perhaps one day people like me might be able to free themselves of the long tether and put away those heavy portable tanks.

One of my visitors this week is a brilliant man whom I've known since he was a brilliant boy, before we started kindergarten. Stefan agreed that technology needs to catch up in order to adequately power a tiny oxygen concentrator, but it's not out of the realm of possibility.

So go forth. Make the big bucks and help millions of patients who like me are tired of feeling like an animal on a lead. And make sure my friend Deb gets a commission out of it, will you?

WHEN THE RUBBER HITS THE ROAD
Friday, June 28, 2013

Not one of us can escape the reality that our lives will come to an end. We'll all die, whether it comes quickly without warning, or we're given time to deal with what's to come.

Given that it's something we all must experience, why is it so difficult to talk about?

I should clarify that. It's become commonplace to see advertising for life insurance, cemetery plots, funeral services, and crematoriums – the death part. When death is seen as something not to be worried about until far off into the future it doesn't seem so ominous to most.

What we seem to struggle with is the time leading up to death when it's known to be not that far off. On one hand, we're encouraged to write a will, appoint powers of attorney, and decide what we would want for ourselves should serious illness be something that we're faced with.

Does it matter what we want for ourselves? It ought to. In my humble opinion, it ought to matter very much. I believe very strongly that we should have a say in how we want the end of our lives to play out. Whether your wish is to have every reasonable measure taken to prolong your life, or your wish is to have little to no intervention to alter the course of your illness (or something between the two), you have a right to speak up for what you deem to be best for yourself.

When dealing with end of life, so many choices are already taken away from us. Serious illness can rob us of our physical abilities, our mobility, our sense of wellbeing, our security, our freedom, our livelihood, our finances, our dignity, our dreams and plans for the future, and even the company of our family and friends while we're still here. I personally have been hit on each of these fronts – on some harder than others. And serious illness can, and likely will, offer significant consequences in the lives of our loved ones. I need only look into my daughter's eyes to see how deeply it hurts her to watch me deteriorate in this way, and recognize how my illness has turned her life upside down.

If I haven't yet made myself clear, I am a strong supporter of end-of-life options. I embrace the possibility of a gentle death for myself. We know with certainty that I'm not going to get better – every week that passes becomes more challenging. My daughter and many close friends have made it known that they understand and support my position on the matter. The difficult events of the past week (a meeting with my palliative support team, and numerous conversations leading up to it) have only strengthened my conviction for a gentle death to be an option available for all Canadians at end of life.

Recent announcements by the Ontario government suggest that this province may soon follow in Quebec's footsteps (where introduction of the bill to the legislature was welcomed with a standing ovation) in bringing forth legislation to permit physician-assisted death. I applaud this move, as do many other Canadians, if the polls are accurate.

Wherever you sit on this issue, I would encourage you to watch a movie entitled, *How to Die in Oregon*. Not yet available on Netflix Canada, but it can be rented/purchased on iTunes. If you're visiting me and want to see it, I have a copy and would watch the movie again. I'll provide the tissues.

Even if physician-assisted death is not what you would choose for yourself, is it something that as a society we want to deny to those who are suffering with terminal illness who desire a gentle end to their suffering?

I'm not even sure if a physician-assisted death is what I would choose for myself if it were available, but I would find great comfort in knowing that it was legally available should I feel unable to tolerate the circumstances of my illness any longer.

This is a contentious issue, and I wish no disrespect to anyone whose personal beliefs are contrary to my own. I do ask however to be respected for my own experiences of walking in these shoes. When the rubber hits the road, you may (and perhaps unexpectedly so) find yourself wanting to have options available to you should you be dealt a terminal prognosis coupled with unrelenting pain and suffering.

FLOATING
Tuesday, July 02, 2013

I write about the good, bad, and ugly of progressing through this illness. Tonight, I bring to you the stoned. Yup, this new medication has me completely whacked-out high. It's not doing a thing for the pain yet; I've been told that adjusting to this new medication (Gabapentin) could take a few weeks.

I have mixed feelings about trying yet another medication that is experimental. Gabapentin is used for nerve pain and we'll have to wait and see if it's at all effective for bone pain. In the meantime, I'm feeling doped-up and sleepy. At least one good thing has come out of it; I've had a few nights of decent sleep.

It's perplexing to me why anyone purposely takes drugs to get high. I don't wish to pass judgement, do whatever floats your boat as long as others aren't hurt in the process. I, however, quite detest knowing that my brain isn't working with all pistons firing. It's distressing to know that my judgement is impaired; that I'm not able to fully take in all that is going on around me right now.

It scares me silly that Erdheim-Chester disease can spread to the brain. If given the choice between having brain impairment or the physical bone pain that I experience, I'll keep the bone pain without hesitation. It's frightening to think that one day I might experience both.

An important component of my care plan is knowing that I have two people whom I trust implicitly as my powers of attorney for my medical care. These are people who love me, and will do whatever is necessary to ensure that I'm as comfortable as possible if I'm unable to make decisions for myself.

Before posting this, I'll be having it proofread to make sure that I'm not offering drivel to you. Then I can go back to staring at the wall for a few hours. I do hope this phase passes soon; I really do have better ways to use my waking hours.

BRINGING THE OUTSIDE WORLD IN
Wednesday, July 03, 2013

My nurse Annelies was here for her regular visit this afternoon when we heard the distant rumble of thunder. Although I was in the midst of my medication-induced haze (which wears off after four or five hours, I'm losing my patience with this adjustment period!) I smiled broadly. She asked what had brought the grin to my face.

I explained that with endless days looking at the same bedroom walls and a small patch of sky in my sightline through the window, a thunderstorm was something to be welcomed – a change of scenery as dark clouds roll in; the smell of the lightning; the crackle and boom of the thunder. I've always loved thunderstorms. Since I was old enough to let myself out of the house, I'd head straight for the front porch or balcony to take in the drama of a storm.

Of course I can't run outside anymore when a storm approaches, but I love that if she's here, my daughter will watch the storm with me through that small patch of window, hoping that we'll catch a glimpse of a lightning strike.

My daughter does some truly amazing things in trying to bring the outside world to me. She's always had a rich vocabulary and she uses it to describe with as much detail as possible what she knows I would have enjoyed seeing for myself, but can't.

We have two cats now. Scrabble, whom I introduced to you when I adopted him in November, and Mia, who was Suzanna's faithful companion during her second year away at university.

The two cats don't get along. Plain and simple, Mia wants nothing to do with the younger, rambunctious Scrabble. We've had to get creative to allow each to have his or her own space in this small apartment.

Occasionally the two find themselves in close proximity, often under some rather hilarious circumstances. Suzanna runs for her phone, documents the moment with a snapshot, and comes running to show me.

It may seem like a small and perhaps insignificant gesture; to me these glimpses of the world outside of this room are very much appreciated. I hear the constant hum (in reality a whole lot louder than that) of life going on in a world that I'm unable to participate in. Normalcy can sometimes seem so very far away. Trying to remember what it was like to walk up a flight of stairs effortlessly, to drive to a photo shoot, to chop ingredients for a favourite recipe. What did it feel like to put on a favourite outfit and walk around in heels, to throw a ball back to the neighbour's son, to sit at a table for a meal? Those moments seem so very far away.

I could allow myself to be miserable in remembering all that I can't do, instead I try (and usually succeed) in appreciating what Suzanna and others can show me of their world. Please keep it coming, reminders of the outside world are what help me to cope with being confined within these four walls with my view of a small patch of bare sky.

And for those times when I'm not successful in pushing away the reminders of what is no longer possible? My daughter quickly comes to me with a kiss for my forehead, expressing her wish to make it all better if she could. At those moments, the outside world melts away and all that matters is right in front of me.

SIX DAYS WERE ENOUGH
Friday, July 05, 2013

Another medication experiment gone awry. The Gabapentin proved to be an abysmal failure. Not only did the pain increase (the bone pain remained, and in addition I developed pain similar to the shin splints I experienced back in my very short and rather insignificant track and field heyday, doing hurdles), but I also zombied out for long periods of time between doses.

The clincher for me happened yesterday when I found myself so out of it that I was unable to reach for the phone when my Sue called from out west, where her job currently has her stationed. It wasn't exhaustion; it was the inability to figure out what was ringing and what to do about it. I was so stoned that over the course of the week I couldn't have told you for the better part of my waking hours whether it was morning or afternoon, whether I had just woken up or was ready for bed, if I was hungry or had just eaten. Poor Suzanna was almost as frustrated as I was with my lack of awareness and my inability to focus on anything more complicated than the hem of the bed sheet, save for a few hours each day as a dose would wear off and I readied myself for the next one.

A totally unsatisfactory condition for me to be in, this is not a state of mind I wish to visit – much less live in, if given a choice. I understood that disorientation might come into play for the first few days, but it was only getting worse and dangerously so. The last thing I want for myself is to become unable to communicate with my daughter and friends; this last week brought with it a deep sense of isolation.

I've brought forward my views on dying with dignity, and this is another instance where I believe that each patient should be allowed to make choices best suited for them. The acceptance and refusal of treatments should be a major part of this discussion.

Are the patient's wishes always respected? I'm saddened to say that from personal experience this is not always the case. Far too much of whatever energy I have available is spent discussing this issue with others who have a say in the direction of my care, but don't have to live in my shoes. Let me add that the majority of my palliative team are supportive and nurturing, but there are a few horizons yet to be broadened.

For now, I need to deal with the disappointment that yet another pain-relief strategy hasn't worked. I'm used to this and have learned not to set high expectations, however, it's impossible not to feel some sadness over yet another medication that didn't help.

LEARNING HOW TO DO THIS
Saturday, July 06, 2013

About two years ago, a client, who has since become a good friend, called out of the blue.

She'd heard that my health was poor and wanted to extend her support and friendship, for which I'm grateful. We spent several hours on the phone that evening, and after catching up, she offered a suggestion for a TV show that I might enjoy watching called *The Big C*. She cautioned me that although a show about a woman dying of cancer might seem like a strange recommendation for someone in my state of declining health, she was certain that I would appreciate its message.

Spoiler Alert – if you haven't watched the show and wish to, you might want to stop reading at this point. Or not. That's the nice thing about getting a heads up; you can make your own choices. Not a random thought, it does have relevance to the rest of this post.

I've watched Seasons 1-3, laughing and sobbing my way along. There have been so many moments that have resonated with me, and some that I wish I could have related to. Some episodes needed a second or third viewing, in order for me to look past my initial gut reaction.

Cathy Jamison (played by Laura Linney) is dying, and is keenly aware of how limited her chances for survival are. She's mother to an only child, a son close in age to Suzanna. She has a husband who stands staunchly by her side through thick and thin – even though that road isn't necessarily travelled at the same speed by the two of them. The overwhelming weight of me doing this without an adult partner can be crushing (my best friend's unrelenting support notwithstanding, but there is a difference that she herself knows leaves a hole). For that reason, the show has been especially hard at times to digest. Suzanna is of tremendous support to me but I can never lose sight of the fact that she is my child, and it's up to me as her parent not to look to her for comfort when I am afraid. She has already had to grow up way too quickly, and bears more responsibility and fear than I would ever want anyone to place on her. Least of all me, yet here we are.

I've learned how to do much of this from Cathy Jamison. Learned how to ask for help, learned how to grieve, and learned how to make choices that are best for me and my daughter. Learned that it's okay to challenge my medical team when I need more information or something doesn't seem quite right. Learned how to answer questions (or sometimes how to dodge ones I'd rather not address), learned that unconditional love is indeed what rescues me when I'm feeling weakened, ugly, and diseased.

There's no question about it – this all sucks. The circumstances have little wiggle room, but my attitude is completely within my control.

I'm in the process of downloading Season 4, the last in the series. Eight hours of what is bound to be a roller coaster ride for me, I'm planning on tackling the last of *The Big C* in one go this evening while Suzanna is out. She doesn't need to watch as I process this, it likely won't be pretty.

I've already tripped upon a season finale spoiler online; Cathy's fate is much what I had expected. I'm not upset by this discovery; in fact I think it helps set me up for being able to relate more closely to her character. What additional lessons I'll have learned by the time the final credits roll remain to be seen.

I'm prepared – a full box of tissues and an open heart. Much emotion has been building up over the last few weeks with events that haven't gone well. I suspect that this will be just what I need to release it. Heads up.

THE FINAL SEASON
Monday, July 08, 2013

My *The Big C* marathon a few days ago? I'm grateful that I was mistaken in that it was only four hours, not eight. I don't think I could have handled more; I doubt there was a tear left in me to cry out. In the first half hour alone, I hit pause three times to give me time to deal with my feelings about the storyline.

What did I get from the final season? A somewhat diminished feeling of isolation, yet at the same time very much a heightened one. It sounds contradictory I know.

I could identify very closely with Laura Linney's character and the ordeals she faced; it was astounding just how many correlations there were to my own life. It felt like the writers had crawled into my head and it was more than disconcerting to watch what felt like my own life unfolding. Or perhaps more accurately, folding.

I cried uncontrollably when the main character was acknowledging the utter sadness of what she will miss in her child's life. With that came the reminders of my fears about who will be there for my daughter when I'm gone, when so many seem to have difficulty being around our situation while I'm still here. My disease may not be contagious, but I suspect that the fear of death just might be.

The hardest part of watching the end of the series was how prolonged the dying process was for Cathy Jamison. She would be in a great deal of discomfort and pain, looking like it was close to the end – yet two months, four months, six months later she'd still be hanging in.

Even when Cathy decided that she no longer wished to continue treatment; that she was in every way ready to let go, her body still didn't release her. I don't think that anyone who isn't living this scenario can understand the mental fatigue that comes with living like this.

For those of you who might be thinking, geez – Sandy's still here? I thought that her prognosis was supposed to have her on her way out quite a while ago?

It's not for lack of letting go. Although I sobbed harder than I have in a very long time at the final scene (if you know my family situation you'll understand why it was a heartbreaker for me), knowing that everyone close to Cathy could finally pull out of the limbo that they'd been in for years brought to me a sigh of relief.

Going forward, we have to do better for our dying. Although Cathy had advocates in her husband and brother and I'm doing the legwork myself, she, like me, ran into brick wall after brick wall with bureaucracy and others' fears of bending the rules in the name of compassion. Truly, we must do much better than this.

UNFINISHED, IMPERFECT WORKS
Wednesday, July 10, 2013

I've always admired Dustin Hoffman. With every interview I see, I think more highly of him as a person. He's an actor who has the courage to use the voice given to him as a celebrity to speak out on issues that concern him; a man who isn't afraid to point out his own flaws and foibles. A man who isn't afraid to show that he's as human as the rest of us.

I watched a video clip a few days ago, from an interview from last year in which he spoke about his preparation for his role in the movie, *Tootsie*.

If you haven't yet seen this clip, I'd encourage you to do so. Although he's speaking to the issue of how women are measured on their perceived level of outer beauty, it's a discussion that could easily be about biases in regards to race, sexuality, and disability.

It's days since I first watched it, and I'm finding it difficult to let this one out of my head. Wondering what wonderful souls I might have missed out on getting to know in my lifetime because I made snap judgements for whatever reason.

Many a time I've found myself in the position of being deemed lacking by someone else; who hasn't? I could give you numerous examples, but you probably have many of your own to draw upon. Not beautiful/handsome enough, not smart enough, not clever enough, not the "right" colour, not of the "right" faith, not of the "right" sexual orientation, not of the "right" level of income or education. The list goes on.

My physical disabilities proved (in the outside world) to be yet another reason to be overlooked and dismissed. I don't miss that at all. To many strangers, I was deemed unworthy of being acknowledged or being looked in the eye.

I generally would think to myself that if I had been dismissed so easily by a stranger for not being "enough" of whatever, then that person wasn't worth knowing.

And then there are moments like when I watched this video and I am reminded that everyone has room to grow their appreciation of others. (Whether they care to take that opportunity to expand their hearts is another matter.) I appreciate that Dustin Hoffman was humble enough to admit that he could have done better, and that he intended to do so going forward after his experience. Isn't that called growing up? I'm grateful to have friends who have the wisdom to know that none of us ever truly finish that process. The learning about ourselves and the world beyond never ends.

LINES IN THE SAND
Sunday, July 14, 2013

I can't remember which show I was watching last week when I heard a police officer, speaking about a suspect in a murder case who had cancer, say to another, "Don't let him surprise you, he's dying and has nothing to lose."

It turns out the suspect wasn't the culprit, but that line has stuck in my head and has come to mind when faced with a few dilemmas over the last week. Does the fact that I'm nearing the end of my life influence my actions and decisions? Certainly in regards to choices I have to make about my medical care, it's been a very busy week on that front with more ahead in the coming days.

I'd told myself that I was never going to be in a hospital again if it could be helped. But a doctor has proposed a high-risk procedure that could ease my pain, and I find myself leaning towards going for it. It does mean revising my plan to avoid hospitals, but given a rather compelling possible beneficial outcome, it deserves discussion between me and my daughter. I'll share the details once we've made a decision. For now, we need to weigh the pros and cons presented by my medical team without any outside influence.

Knowing that I have limited time dictates evaluation of personal situations as well. I'd like more of what makes me happy, and a whole lot less of what makes me unhappy. Who wouldn't? This week, I was presented with a surprising number of options, given the limitations that my physical disabilities throw in my way.

My friend Deb I were so wrapped up in great conversation this afternoon that we lost track of time. She found herself running late in picking up a family member. As she reached for her phone, Deb said that the family member would understand the delay, given that it was me who was being visited. I jokingly added, "The dying person trumps all."

Not that I should take precedence over others; I'm still the me who wants to make everyone happy and not raise any conflict. But I have, and will speak up because my lines in the sand are moving. Some are being drawn in more firmly, other erased. What I'm not prepared to do anymore is let someone else tell me where my lines should be drawn – that I've done far too much in my life. I have nothing to lose anymore, except for my inner peace if I've not spoken up for what I believe to be the best for me and my daughter.

BITE BY BITE
Monday, July 15, 2013

One rough day, or rather another rough day. It's been weeks of intermittent, low-grade fever and chills on top of the other shenanigans that my body has been up to. (And enough with the hiccoughs already!) It truly can get quite tiresome.

My friends and volunteers consistently offer to bring me whatever edible treats might appeal to me, yet I can't think of anything in particular that I want. I did have one coincidence a few weeks ago. Minutes before a food volunteer arrived, I told Suzanna that I was hankering for some mashed potatoes – lucky me, that was exactly what the volunteer had prepared. Serious comfort food. Seeing as I'm mostly on soft foods and liquids now with a wonky esophagus that doesn't always cooperate, a little butter (okay, a lot of butter) is a welcome addition to help slide spoonfuls of mashed potatoes on their way.

This evening, I passed on Suzanna's offer to prepare dinner for me before she went out for a few hours. The thought of food just doesn't appeal to me. Some of you might want to suggest that I should eat anyways, but I know from experience it's best to leave well enough alone. My body will tell me what it needs – I have to trust it.

Others have expressed regret on my behalf for the foods I've had to give up either due to allergies or a rapidly expanding list of intolerances, but surprisingly I generally don't feel deprived. Who knew there were so many varieties of delicious soups on offer?

I can think back fondly on foods that I've enjoyed over the years without feeling upset about missing out. It's not difficult to remember the tastes, textures, and aromas – I was without doubt someone who lived to eat, rather than having eaten to live.

A NIGHT I DON'T WANT TO REPEAT
Friday, July 19, 2013

I jinxed myself when I wrote last week that I had hoped to never visit a hospital again. That's exactly where I found myself two nights ago, in the dreaded emergency ward. I'd been able to stay out of there for almost two years, but unfortunately my body conspired against me.

It was a very difficult decision to make in the middle of the night. (Suzanna was away at her father's for the night, upon my urging to give her a break from caring for me.) I'd been feeling particularly unwell for the previous few days; a fever that's stuck with me for weeks was getting worse. The chest pain had migrated to a new spot in my chest, and dehydration was setting in. By the time I called for help, first to my on-call nurse who recommended that I call 911 immediately, it was hard to even blink my eyes or swallow for the lack of moisture in my body.

What happened next might seem funny in the future, but not just yet. The paramedics were given my lockbox code to get into my apartment; they said that they'd had to fiddle with the lock in order to get in. Once they'd gotten me settled into the stretcher, an IV running (finding a viable blood vessel was fifteen minutes of stress – more so for them) we tried to leave the apartment. The door wouldn't open.

A second fire truck/team had to be summoned to break the door open from the outside to let us out. A very long fifteen minutes for all of us. In my experience, I've never seen an emergency professional lose their cool in a stressful situation, and these gentlemen never let on if they felt for even a moment that they were losing control of the situation.

Feeling so ill, I didn't care in the least that we were leaving the apartment open. I just needed to feel better if it were at all possible.

Our local emergency department, save for one very impressive doctor who took over my care in the morning, lived up to my expectations based on previous visits to that ward. It didn't start out well, the first doctor to see me was the same one who three years ago, after I landed in emergency with severe breathing difficulties, asked me if I had "decided" that

I had ECD by researching symptoms on the Internet. Coincidentally, one of the paramedics who picked me up this week remembered that he was also with me on that night three years ago. He was so sweet on both visits, this time holding my hand while his partner did my intake work with triage.

While the ER was letting me down, my body wasn't exactly living up to my expectations either. One nurse was able to get a small amount of blood out of a vein a few hours after I arrived but the quantity was insufficient for the lab. Four nurses then made a total of close to twenty attempts to access a vein without success, until the second doctor finally put a stop to it. It didn't hurt me, but he just couldn't watch it any longer. Who knew that they could try to draw blood from a thumb?

I could write chapters on what went wrong at the hospital that night and yesterday. Firsthand experience as to how my palliative status altered what many will already know to be a challenging situation of visiting the emergency department. The worst part was the look in my daughter's eyes when she arrived the next morning, seeing firsthand the pain and indignities that I was experiencing. There's fear that this visit might not be the last to the emergency ward, despite my wishes to avoid it. If I thought that I dreaded it before, it's nothing compared to how much the thought of a return visit scares me now.

THE WICKED NIGHT, PART 2
Sunday, July 21, 2013

I mentioned a few days ago that I'd had a rough time at the local emergency ward. In hindsight, another lesson for me in learning how to do better in asking for help.

Let me first say that I'm well aware of the fact that hospitals are understaffed. Many team members have to cut corners in order to get to all the patients. There are fewer checks on the patient, hygiene and health safety protocols are compromised, or information isn't passed along or documented appropriately. Charts not reviewed thoroughly. (I have serious drug allergies, if I hadn't been somewhat on the ball Wednesday night, things could have been even worse!)

Let me also add that it was my decision not to ask Suzanna or a friend to meet me at the hospital in the middle of the night. Many have offered to come if I need them, but my wish to allow the people I care about to get a good night of sleep won over.

I was admitted with severe dehydration, brought on by ongoing renal issues. I know my body well enough by this time to know exactly what I need. Rehydration (by this time I was well beyond doing this orally) and anti-emetics to get the nausea under control. I take some responsibility, my anti-emetics have an uncomfortable side effect and I held off too long with taking them at home, hoping that'd I'd rally. It's a simple equation, and not to get graphic, but output of liquids greatly exceeding input equals trouble.

The IV drip had been started by one of the paramedics while I was still at home, at the hospital a nurse moved the saline bag to a stand well above my head.

I was placed in a room by myself with a heavy door; no monitors, no call button. I was too weak to get up in the first place, and my IV tube was not long enough to get the door open by myself anyway. Over the course of a few hours, when I realized that the level on the saline bag was not dropping at all, I resorted to calling for help. I just wasn't feeling that all-too-familiar coolness of the saline solution flowing into my vein. On top of that, my blood was flowing up into the tube.

When a nurse finally arrived, he dismissed my concerns – telling me that because of my cardiac issues they had me on a very slow drip.

An hour later, I again called for help, shouting into the hallways at 3 a.m. as much as my weakened voice would allow, insisting that things were not okay. If I thought that I was dehydrated earlier, I knew things now had potential to become critical. I had missed my dose of cardiac arrhythmia meds on top of it, something I've had stern warnings in the past not to mess with. Again, I was told I was being impatient.

It wasn't until another hour later when a different nurse came by to make a second unsuccessful attempt at gathering a blood sample that she actually looked at the IV tubing and bag. I'd indeed been not getting fluids, or the anti-emetics that began to help me feel a bit better not long after, when they finally started flowing.

It was when I had a bit more strength that I had the courage to address what had happened directly with the first nurse. We ended up having a long conversation about, speaking for myself only, my needs as a palliative patient. I spoke about how the emergency ward was truly the very last place I wanted to be, and that given a lengthy serious illness, I had a pretty good idea of what I needed. I needed measures taken to make me feel more comfortable so that I could go home again. What I heard in reply was a plea to speak up on behalf of the nurses, to help their cause. Sorry friend, I really feel for you – but my energy has to be directed towards my own care.

What happened in between was simply awful. I pray that it was my last visit to emergency. When a patient considers that in the future, the lesser evil to be possibly dying at home in a great deal of discomfort and mess – there is something really wrong with the system.

I've just passed what I've come to learn by experience to be the critical seventy-two hours after discharge from the hospital. This is the time during which if I've picked up an infection in the hospital, it would have likely shown itself.

If there is a next time, I apologize in advance, but I will be asking someone to come with me. And I'd encourage any of you to do the same, instead of trying to not be an inconvenience to a friend or family member. I've said it before and I'll say it again – it's too risky to go through the system without an advocate.

A special thanks to my wonderful neighbours, who upon learning of my trip to the hospital via my blog, wrote me a lovely note, insisting that I need go no farther than one door down when I need help. Angels everywhere.

IN EVERY SENSE
Thursday, July 25, 2013

Thank you to the friends who expressed concern when this blog got quiet this week. Some physical and personal challenges have been exhausting me. Allow me to share some brighter highlights, which did an excellent job of chasing away the tougher moments of the past week.

A few visitors truly brightened my week: Deb, who I'd not seen in a very long time, with distance between us having been a major obstacle, and Kristee, who shared her birthday with me yesterday.

Not to mention several friends, old and new, who made it clear that they could be called upon to accompany me/Suz to the hospital should I ever need to go to emergency again. My account seemed to have scared some of you almost as much as it scared me (and I'd even left the worst of it out to spare you the uncomfortable details).

On that note – let me once again say how much I appreciate my palliative nurses, most of all my lead nurse, Annelies. Upon hearing of my ordeal at the hospital last week, she spoke with my doctor immediately to order in supplies so that we can accomplish rehydration here at home the next time I get into trouble. I thought I was fairly well educated on medical protocols; I was delighted to learn that if a vein can't be located, rehydration can be done through a subcutaneous needle into the fatty tissue instead. That part I can provide, I'm not exactly packing abs of steel these days! I guess I'm not as prepared for my med-school entrance exam as I had thought.

A NEW HOME DECOR ITEM
Sunday, July 28, 2013

With my nursing team's persistence in making sure we do our best to keep me out of the emergency ward, I received a delivery last night at dinnertime (on a Saturday no less) of the IV equipment. When the palliative team comes through with help, they go all out!

Suzanna met the delivery person at the door, and in came a rather substantial IV pole and several large boxes. She hasn't opened the boxes yet, save for putting one bag into the fridge as she'd been directed to do.

As curious as I am as to know what's inside (I would have thought that several bags of saline, tubing, and syringes could easily have fit in half of one of the large boxes), I'll leave it to my nurse to sort through when she visits tomorrow.

I'm grateful that I'm being looked after so well, but several thoughts come to mind. Where on earth are we going to put all these supplies? Every nook, drawer, and cupboard has been filled. The oxygen concentrator and tanks already take up floor space; my crisis kit has taken over the fridge. There's just nowhere to put two huge boxes of more supplies.

The second thought is how this apartment long ago stopped looking remotely close to a normal home. Not that it ever truly did; I didn't have the strength to properly unpack when I moved in last September, so much remains in boxes. From the moment of approach to the front door where a sign boldly states that oxygen is in use, the apartment shrieks out that a sick person lives here: a wheelchair at the entry, machines whirring, oxygen tubing snaking down the hall, safety devices in the bathroom.

Now the IV pole. I'm not even sure how it's going to fit into the bedroom, much less wheel through the doorway into the bathroom. The simple answer is that it's not – I'll leave that to your imagination as to how we're going to tackle that dilemma.

The one thing that makes this all manageable in my head today is the knowledge that the IV is not meant to be a permanent measure at this time, only as an occasional procedure when I need rehydration. At least I'm praying that it's occasional, that's up to my kidneys to decide how that plays out.

What to do with the IV pole when it's not in use? Well, we've let our imaginations run as to how to incorporate it into the apartment decor.

Coat rack? Drying stand for fine washables? Year-round Christmas tree? Hang cured salamis from it? Magazine rack? Monkey bars for the cats? Monkey bars for me?

As much as I appreciate that my team is trying so hard to keep me here at home as long as possible, today everything is just a little too much in my face for my liking.

SLEEPY TIME, SORT OF
Tuesday, August 06, 2013

I've been reminded a few times today that there's been a longer than usual break since my last post. I'm still here!

There's been quite a bit going on around here, though nothing that I felt particularly moved to write about. The IV pole and pump that had been delivered were taken away again just a few days later. (Funding was not approved for full-time residency of the equipment in our apartment. Where oh where will I now hang the cured salami?)

Tomorrow morning more medical supplies arrive – catheter kits to be implemented as needed. Probably more than you really needed to know, but that's my reality. This isn't pretty and certainly isn't much fun. It gets less enjoyable with every week that passes.

In preferring to avoid getting into the unsettling details of my physical health tonight, I thought I'd dive into my "blog notes," emails that I've sent to myself when a blog post idea occurs to me but I'm not in a position to write it up at that moment. Usually because it's in the middle of the night and I'm trying hard to enforce a no-technology rule between 3 a.m. and 9 a.m. I may be wide-awake, but it makes my friends feel better if they believe I've had a decent night of sleep. Mind you, in emailing myself I did utilize technology so I'm obviously not doing a great job of sticking to my guns.

Note from July 16th, time stamp of 4:34 a.m. "Not finishing bubbl witch." (sic) I read this over a few times wondering what I might have meant. (I never said that I was coherent in the middle of the night.) I finally remembered, but it's an irrelevant point to me at this moment.

I do get a few hours of sleep each night, yet even then it appears that my mind is keeping quite busy. I remember vivid dreams, but I also talk in my sleep. I have conversations with Suzanna, hearing her end, and replying with no recollection the next morning of what we discussed. We've started recording my sleeping hours. Here's a gem from the other night.

Suz at 3:22 a.m. heard, "Are you trying to wake me?"

"No, why?" she asks.

"It sounded like a thumb trying to wake a finger."

If anyone knows what a restless thumb might sound like, do let me know. We're days later still laughing when we think about where that exchange might have gone had I kept talking. There's plenty more where that came from, I'm sorry to admit. Conversations about fried chicken (surprising coming from me, I have an anaphylactic allergy to poultry and haven't eaten it on purpose in about twenty-five years), about potential death brought on by my arm that fell asleep, asking Suz if she's cooking Chinese food (she wasn't, apparently I misinterpreted the stink of skunk wafting in from outside) and then telling her I was too tired to chew any food anyway.

Tonight? Talk of travel would be a nice change. And so would remembering it.

LESSONS FROM A FRIEND
Saturday, August 10, 2013

Last year for my birthday, my daughter gave me a gift of the audio book version of *The Five People You Meet in Heaven* by Mitch Albom. I often think about the messages of this book, and on another by Mitch Albom entitled, *Tuesdays With Morrie*. If there's one upside to a slow demise, it's the opportunity to reflect on one's life experiences. Where have I found my purpose? Did I find it at all? Did my actions during this lifetime make any difference?

Before I go on, I'd like to make it clear that I'm not looking for answers to these questions from anybody other than from myself. I'm not seeking validation; there are other reasons for this post being written.

Should I have the privilege of ending up in Heaven, there are a few people I'd like to meet up with again. One is a woman I knew many years ago for a relatively short time. I'll call her Sarah.

When I had just turned twenty (just a few months older than Suzanna is now) I found myself having trouble walking. My legs would buckle from underneath me at the most inopportune times. I was often feeling weak, my balance was off, and I was experiencing odd vision problems combined with episodes of vertigo.

I was, at the time, attending my second year of university. It would have been reasonable to suggest that stress might have been a factor, I'd not had any financial support to attend school from either my family or from student loans. (Thankfully, the rules have since changed. At the time, even though I'd already been living on my own for several years and was completely independent, my father's level of income as reported to Revenue Canada rendered me ineligible for education loans.) I was not only attending school full-time, I was also working a minimum of forty hours a week, waiting tables at a pizza place to make ends meet. I'm not sure how he even fit into my life, but I was also maintaining a relationship with a boyfriend who'd been an important part of my life for the previous two years.

After I made a few visits to my doctor, the doctor determined that we were dealing with more than just exhaustion. I was admitted immediately to the hospital for tests and observation. I've previously mentioned that I've had health issues throughout my adulthood; this is where it all began. Who is to know whether this was the early manifestation of Erdheim-Chester Disease? I suppose an autopsy will offer more information as to the history of this illness in my body.

As is the case now too, hospital beds were scarce and the only spot that could be found was in the pediatric ward. Not having any private insurance, I ended up in a four-bed unit. Two of the other patients were in their early teens; the fourth occupant was another adult who'd also landed in the kids' ward thanks to a bed shortage.

This woman was in her mid-twenties, blond and slight, and the day I arrived had just come out of major surgery. She was obviously in a great deal of pain for several days afterwards, and it wasn't until later in the week that I'd learn more about her. I'll call her Sarah to honour her privacy.

Sarah had a doting husband who would be at her bedside as often as visiting hours would permit. Other members of his family would often stop by, hoping that they could tempt her appetite with delicious treats.

I'd learn, once her pain had subsided a bit, that Sarah had cancer. She was a DES daughter, the cancer brought on by her mother having been prescribed a drug during pregnancy that had been believed to lessen the chances of miscarriage. It was discovered in the early '70s that this drug was linked to a high rate of cancer in the daughters of these pregnancies. Sarah was one of the very unlucky ones.

She and I ended up being in that hospital ward together for almost four weeks. It's not important to this story, but I was diagnosed with probable relapse/remitting type Multiple Sclerosis – a diagnosis that I carried for over twenty years until ECD was confirmed. Those weeks in hospital consisted of multitudes of diagnostic tests with plenty of time in between them, waiting for results. During those long hours, Sarah and I shared many lengthy and complicated conversations.

Sarah had had a radical hysterectomy, in hopes of removing all the cancerous cells. Her time spent in the hospital was in recovery from the surgery with no further treatment plans. Ultimately, she wanted to go back home to the tiny apartment she shared with her husband.

To ease Sarah's discomfort, the nurses would draw a bath for her and Sarah would invite me to keep her company at the side of the tub. In the bathwater, she told me all about her life. Since she had a few years on me, I thought her worldly and wise and was honoured that she trusted me with the details of her life. Looking back, there were so many similarities in our life experiences that it feels as if we had been destined to meet.

Back in our room, things were different. We were kitty corner across from each other, and with the other patients in the room, communicating was difficult. Between facial expressions, hand gestures, and occasionally with hand written notes passed between us, courtesy of the nurses, our friendship strengthened. This is, of course, well before the time of texting and emails; I can only imagine how furiously rapid the communication would have been, had today's technology been available at the time.

Once we were both released from the hospital, we kept up our relationship. In the first few months, I would visit her and her husband often. Sarah loved to knit, and would always have her hands busy with her latest creation as we caught up. She, her husband, and his family were a welcoming clan; I was often invited to family events with his parents and siblings.

A few months later, I raised the white flag on my education. I'd fallen too far behind in my classes after a month away, and realized that there was no possible way to maintain both full-time school and full-time work. I left university, and with what was remaining in my stash of accumulated education funds, I set off to backpack by myself across Europe.

My first destination was Paris, a city I wish I'd had the opportunity to get to know as well as I came to know Toronto, but I'm grateful I got there at all. Three times in fact, the second trip being important to this story. On my European adventure, I also visited my mother and her boyfriend, who were living in Italy at the time, and I stopped in to spend time with relatives in Germany too. The rest of the time I spent getting the best possible value from my Eurail pass. (Do they still have those?)

After some months I returned, only to find that my boyfriend of close to three years wanted to end our relationship. Absence doesn't always make the heart grow fonder, and in hindsight I can't blame him, we were on very different paths; his well-defined, mine uncertain.

For a while I felt afloat, not knowing what road to follow. Wallowing in my uncertain future, I abandoned many friendships, including the one with Sarah. There would be the occasional phone call and she'd often invite me to visit but I rarely did. Sarah was not doing well and I was afraid to see her, afraid that I'd say the wrong thing. Confident that her loving husband and his wonderful family would be looking after all her needs, my excuse was that my visits would exhaust her.

Jump forward another year. By this time, I'd taken a course to be certified as a travel consultant, was working for an agency, and was in a relationship with the man that would become my first husband, and Suzanna's father.

Professionally I was doing well. The pay was lousy but at the time, the travel benefits for agents were fantastic and I was taking full advantage. Through an incentive offer at work, I'd earned two weekend trips away; one to London, England and the second to Paris. The fact that the trips were separated by only three days back in Canada seems, in hindsight, ridiculous. To my early-twenties self – it was adventurous and beyond exciting.

After crossing the Atlantic four times in the space of eleven days, I came back from Paris giddy, but thoroughly exhausted. Yet as soon as the plane touched the ground, I felt something nagging at me. I couldn't put a finger on the reason for the uneasiness.

I made my way back to my apartment, and for reasons I'll never understand yet am so grateful for, I opened up that day's *Toronto Star* and was drawn to the Death Notices. There was Sarah's name; the second night of visitation at the funeral home would be drawing to a close in less than an hour and a half. I quickly changed my clothes, splashed water on my face and headed to midtown from my northwest Toronto apartment.

The look on Sarah's husband's face as I entered the room is still as clear as can be in my mind, to this day. He rushed over, hugged me so tightly, and told me that he'd been trying to reach me for over a week, but didn't have the correct phone number. Sarah had wanted to tell me herself that her death was likely to occur within a few weeks, that she'd wanted to see me before she died.

Rarely a week goes by that I don't think of Sarah. After more than twenty-five years, it still rips at my heart that I'd let our friendship lapse, that I wasn't there for her.

I pray that I do get to see her again. That'll I'll have the chance to tell her what she meant to me, that I loved her. That I had been scared of losing her and avoiding her was the only way I could handle my sadness at the time.

I pray that if I get the chance to see Sarah again, she won't be holding resentment against me for not being there for her at the end. That she'll allow me to tell her that she mattered, and that she taught me lessons that continue to slowly sink in to this day.

Although I never knew Sarah as a "healthy" person, I remember her for her dignity, inner strength, and wonderful sense of dry humour. I'm also grateful that I had the opportunity to see her stubbornness, to learn what sorts of things annoyed her (including me at times!), and to hear stories of her childhood that helped her become the Sarah I only came to know in her last years.

She was so much more than just her cancer. The reality is that I'd never have met her if it hadn't been for her illness, but she let me see beyond that.

I've wanted to write about Sarah ever since I started this blog, I'm not sure why now seemed to be the right time.

I tell this story not because I want to make anyone feel guilty if they've been uncomfortable about getting in touch or visiting. I tell this story because I've stood in the shoes of being overwhelmed by the reality of an illness relentlessly attacking someone I cared about.

I can't predict with any certainty how I'd react if someone else I cared about was diagnosed with terminal illness. I'd like to believe I'd go about things differently, but even being in the position I am now – I just don't know. That's as honest as I can possibly be on the matter.

THURSDAY
Tuesday, August 20, 2013

It's my birthday in two days. I mention this not because I want to drop a hint for you to wish me a Happy Birthday on Thursday, I mention it because I'd rather you didn't.

I'd prefer to ignore the day entirely, and if it weren't for a loving daughter who insists that the occasion be marked in our own way, I would be passing the day as any other.

What complicates things a bit is that Suzanna's birthday falls on the next day; Friday. That day, her twentieth birthday, is of course much cause for celebration. The two birthdays have been intertwined for two decades; it's hard to pull them apart.

We've come to a compromise; she and I. Suzanna booked both days off of work. Thursday will be just for the two of us. No nurses, no PSWs, no visitors, and this may seem unreasonable – no calls, they'll be going to voicemail.

Just the two of us. My birthday wish is to spend my day with my very favourite person. Not celebrating, just being. Spending time with my daughter makes me happier than anything else possibly could, and I expect that she and I will have a lovely day – but I just don't think I have it in me to be wished a Happy Birthday. It's just not going to be a day I wish to be congratulated on.

I don't mean to be petulant, unkind, ungrateful or disrespectful towards friends and family who might normally get in touch. It's just what I need to do for myself and Suzanna. For this last round of birthday togetherness.

Perhaps you might think I'm being pessimistic. What I'm being is realistic. I'm just not going to get to fifty, I'm thoroughly amazed that it looks like I'm even going to get to forty-nine after what my body has been doing to me over the last few weeks. Unless, of course, there's a nasty turn over the next few days, and I don't even make it to forty-nine. I pray for Suzanna's sake that my body doesn't betray us. Wouldn't that just be the ultimate kick in the pants with wanting so badly to be here for her as she leaves her teens?

Suzanna's birthday is another matter entirely. She and I have the morning together, and then James, her dad, and her friends will be making sure that she makes merry. I wouldn't have it any other way. I can't join in but my thoughts will be with her throughout the afternoon and evening.

As much as it has been a fun story to tell over the years about how I went into labour on my birthday and she, apparently, was so determined that she have her own special day that she wasn't born until 9:38 p.m. the next evening – I wish so much right now that our days weren't side by side.

If you happen to be thinking of me on Thursday, instead of getting in touch you'd be doing me a great honour by sending a wish into the wind for my daughter. A wish for a wonderful future, a wish that all of her dreams come true. A wish that the person I have loved most of all has plenty of very special birthdays ahead of her.

A wish that life gives back to her what she has given to me. If that happens for her, she'll indeed be a very lucky woman.

WE GOT THERE
Friday, August 23, 2013

This post goes out not a minute prior to 9:38 p.m. EDT. I'm afraid to jinx something so very important to me.

For those friends who were quiet on my birthday; my heartfelt thanks for honouring my request. For those who reached out to me with cards, emails, phone calls and other surprises – I dearly thank you as well. I appreciate the thoughtfulness from all, in respecting that Suzanna and I were "off the grid" yesterday, in not answering the phone, door, or checking in online.

It was our day, and it was amazing. I didn't go any farther than the ten feet to the bathroom, yet it was easily my most fabulous birthday ever, thanks to my daughter.

Today it's her birthday, her twentieth. She's out celebrating with friends tonight, and hopefully having a wonderful time. I can't wait to hear the highlights of the evening when she rolls in at, well, whenever she's ready to roll in.

Turning twenty isn't typically one of the more celebrated milestones. At eighteen she could vote (and adopt a child apparently!), at nineteen;

legally drink. She's looking forward to her champagne birthday when she turns twenty-three.

Twenty is an important one to me for a different reason. I just couldn't bear the thought of leaving behind a daughter while she was in her teens, and if this post goes up tonight – it means that we made it.

In many ways, she had to become a responsible adult well before now, due to our circumstances (whatever the legal interpretation of adult might be). She's had many experiences that few her age can relate to. She's risen to the occasion time and time again.

Yet despite her maturity, the "teen" at the end of her year of age had riddled me with anxiety. I've had this hanging over my head for months; would I still be here to see this milestone? What would it take to be here with her today? Would I have failed her if I wasn't?

Whatever blessings, faith, determination, and luck were at play, I'm privileged to be able to wish my beautiful and amazing, no-longer-a-teenager as of 9:38 p.m., grownup daughter a birthday to remember fondly.

A REALITY CHECK
Friday, August 30, 2013

I changed the header for the blog. Not only was my listed age no longer accurate, the description had been making me cringe for months: "Trying to maintain a productive and happy life despite being diagnosed with a serious systemic illness with no cure and a poor prognosis."

That sentence was written over four years ago at a time when, with modifications, I led what might have looked from the outside like a fairly typical suburban life – a quality of life that I had anticipated would gradually change as my health declined.

You'd think that in taking four years to get to where I am now that the changes would have seemed gradual, but that's far from the way it feels.

In reality, it's been more like hanging on to a series of ledges leading to the inevitable last one – gripping the edge of each as tightly as I could before having to let myself drop to the next level.

I wanted to keep believing that instead of steep drops, it would be a staircase on which I could occasionally climb back up a step or two to visit for a short while before a permanent change in status.

It's just not the way it's worked out. Talk about some harsh life lessons in accepting realities; the "glass half-full" approach I've always tried to adopt could only take me so far. There's a limit to how much shine anyone can put on a tough situation, regardless of how much of an optimist they might be.

There will be no miracle cure for me – there will be no remission. This only gets more difficult until it stops altogether. I no longer utter the words I used to say at the end of a particularly difficult day, "Tomorrow will be better." Those words have become as useless to me as the physical body I inhabit.

It's not that I'm giving up; rather it's acceptance that I'm no longer strong enough to hold on to a particular ledge anymore. Another day, week, or month passes – another ledge to let go of.

And with a little lot of help from my daughter and my friends, finding the strength to look towards that final ledge. Averting my eyes won't make it disappear.

BLOGGING FORWARD...
Wednesday, September 04, 2013

I wasn't sure what to expect when I started writing this blog over four years ago. Putting one's personal details, thoughts, and opinions out there has its risks, but as it turns out, it's also had many delightful outcomes. The blog has brought me new friends, a great deal of support, and many smiles along the way. For these positive outcomes, I'm very grateful.

I want to thank two members of my palliative team in particular, who this week reminded me of why I started this blog in the first place. It was to keep my friends informed of my health without repeating the same information over and over again – and over the last few months that's exactly what I found myself doing again while I went into a "protective" mode. Many readers have also let me know that the blog has been helpful in dealing with their own serious illness, or that of a loved one. I'm honoured to know that my words might have brought comfort to others along the way.

So here's the scoop. I'm not doing well. A few weeks ago I was diagnosed with congestive heart failure, causing significant additional breathing problems not eased by increasing the oxygen. Fluid has been building up in various areas of my body. (Lying on my back almost 100% of the time might give you an idea as to how gravity has been playing its part.)

Daily medication "drains" the fluid for a few hours each morning. Not to be indelicate, but if you have an idea of the pain and discomfort involved for me in getting up to go to the bathroom every few hours – you can multiply it significantly when I require usually more than ten or fifteen bathroom visits in the space of two hours. By mid-afternoon I'm in so much pain that it wouldn't take more than mere suggestion to agree to have my legs amputated.

The PSW visits are the worst. Hobbling around the corner to lie down while she changes the bed sheets is agony. One might suggest, instead, sitting up nearby for few minutes in a chair, but that's even worse. Sitting up gets me shaking so badly from weakness and pain that I end up near tears.

With my palliative team we've come to the decision that the pain management protocol I was going to try in hospital (mentioned in a post a month or so ago) is no longer in the cards. I'm simply too weak to travel there to give it a try. It was risky to begin with, but my declining health has further shut the door to that experiment.

We've declined the food delivery service; unfortunately my appetite and ability to swallow have both significantly diminished. The volunteers were so very kind in trying to prepare meals that might appeal to me, but unfortunately little does these days. It's easier to let Suzanna shop for herself; she's a great cook and I get the benefit of the wonderful aromas.

The tables have turned on my sleeping habits as well. For the longest time it was standard to only get four or five hours of sleep, now I'm asleep far more than I'm awake in each twenty-four hour period. The upside is that I have fewer hours now that I need to fill with mental stimulation. That had been becoming quite a challenge, with bone pain often succeeding at thwarting my attempts at mindful distraction.

This post isn't meant to make anyone feel sorry for me; to me it's righting a situation that has been out of whack for some months. This is what my days are like, it was time to stop pretending that it's one wondrous and humour-filled day after the next.

It was time to get back to representing things as they are. With that comes a hope that there is understanding as to why I've become quite lousy at returning emails and phone calls, and why I've been cancelling a lot of visits lately. I'm feeling nothing less than miserable much of the time, and we're now faced with tough decisions as to where we go from here.

Despite any negativity that came along, it doesn't for one second change the positive aspects that writing this blog for over four years has brought to me. Thank you for the support, concern, and well wishes. I hold them dear.

AS ANOTHER PAGE TURNS
Saturday, September 07, 2013

It's been one very long year.

Fifty-two weeks ago, I moved into the apartment we're living in now. It seems like a lifetime ago, yet the details surrounding that weekend are still fresh – at times somewhat raw.

Suzanna and I had lived for the previous three months with dear friends who had given us a wonderful home when we had nowhere else to go.

I was going to try to live as best I could, independently; Suzanna was heading back to university. We had no idea that although I was struggling to move about (the one thing I wasn't going to miss about our friends' home was the staircase!), we didn't anticipate how quickly my health would decline. By the end of December I needed a wheelchair, was on oxygen, and was very close to being confined to bed, due to weakness and pain.

Since last year, I've lost my ability to walk more than a few steps at a time, can't prepare food for myself (even swallowing is not always successful) and often need help with dressing. A few weeks ago, Suzanna fashioned a way for me to pull myself out of bed with a belt, since I'm unable to lift myself up without assistance anymore.

There is so much that I've lost in this last year, a bitter pill to swallow for someone who has prided herself on being independent, resourceful, and responsible. I had a lifetime of being the person who could be relied upon to come through in situations thick and thin.

It's at times humiliating to need this degree of assistance, and to need more as each week goes by. This week I have a meeting (as has been the case for the last six months, here in my bedroom) with my doctor, case manager, lead nurse, and my daughter as we try to figure out what's best for both me and Suzanna. We have some disconcerting territory to cover; decisions to be reached over recent developments that we can no longer pretend aren't as serious as they truly are.

That's all more than enough reason for this past year to feel like it's gone by very slowly.

But then, I look at other reasons for this year to have felt so long. Friendships lit, rekindled, and nurtured. There are valued friends who have been a part of my life for many years, yet also new friends who came into our lives just in this past year – and in the best of ways feel like they've been around forever.

I've had the most incredible past four months with my daughter, who paused her education to come home to look after me. It's been easy to forget that she lived away from home for sixteen months in the last two years; our relationship certainly didn't suffer for the miles that separated us. Despite the sadness that sits on us with her not returning to university with her friends this week, she assures me that she not for a second regrets her decision.

We know that this comes to an end, and we pack as much love as we possibly can in this time together. It's an unspoken commitment between us; squeezing in what we can of what the next thirty or forty more years ought to have been allowed to us. Life really sucks right now. We acknowledge it now and again, and then move on to appreciating that for now, we still have this time together.

The hardest year of my life has also turned out to be the sweetest in so many ways. It's one very long year not because of the hardships, but because of just how much care and love has been squeezed into it. I'm one very lucky dame.

BREAKING BAD-LY
Wednesday, September 11, 2013

Even with knowing that the end is getting closer, there are still surprises to be had. The final half-hour of my case conference yesterday brought a few I could have done without.

In attendance were my doctor, lead nurse, case manager, and Suzanna. And of course me, reclining on the bed wedge like a lady of leisure. Except I wasn't playing the part very well I'm afraid. As always, I was in great pain, and my effort to breathe was hindering communication. Words needed to be chosen carefully, and the listeners needed to be patient in waiting for me to catch enough air to get my thoughts out.

The bulk of the meeting was spent reviewing logistics in keeping me here at home as long as possible. More equipment, more meds, setting baselines for when it's time to go elsewhere. Details on the elsewhere part I'll save for another post; we're all still hoping that I'll have a peaceful passing in my sleep with my daughter at my side. Maybe not what everyone would be comfortable with, but Suzanna and I both hope that this is the way it ends.

An hour into the meeting, Suzanna excused herself for an important matter. (Maybe I can twist her arm into writing about it sometime.) I'm very proud of the strength that she has within her to share her limited energy with someone else who also needs her right now.

After she left, the conversation took an interesting turn. I suppose that the others felt more comfortable with Suzanna being absent when they told me how much my physical appearance had changed since each had seen me last. The observations were shared gently, and with concern not to offend – but I did need to hear those truths. For so long, the outside didn't match the way I felt on the inside – it was validation for me that this is not just a bad nightmare (as hard as Suz and I often wish it were).

The case manager then went on her way, leaving my doctor and nurse to do a quick examination. Without them even touching me, the first observation is that my body is drawing energy to my core, with very pale and cold extremities.

My doctor listened to my heart, and confirmed what I already knew. The heartbeat was weak and irregular; pulse very slow. It's one thing to notice when a heartbeat is unusually strong, yet there's an odd awareness, like an echo in an empty room, of when there's an absence of a normal heart rhythm.

Feeling around my abdomen to check my organs, my doctor came across a few surprises that could indicate some upcoming challenges; masses that weren't expected. Not unexpected with Erdheim-Chester, yet the location's a bit of surprise for me. It's been well over a year since my last CT scan so we can't really be sure of the sizes, but the fact that they could be felt through my skin alarmed me a bit.

We both however had quite a shock when the doctor was palpating ever so gently just above my left kidney, and a rib gave way. I wouldn't say it hurt, it sent a shiver up my spine like listening to fingernails dragged against a chalkboard.

Tentatively checking other ribs, it would appear that at least a few have broken or softened due to bone tumours. As has my collarbone (which I'd already known has been significantly infiltrated since my pre-radiation bone scan last summer).

Then came the words that, as I think back, feel all jumbled and impossible – no more hugs. If a rib could give way with so light a touch, there's a strong likelihood that even a gentle hug could break more bones.

I'm a hugger with my loved ones. To excess at times, I'll admit. There are times when my daughter would be leaving to go back to school after a visit and I'd hug her as if my life depended on how much love I could transfer to her in a squeeze. Coming home was the same; I wanted to make up for the hugs we'd missed while she was away.

When my daughter was small, bedtime was accompanied by a, "Hug, kiss, and a squeeeeeeeze!" That was my way to not only justify a second hug, but to prolong it for as long as that last breath of air would allow.

I'm going to miss the wonderful hugs that my friends offer me; I've always gotten great comfort from them. It's going to hurt to tell them that I can no longer participate in our usual ritual when greeting each other or saying goodbye.

As for my daughter, I can't even go there. We'll figure something out to maintain the physical contact that is so important to our relationship. She deserves as many hugs from her mom as she could possibly want

– the delivery however, going forward, might look a little comical to the outside observer.

Although I expected much of the territory that we covered in yesterday's meeting, I still left feeling blindsided. Another ledge from which my fingers have lost their grip. How many more ways can a body and soul fracture until they become indistinguishable from a pile of shards?

FINISHING OFF THE BAR OF SOAP
Tuesday, September 17, 2013

A few years ago, the final Christmas spent with my ex, my husband gave me a gift that might sound a bit strange. Coloured tissue was tied with a string and inside were several dried-up slivers of soap and a few nearly-empty tubes of toothpaste.

My thriftiness had been a running joke in the household, and the gift, at the time, did make me laugh. It was a very short-lived giggle; the evening spilled over with awkwardness knowing that my husband had chosen to leave the marriage and would within weeks be moving out.

Not to say that I don't appreciate high quality goods and services and accept that they're priced accordingly. The point that was being reiterated with the gift was that I didn't care for wastage of whatever item good money had been spent on. I admit that I could be a nag about food being eaten up before it spoiled, or getting annoyed at finding toothpaste in the bathroom garbage that had more than a few good squeezes left in the tube, or soap being replaced while the current bar still had a few days of usefulness left in it.

This thriftiness didn't grow out of the period when I'd left home as a teen and ate ramen noodles meal after meal, out of necessity; it had come much earlier from the lessons learned from a mother and her sisters who'd been young girls in Germany during World War II. Food and provisions at times were scarce, and no matter how poor the condition, the item was used or eaten.

The experiences of one generation passed on to become habits of the next. I smile when my daughter also tries to get the very last bit of toothpaste out of the tube, or when I go into the shower and a usable sliver of soap waits for me to finish it off. Or when she reminds me that there's food in the fridge that needs eating up.

My need to finish things off is making life a bit complicated. As much as I'm trying, I can't clean up all the loose ends that I'd like to before I go.

Including this blog. It's been gently suggested by a few friends that I write my last entry in advance, to be posted by Suzanna after my passing. No matter how hard I try, I just can't do it for the tears that flow. If it hasn't yet come across in the last few years of writing this blog how grateful I am for the blessings in my life, I haven't done a very good job and wouldn't expect to be able to sum it up in just one post.

My plan is to wrap the blog up over the next few weeks. It's time. There are some things I'd like to share before I stop writing here, some things that might surprise, delight, or sadden you. I need to tie up this loose end, to give you an ending to the story as best I can. Suzanna has promised that news that I can't share myself will be posted; it saddens me when I read a blog written by someone who's terminally ill and it ends suddenly with no news of what happened to the individual I grew to care about.

I can't do that to the many of you who've faithfully followed my blog over the last years. We won't leave you without the final chapter.

PUTTING MINDS AT EASE
Wednesday, September 18, 2013

I'm overwhelmed by the very thoughtful, terribly kind, and beautiful supportive notes being sent to me here on the blog and privately. I haven't been able to give any of them the proper reply that each deserves, please know that I read and cherish each one. At a time that can be isolating and frightening, I do not feel alone. Thank you for giving me this gift.

I don't mean to be alarmist, but it has to said that although I have a few specific subjects that I'd like to write about while I'm still here, it's not guaranteed that I'll get to them. Little in this life is certain; this is a lesson I keep being taught over and over again.

There are two questions about Suzanna that get raised over and over again, and I'd like to answer them now so that I can set some minds at ease.

Although there is not enough known yet about Erdheim-Chester Disease to be 100% accurate in my answer, there is no evidence to suggest that Suzanna or her future children are at risk for acquiring ECD. None of the diagnosed patients scattered around the globe have been found to be even remotely related to other ECD patients. This knowledge helps me sleep at night.

The second question I'm often delicately asked is if Suzanna will be okay financially after I've passed. Bluntly, yes. My life insurance coverage will allow her to complete the university education she wants and deserves.

I feel better putting that out on the table, I hope you do too.

ONE THING THAT'S KEPT ME BUSY
Tuesday, September 24, 2013

Many surprises and opportunities have fallen into my lap over the last six months; it's hard to imagine that so much could happen within the confines of the four walls of my bedroom. Outside of telling close friends, I'd decided initially that I was going to keep fairly quiet about two of the projects until they were completed. As things are going, my chances of being around at the time of completion are getting slimmer and I'm being graciously guided as to what information I can share while I'm still here to tell you myself. Sounds a little mysterious, doesn't it?

Followers of my blog might remember that I had a pacemaker implanted about ten years ago. I'd been diagnosed at the time with vasovagal syncope. Sudden and significant drops in my heart rate were causing me great discomfort, often resulting in me ending up on the floor in a faint, or near faint. Injuries were a common occurrence; sharp corners on furniture had a way of leaping into my path. This condition was preventing me from leading a normal life; I couldn't drive, work, or take care of my daughter in the ways I would have hoped.

Thankfully, the pacemaker returned me to a fairly normal life for a few years, until I was diagnosed with Erdheim-Chester Disease in 2009. If you've been following the blog you'll have a fairly good idea how things progressed from there, cardiac issues continuing to be of major concern.

When I signed my Do Not Resuscitate order early last year, I had to give pause as to how my pacemaker would be handled. As I mentioned a few months ago, I'd already decided that I wouldn't have the pacemaker replaced when the battery died.

Two concerns quickly came to mind. The first, if my daily health issues were already so challenging, what would they be like with a non-functional pacemaker on top of that? Knowing my triggers of ten years ago, even getting out of bed to go the bathroom would be out of the question with an expired pacemaker battery. I also had to consider that ten years ago, I was in otherwise better health; a much sturdier state than I am in today.

The other concern was whether the pacemaker is keeping me alive artificially. Might I have already died if it hadn't been bringing my heart rate back up again after every crash? The data downloaded from my pacemaker over the last ten years tells us that I average at least forty major drops a day.

A year and a half ago, I set out to have my questions answered, in preparation for a time that might come when it could appear that the pacemaker was the only thing keeping me alive. What rights did I have as the patient to have the pacemaker turned off?

The path has been a complicated one. The charter of rights of Ontario clearly states that I have the right to have the pacemaker turned off, in the same way respiration or dialysis treatment can be refused. On paper...a clear option, but not so clear in practice.

About six months ago, I was speaking at length with a member of the Ontario Dying With Dignity association about my questions and concerns, when she asked if I might consider speaking with a representative of the CBC whose team was producing a documentary on end-of-life issues facing Canadians.

I did speak with the CBC and was asked if I would consider participating in the documentary, and I agreed with one stipulation. My daughter Suzanna had to be fully supportive of my involvement. It would be another four weeks before she was finished her exams and I didn't want to raise the idea of my participation until she had cleared her plate.

The documentary is scheduled to air sometime in November, which will tell you that Suzanna did indeed give her blessing to the project.

There a few points I'd like to raise. First, the CBC team has been absolutely wonderful to work with. Not only have they been very appreciative about how much energy this project has taken out of me and make every effort to lessen any burden on me, they've been at every point very respectful and compassionate towards me and Suzanna.

I'm going to use the term "dying a gentle death" as a way to describe what I've been trying to achieve for the end to my own story. Each of us will have our own perspective and feelings on the issues of when modern medicines and medical procedures ought to be used to try to extend life, and we will also have our own thoughts on when it's appropriate not to intervene.

My decision to participate in the documentary comes from a desire to allow other Canadians a chance to, "walk in my shoes." You may find yourself agreeing or disagreeing on some of the points raised and to that you're perfectly entitled. What I do ask is that if you feel compelled to speak out on whatever your position might be, that your comments please be directed to those in our government who can speak on your behalf.

Suzanna and I are trying to do what's best for the two of us. Despite going public with our story, ultimately, for us this about a mother and daughter who love each very much. Neither of us wants the other to suffer beyond what we feel we can handle.

A side note: It took me a few weeks to find the words and the courage to share this post. Two emergency calls for help this past weekend had me and Suzanna again revaluating time lines and decisions, encouraging me to share this information sooner than I might otherwise have done so. It was my wish that you hear about the documentary from me rather than recognize my name spoken on your TV one evening a couple of months from now. I'm grateful to my CBC team for giving their nod to sharing this news before the piece is complete.

UNCONDITIONALLY
Thursday, September 26, 2013

I'm fudging the truth when I tell others that I'm recovering from the events of last weekend, when Suzanna twice had to call for emergency help for me. Who am I kidding? I'm not recovering; it's just further decline and there's no escaping that reality.

When I had a visit from my doctor two weeks ago, she and I had a frank discussion about what the immediate future might look like. The hardest part was sharing my doctor's thoughts with Suzanna when she arrived home a few hours later. In the oceans of uncertainty surrounding the final stages of this illness, Suzanna grasps for the small amounts of definitive information we have. I hide nothing from her; it simply doesn't work in our relationship to have any secrets between us.

Suzanna immediately made a decision to take a leave of absence from work, choosing to finish out what was left on her schedule so that her employer wouldn't be left in a bind.

It broke my heart. Not only had Suzanna postponed university for me, she was now giving up the one thing that guaranteed her a respite from what she faces every day here with me.

After the events of this weekend, she felt that she didn't want to be out of touch for any length of time. At work, her phone was accessible only at break time; the idea of me not being able to reach her immediately if I needed help was too much for her.

Thankfully, her employer was compassionate and understanding, ensuring that they would find staff to take on the remaining shifts on her schedule.

The closer we get to the end, the more surreal it seems. The more we feel cheated out of what ought to have been ours to share as mother and daughter. I'm going to allow myself to be boastful; I think I would have made one very loving and kickass, fun grandmother!

Suzanna mentioned that when she does go back to work, everyone there will know what has happened to allow her to be there again. She wondered how she'll handle the comments from well-meaning workmates. The same will apply when she returns to school; she'll go back only because she lost her mother.

In our usual fashion, we try to find a smidgen of humour in all the sadness. We joked that she goes back into the world as "half orphan," but we both know it's not nearly that simple.

Throughout Suzanna's life, I've kidded her that I knew her better than she knew herself. As many parents do, we so intimately know the patterns and habits of our children as to often predict with great accuracy how they will react in a given situation. Even today, there are times that she'll look at me sideways, wondering how I could have known what she was about to say.

Over twenty years together, the tables have turned. Suzanna has come to know me better than I know myself. She has a knack for pinpointing what's at the root of whatever is eating away at me, often before I figure it out for myself. This is something that I've come to realize can only happen when you trust completely in someone's love for you. I find great comfort in thinking that that my daughter has trusted me enough to let me know who she is, and that her unconditional love for me has allowed me to be human too.

MY GUIDE TO GETTING BY
Monday, September 30, 2013

As I come close to finishing off this blog, there are a few thoughts I wanted to share: Words I've tried to live by, ideas that I felt compelled to explore, concepts that I aspired to incorporate into how I act and speak.

Some old friends from my office work days might remember that I could be depended upon to have a motivational "Thought of the Day" calendar on my desk, anyone was welcome to goof around with the magnetic word tiles I'd arranged on my file cabinet in a quest to inspire, and I had a lending library of motivational books on the shelf. Yes, I was one of those annoying people.

And I'm not yet done with being that annoying person who tries so hard to see the upside of every situation and to recognize the best in every person.

So here comes my list. I take credit for none of these ideas; I've borrowed and revised as I went along to see what worked for me. Sometimes success came along, other times crashing disappointment. Life?

What we put out into the world gets reflected back. If you don't believe me, spend a day offering every single person you come across a genuine smile and see what happens. It's magical.

On that note, smiles and a kind word are contagious. Nothing can convince me otherwise.

If your intuition has served you well in the past, keep trusting your gut.

Work hard, be nice. (Quote by Rafe Esquith, Los Angeles teacher featured in the film *Hobart Shakespeareans.*) Not only does it cover karma and The Golden Rule succinctly, it sums up the guiding principles of pretty much every religion quite nicely, doesn't it?

We all make a difference. We can have a positive influence or a negative one; we each hold the power to shape the lives of others. It's a tremendous responsibility to be taken seriously.

Listen to children. Amazing insight can be found in the most innocent of observations.

You can choose your family, and define for yourself what that word means to you.

If a doctor or teacher gets high ratings on Internet rating sites, you can bet that he or she is also someone very special outside of work too. (I had to add that one, I delight in the fact that I've yet to be proven wrong on this!)

Walking on eggshells is just impossible. Any relationship that required me to do so is gone for good; I always ended up crashing through.

Giving the benefit of the doubt doesn't always end well, but it wins out most of the time.

"The first time someone shows you who they are, believe them." Maya Angelou

"Once a word leaves your mouth, you cannot chase it back even with the swiftest horse." Chinese Proverb

There is a big difference between sympathy and empathy, there are times and places for each. The first is closer to pity, the second essential to the human experience.

And to finish, my hardest lesson. I can't make everyone happy. Goodness knows I tried.

MEASUREMENT
Friday, October 11, 2013

There are all sorts of reasons why I haven't posted for a week and a half; none of them make me particularly happy. I wish I could tell you that it's been a whirlwind of friends coming through our door keeping me entertained, when in reality I have to turn down just about every offer of a visit because I'm too exhausted for conversation most of the time.

As much as I wasn't pleased that Suzanna had to give up her job to keep a closer eye on me, it's been a great relief to have her near. I can do less and less for myself with each passing day as I get physically weaker. Moving my laptop to my lap has become a two- person job if one of the persons is me. Even holding my wrists up to my iPad propped on my chest for more than a few minutes has become too difficult. With this knowledge you might forgive me if my emails have been short and to the point, if they come at all.

In case you're wondering, this post is being dictated, with breaks for giggles at the strange interpretations that the auto-correct feature has offered up.

My diminishing strength can't be ignored. Suzanna had set up a belt to help me pull myself up to get out of bed to use the bathroom. This worked for several weeks until I lost the strength to sit up on my own. Her hand has to either help pull me up from in front, or push my back to get me past the point at which I find myself stuck.

The hardest part of all is at times losing my ability to speak. My thoughts are lucid, what I would like to say is clearly formed in my mind but turning that into spoken word eludes me more often as the weeks go by.

I'm frustrated; Suzanna is frustrated (although she tries so hard to not let it show). It embarrasses me when I struggle through a discussion with one of my care team members (I can't reschedule them as I do with friends when it's a particularly hard day), hoping that they can see in my eyes that I'm still on top of my game mentally – it's just the output that is filled with gaps and missteps, at the very least a much slower pace than my usual rapid-fire banter.

My short-term memory is also faltering; poor Suzanna often has to tell me the same thing several times over. Thank goodness she's around when my nurse asks me how the previous day went; the days run into each other as one blur. And please don't ask me what my last meal was. Half the time you'd see me defer to Suzanna for the specifics.

A few nights ago, I was teary and filled with self-pity over my diminishing abilities. I've been able to do so little for myself for so long; I've been dearly hoping that a fatal heart attack would save me from these indignities. Suzanna gently held my hand and asked me if it was just now truly hitting me that I was going to die? My girl knows me all too well – I nodded through my sobs. There was some truth to her thoughts despite me having had years to get used to the idea.

Trying to be stoic is bloody exhausting. Trying to hide how awful I really feel can be excruciating. The realities of what I'll be missing out on in the lives of my daughter and loved ones hit fast and hard these days.

I think a lot about how much I will miss the people I care about. Maybe it's a ridiculous idea that I will be missing them after I'm gone, but for now it's a comforting measure of how just many wonderful people fell into my life and how much I care about them.

WHAT I CANNOT KNOW...
October 16th, 2013

A few weeks ago, I experienced a few rougher days, one of them requiring the assistance of 911 paramedics. I was that night made aware that I'd been unconscious at one point, but it wasn't until almost two weeks later that I heard something about the events of that evening that I hadn't been told at the time. I still can't quite get my head around it, and I wasn't sure that I wanted to write about it, but here I go.

I'd had a bad spell with an erratic heart rate, in which my heart was racing for over an hour at over 160 beats per minute. Earlier in the day, it had been quite low – it was becoming evident that my pacemaker wasn't quite behaving the way it had been programmed to kick in if the rate dropped below 60 beats per minute.

The paramedics had come and gone. Although my heart rate had been very high for several hours and they insisted that I ought to be taken to the local hospital, I had refused and decided to deal with the consequences, whatever they might turn out to be.

An intravenous line had been started by one of the paramedics; my veins have become very hard to find and he wanted to give it his best shot to at least give me some hydration and easier delivery of any medications. I was on the left side of the bed, and of course the only vein that seemed viable was on my right arm. He asked my daughter's permission to crawl across her side of the bed to get the job done. At the same time, in an effort to keep my spirits up, he joked that he could just stay put in the bed to keep an eye on me all night. Not only do our local paramedics do a great job of finding that shy vein, they seem to all have a wonderful sense of humour.

My visiting nurse was adjusting the IV drip when I lost consciousness. When I awoke, my nurse was asking me if I knew where I was, and Suzanna was on the other side, holding my hand with a look of relief on her face.

I remember my first words were to tell them both that I had sunk deeply into the foam of the mattress, and wasn't that bizarre? Then I proceeded to tell them that I'd had a dream that I was flying very high over the city of Paris. The streets were empty except for Suzanna running through them, in a flowing red dress. In the dream I was too high to make out even the most obvious of details yet I knew it was her. I remembered thinking that although I have a great fondness for Paris; I really wanted to be flying over New York City. The location changed in my dream, yet Suzanna still ran below me and somehow I knew that she had joy in her heart and was running towards something that would make her happy.

The nurse had told me that while I was unconscious, she and Suzanna had been imploring me to answer their questions. Suzanna had been asking me to squeeze her hand if I could hear her, but I hadn't responded to either of them. What seemed curious to both of them is that I'd had a big smile on my face, even though moments before blacking out I'd been in great distress.

It wasn't until later when Suzanna was telling someone else the story, that I heard details of that evening of which I'd been unaware.

Had I been asked, I would have said that my dream had lasted perhaps twenty to thirty seconds. It had ended too soon. I had felt peaceful for the first time in forever, and I'd been completely without pain.

It turned out that I'd been out cold for closer to five minutes. I confirmed the details with my nurse on her next visit; she told me that while I had been unresponsive, she was getting ready to tell Suzanna that this was likely the end. It was likely the semi-functional pacemaker that had brought me back.

Suzanna told this story with a sense of calm. She said to me that she couldn't have imagined a nicer way for her mother to leave, with a big grin on her face.

I can't know for certain what happened in those five minutes, but if I get to leave this physical body with such beautiful and peaceful thoughts, with my beloved daughter holding my hand, and without any pain, I'll take it. Knowing that it's also what Suzanna wants for me makes it the most desirable wish I could possibly hold right now.

THE REST OF HER DAYS...
October 18th, 2013

Suzanna has been excitedly sharing some thoughts about her future education plans, and I couldn't be happier that she's comfortable sharing them with me.

It is of course difficult to think about not being around to see how her life plays out, but there is also great joy in hearing her ideas. She's been studying molecular biology and genetics, and has three years to go in her Bachelor of Science program. My illness has so far taken her three semesters off-track in her four-year program.

After she finishes her first degree, it's Suzanna's plan to do her master's degree. Having conducted research about her options for universities offering her program, she has her heart settled on a university in Australia for a two-year program.

The plan may change one hundred times between now and three years from now, but the fact that she is making plans puts me at peace. Although there is a pall of sadness over us with my declining health, there is also sunshine to be found as we peek through the clouds to glimpse at what her adult years might look like.

Acceptance of what is to come over the next few months seems to soothe us both. We have a clearer picture of how things are likely to happen, what our options are, and who holds the handles of the safety net that waits beneath us.

Despite much of this being frightening and uncomfortable, acceptance gives us what we need in our hearts right now. I can stop fighting so hard, knowing that my daughter will be okay. My passing will of course hurt, but I can know that as a mother I did my job; I helped to prepare her to embrace the opportunities that lie ahead and helped prepare her to face the challenges that force their way into life.

She is strong – much stronger than I was at her age. Understanding that I trust her to make good decisions, she gains more strength in being able to talk to me about her future. She knows that I offer my blessing to follow her heart and allow her intuition to guide her.

I was here long enough to see for myself that she's become a very capable young woman with a bright future ahead of her. It's not a matter of no longer being needed by my daughter; it's a matter of her showing me and the rest of the world that she trusts herself enough to move past the loss of her mother. She's going to be okay, and I couldn't be prouder.

MOM'S LAST CHAPTER

The last few months of my mother's life were eventful, to say the least. Despite many months of careful planning, so much could not have been anticipated.

The CBC documentary aired on November 25th. During the weeks leading up to the airing, Mom and I oscillated between excitement and anxiousness in anticipation of what we would see. She had not seen the parts I had filmed, and I had seen only minimal portions of what she'd had to say. At 9 p.m. on November 25th, we lay beside each other in Mom's king-sized bed, held hands, and watched.

We didn't look at each other the entire hour. I knew I would burst into tears if I looked at her. We made it to the end with a few tears, but luckily not so many that we couldn't see the screen – a more frequent occurrence in our household than one might think!

We felt so proud of each other for what we had accomplished with the help of the CBC team. Telling Mom's story and the story of our family's struggles through these last years of her life was a cathartic experience. The responses from friends and the public were overwhelmingly positive. Mom had wanted to be here for me when it aired, so she could help me through any negative reactions. Thankfully, there were very few.

I have not been able to watch the documentary again since her death. I'm not sure whether it is because I'm scared it will make me miss her more than I can handle right now, or if I'm saving it for a day when I really need to see and hear her voice again. It will be there for me when I'm ready, as a powerful reminder of how much she loved me and how brave she was.

A few weeks after the airing of the documentary, we set the wheels in motion to go to the hospice. Mom's dear friend, Sue, flew from Halifax to help us through the process, making calls and arrangements to ensure the transfer would go smoothly. Unfortunately, plans for the hospice fell through at the last minute as there wasn't a vacancy for Mom as had been expected.

We now had to scramble to find a place for Mom. It was becoming more apparent that she was in too much pain and discomfort to stay at home much longer. Dr. Downar, whom we had met through the CBC taping, became a wonderful support to my mother and me during this time. Within days, he arranged for Mom to be transferred to the Intensive Care Unit at the Toronto General Hospital. Although we'd had most of Mom's things packed days before, everything happened so quickly that night that we all felt a little out of control.

It was heart-wrenching to watch Mom say goodbye to our apartment for the last time; the place where we had shared so many laughs and late nights and good memories. The hardest part was watching her say goodbye to Scrabble – the best boyfriend ever – before he went off to the kennel to be boarded for a while. It was a sad day of good-byes.

Mom was settled into her hospital room quickly and by seven o'clock that evening, Dr. Downar had placed her on Fentanyl to help manage the pain. The protocol went well, without any allergic reactions. This always a concern, due to Mom's many sensitivities and allergies. Fentanyl is reported to be 50 to 100 times more potent than morphine. This told us a lot about the level of discomfort she had been living with, never complaining. Relieving some of her pain was such a blessing. Sue and I were thankful to finally see her more comfortable.

It was a hectic few days that followed, caring for Mom and constantly monitoring the screen displaying her vitals. On December 7th Mom followed through on her decision to reduce her pacemaker to a lower setting. I was downstairs having lunch when Sue called to say it was time for me to come upstairs. Coming in to Mom's room, I saw the computer ready to make happen what she had fought so hard for. I held her hand, and without ceremony it was done. Sue and I held our breath, but no big, life-changing event occurred as we had expected it to. Everything was as it had been ten minutes before. Mom's heart was stronger than we all knew, but her body continued to betray her.

A few days later, Mom was transferred from the ICU to the palliative care unit in Baycrest Hospital. We had not expected this step; we thought it would all be over after the pacemaker was turned down. We were now on a different path, and the future was uncertain.

I was a little apprehensive about Mom being moved to a hospital setting. She had always said she did not want to be in a hospital for her last days, so it took me a little time to become comfortable with the knowledge that this was the place where she would eventually pass. '*Eventually,*' however, turned out to be much longer than expected.

In the hospital, Mom had written half a blog post while we were waiting for whatever would happen to happen. Along with my own account, I would like to include her words and feelings in the book:

YOU CAN'T GET THERE FROM HERE
December 30th, 2013

For over three weeks we've waited. Me, Suzanna, and Sue as we held what could only best be described as a tender vigil interrupted by the usual cacophony of silliness, black humour, and dear love that envelops me.

This isn't at all what we had expected. Over three weeks ago, events transpired on very short notice to allow us to take advantage of a spot in the Intensive Care Unit at Toronto General Hospital. We had two hours to pack up anything that I would want surrounding me in my last days.

Dr. Downar (interviewed in our CBC segment) handled quite a number of issues. Firstly, I finally had access to the protocol that would give me an opportunity at long-awaited pain relief. I've been on Fentanyl for the last weeks with great success. How odd to say that I can't even fathom how drastic the pain had become once I'd had a chance to experience life without that intensity. Every few days, the dosage is increased; quite simply, anything I request for symptom management is procured in short order."

It was a long time spent in the hospital for all of us. Christmas passed while we were there; a bittersweet time where I tried to remember it was only another day on the calendar. I felt sad – sad that this was where we were spending our last Christmas together. Mom and I had the perfect Christmas the year before, which we thought would be our last. This year we spent the evening quietly together, not really acknowledging the significance of December 25th.

New Year's Eve came in stark contrast. Our friend, Donna, came to visit on her bicycle. She brought dinner for herself and me, and a lovely container of gelato for the three of us to share. As Mom said, she was dying and didn't have to have a healthy dinner before eating dessert! Donna also brought decorations and bead necklaces and New Year's Eve hats.

We put streamers and beads up around the room and we celebrated in style. The nurses even took part in some fun and wore a necklace or two for their shift that night. It was lovely.

The days, however, were long. Sue and I were both living in the room with Mom, showering every day in the hospital's bathroom provided for family; people like us spending day and night with our loved one. Over the course of the six weeks we were there, that washroom was used only two or three times by anyone other than us. It was not common for family to live in the hospital, especially for this long. Sue and I took turns being with Mom, keeping her company and taking care of her needs. She was rarely alone for any extended period of time.

Sue went back to Halifax for a short break a couple of times, to take care of appointments and to re-energize a bit. I went home on the weekends to regain my sanity, to stay strong for what was facing us. Mom understood. She knew that living in the hospital was not easy. We would be awoken early every morning for medications, and checked on every few hours. We couldn't fall asleep at night until after 12:30 when Mom's medication pump would be checked at the end of each day. During the day, there would be food trays delivered, doctors to see, and all of the normal personal hygiene routines that Mom needed help with. It was hard to adhere to this schedule for such a long period of time, especially with the three of us sharing and sleeping in a small room. Sue slept on a cot on one side of Mom, and I slept in a reclining chair on the other side.

I also carry with me some special memories of this time in the hospital. The nurses were lovely, every day providing excellent care with warmth and compassion. They didn't just care for Mom, they cared for Sue and me too, by checking on us and helping however they could.

We looked forward to the daily visits from the doctor. Dr. Grossman's attentiveness to making Mom as comfortable as possible was so reassuring. She provided any needed medications, but also connected us with people and services that would help along the journey; from therapeutic touch sessions, to all the ice-cream and vanilla pudding Mom could ask for.

The long conversations with staff, discussing the conflicting feelings Mom was having about being around for so much longer than anyone expected, were so helpful. I even received a therapy session while I was there, which helped me deal with my own feelings surrounding the impending death of my mother. A particularly special moment was meeting the art team. They made for us a lovely pillow with Mom's favourite picture of us together on the top. So very thoughtful.

However, the best treat of all was the discovery of the Portuguese custard tarts! From the first sample Sue brought back from the bakery, Mom developed an insatiable passion. We were all a little embarrassed to admit that about 50 tarts were consumed between the three of us (not equally, I have to point out) in the remaining time at the hospital. We have many friends to thank for going on 'custard tart runs' – Those sweet pastries certainly made Mom's last few weeks a gastronomic delight!

Mom and I shared some wonderful afternoons in the time between nurse check-ins and while Sue was out having some alone time in the family sitting room. I would crawl into the hospital bed beside her and we would have a nap, or watch a movie together, or sometimes just talk. We always loved cuddling, but there was something special about those last few weeks. I think she was especially grateful for me walking through this journey with her, and I was grateful for the extra time we had together. Nothing felt right during that time for either of us, in the midst of all the unpredictability, and I think those afternoons reminded us what was important – the love we shared and having each other.

On January 6th, it was decided that Mom's pacemaker would be turned completely off. The rationale was that a ventilator wouldn't be turned to 10% when it was requested to be turned off, so why would it be any different with a pacemaker? Again, we held our breaths as the procedure was done, but again nothing cataclysmic happened. It was such a relief, however, for Mom to get exactly what she wished, and I think it gave her some peace in the final days.

I think that last stage was the hardest for me. I could handle weeks in the hospital – the sleeping on a reclining chair, the hospital food, the noise of the daily activity in a palliative ward – but seeing Mom become someone I didn't recognize broke my heart. She had moments of being herself, but she was often groggy and confused with the additional medications for pain. She slept for long stretches and I seemed to lose touch with my best friend. It was such a lonely time, spending hours at her bedside but not being able to talk with her. I just wanted my mom to be my mom until the very end, but I also wanted her to be comfortable and the heavy medications were the only way. I don't think I fully realized that this would be the last time I would have her with me. I thought there would be more time. I don't think there would ever be enough time.

It was the evening of January 14th when things started to take a turn. Sue had planned to go back to Halifax the next day but that night, everything changed. Mom's breathing changed and it sounded like she was moaning in pain. We couldn't sleep, hearing her sound so uncomfortable, so we stayed up all night. She spiked a fever that the cold compresses couldn't bring down. It was such a long wait to the morning, when the doctor could come in and tell us what was happening. Sue cancelled her flight.

When the head nurse came in that morning, he assured us that Mom wasn't in any pain. She wasn't showing signs of pain such as grimacing, clenching her fist, or furrowing her brow. He wasn't sure why she was making the noises, but it was comforting to know that she wasn't in silent agony. When the doctor came in, she told us that sometimes patients vocalize when they're unconscious, especially if they were talkative people in their normal life. That definitely sounded like my mom!

The doctor estimated that she would pass away within 24 hours. It was hard to hear, but not unexpected, given the change that had happened so suddenly. I was thankful my father arrived and was staying nearby for support. I let Mom know he was there, and shortly after, we began to see the tell-tale signs of someone dying. I would like to believe that she felt comfortable letting go when there was someone around who would take care of me.

Mom's colour was very pale and there was a rattling sound when she breathed. Her breathing stopped for long stretches and started again. This breathing pattern, called Cheyne-Stokes breathing, is probably one of the most unsettling things I have ever experienced. After each pause, Sue and I wondered if it was the last. We sat like that for three hours, until finally Mom took her last breath. I was in total disbelief that she was gone. As I hugged her, I laid my head on her chest and was sure I heard her heart beating. I then realized it was mine. My heart was beating for both of us.

As my dad drove me home, I felt totally empty and alone. I felt like no one would ever love me as much as my mom had, and that I would never learn to be as good a person as my mom was. I was devastated and felt like I couldn't function that evening and for the next few days. I remember just sitting for hours, staring blankly. I couldn't process that my mom wasn't with me anymore. Slowly, things started to return to normal, or something that resembled it. My dad made sure I got out, ate as much as I could handle at that point, and kept me busy.

I am just beginning to realize that my life can go on, and I will be okay without Mom, just like she always told me I would be.

It has been a few months since Mom died, and life is as close to normal as I can imagine it ever being. I still really miss her, but looking at pictures and remembering her feels good – not as painful. I am lucky to have had someone that gave me so many happy memories in such a short time. Looking back, I am glad she didn't die at home. I don't think I could have handled the dying process, and taking care of myself at the same time. I wonder if I would have avoided my own home because of the memories it would have held.

Instead, my home is filled with good memories. Mom took much care in leaving behind many things for me to remember her. She collected pictures from her life, and made special notes on the back of each explaining the context. She collected my childhood pictures, and made videos for me to find after she died, where she talked about funny stories and special memories from when I was young, always reminding me that she loves me. The special possessions she wanted me to have all have tags explaining their significance to her. I recently traveled with a money pouch of hers, which had a tag telling me that she had taken it with her to her travels to Europe and Australia. It is these small things that keep me connected to her.

Two years ago, Mom and I exchanged Christmas gifts and we had both chosen necklaces; completely unplanned. She gave me one with her fingerprint on it with the inscription on the back, "Always my Suzu," her nickname for me. This one I wore for the entire duration of the hospital stay, and the chain broke the night that things went downhill. I was so sad not to have the necklace with me during that time. I had given her one with two hearts on it, referring to the saying we shared when I was a child,

"My heart and your heart." When Mom died, I asked Sue to take the necklace off of her neck since she couldn't be cremated with it, and I put the two pendants from each necklace on the same chain. This is the necklace that I wear every day and it makes me smile every time I look down at it.

I'm a little worried about everything she's going to miss. I'm worried that I won't have anyone to help me get ready for my wedding day. I'm scared of being a mother one day without the guidance of my own. I just have to believe that she gave me the skills to handle all the life changes that come my way. The best things that my mom gave me are not physical objects. My mom gave me something to strive toward, a standard to try to uphold. She taught me to love deeply and without judgment, and to trust that people are inherently good. My mom taught me that it's okay not to be perfect, as long as you try to be kind and work hard. She taught me to be resilient in the face of whatever life throws at you. My mom taught me what it is to love and truly be loved; selflessly and freely.

Because of my mom, I know that I deserve good things and can achieve them. She gave me confidence in myself that will keep me going for the rest of my life. She was the wittiest, smartest, kindest, most optimistic person I have ever known. I can't thank her enough for the twenty years she gave me with her.

I'd like to leave you with something funny she said in the last week of her life, always wanting to brighten other people's days right until the end with a bit of dark humour: "This dying thing kind of sucks, I wouldn't recommend it."

I love you, Mom. My heart and your heart.

LAST RESPECTS

(Editor's Note: Before Sandy's passing, she asked friends to provide "testimonials" for the book to offer their perspectives on her journey.)

Sue Landry
Nova Scotia

Sometimes in life, you are in the right place at the right time. I am so fortunate that I was in the right place 25 years ago when I met Sandy Trunzer, standing outside a hotel during a meeting in San Diego. I didn't know then what a trying road she would travel or the opportunity I would have to see such an amazing woman manage her way through life, and through death. Through this book, *Without A Manual*, you have been equally blessed to share in this journey.

Sandy is someone who has had to endure so much in her own life, yet she has an incredible capacity to forgive. I admire that in her. That is how Sandy chooses to use her energy. The weight of anger is heavy. We all have a pity party sometimes, but she refuses to tie a rope around it and drag it along with her.

Sandy's is a very tough story, but it truly is an inspirational one. Her intent when she started writing the blog, in 2009, was just to offer just musings about what she was encountering. Fighting a rare disease, working to break down barriers in the health care system, and managing her way quietly through the pain is not the life she envisioned but she has had to endure it. Raising her beautiful daughter, realizing her photographic talents, and being thankful for the gifts of friendship and kindness – that is Sandy's story.

There's so much in those blog posts – musings about funny things and musings about really difficult things. The blog is not all negative and black, but she's saying things out loud; just true things that she's seen. It's not a depressing story, even though it is marching down the road to death. She injects a humour everywhere, and she has got a great sense of humour.

Twenty-five years we have been friends. Where has the time gone? We had kept in touch over the years, sharing snippets of our lives. Since she was diagnosed with ECD we've been in a lot closer contact. I guess in the last three years we have spoken every day. Through the magic of Skype and FaceTime we are able to connect no matter where in the world I find myself when travelling. I look so forward to those calls. And it's not doom and gloom. We talk about stuff that all people without any sort of medical problems or medical issues would talk about. We talk about her daughter, and we talk about my husband, our pets –, just normal conversation. Every day that I call, I pray to God that she's going to be there to pick up.

I am honoured to write this tribute to Sandy. That is a tribute to our friendship.

Sandy has not let her personality change, even while she is dealing with a life- threatening disease. We can't even begin to understand how much pain that she is in.

Even now, as she is confined largely to her bed, she wants to participate in life and hear everyone's news; hear about the normal things of life. Her blog began four years ago when she was carrying on a normal productive life as a 45- year- old woman. Although Sandy and I have shared lots of recipes over the years, her blog is not intended to be a list of ingredients or instructions for those working their way through the deterioration of life. There is no right answer. She offers her blog to share some of the things that she's observed or felt as she manages her sickness as she manages her life.

She is focused very much on raising her daughter. Sandy and her daughter have an amazing relationship. This is very tough thing for Suz to go through, losing her biggest supporter and biggest confidante. We all lose our parents, but you don't expect to lose them when you're 20 years old.

Death is an uncomfortable topic for people. We tend to shy away from talking about it. It can be very isolating for those who are experiencing it. It is tough but I am so thankful to be able to be with Sandy during some of the hardest moments, such as the day the funeral director came to make the plans. Sandy insisted that she did not want Suzanna or her friends 'inconvenienced' with the arrangements after she was gone. This is true Sandy.

But you know she takes this all very matter-of-factly. And realizes that she needs to do this and not leave it to someone else. I mean she's been a very, very self-sufficient individual, as long as I've known her. Not to the point where she won't accept help from other people, but she prides herself in being able to handle things herself, and she does an amazing job at it.

Just sitting in bed, there's a lot of atrophying of muscles that is taking place, but thankfully Sandy has her artwork and her pictures around her. They are a very integral part of her. She has real talent. This was evident in some of her earliest work, including a photograph from an old Polaroid that she gave me years ago. This book is not only an extension of her creativity but also of her humanness, of her kindness to all those around her.

I think this book is an amazing legacy. There are many people who will never have the chance to meet Sandy in person, to see her beautiful smile. But thankfully, these people will be able to meet this gentle soul through her words. Suzanna, your mother is an amazing individual, and I see many of her qualities through you.

Sandy is a very unique and special individual, and I am so thankful to know her. It is her gift to me.

Arlene and Fred Faber

Sandy was about 12 years old when we first met. Our beloved dog had jumped through a glass window and punctured his lung. He needed surgery and was starting to recuperate, but also needed someone to watch him during part of the day while we were working.

Entering into the picture was an adorable, intelligent, soft-spoken, and responsible neighbor who lived just a couple of doors away from us. Sandy agreed to take care of our dog whenever we needed her. She was there for us and it wasn't long before we also entrusted her with our two most prized possessions in the whole world; our son and daughter. She soon became our favorite babysitter, often having dinner with us before taking care of the kids, and later spending weeks with us at our summer cottage. She endeared herself to us quickly, entering into our hearts and truly we felt that she was a member of our family. It was a mutual admiration! We had the "best" babysitter and friend in the world and as Sandy has expressed to us, she found a "safe haven" in our home and family.

Over time, as Sandy developed her own life as a teenager, and we moved to a new location, we lost contact with her. As sad as we were that she was out of our lives at the time, we were thrilled when a couple of summers ago, and about 35 years later, through the magic of social media, Sandy sent us a message and we were reunited.

She had become an amazing photographer, mother, woman, and unfortunately, patient. We were sad to learn that Sandy had a terminal disease. Over the months that followed our initial visit, we read Sandy's blogs, talked to Sandy, visited with Sandy and were amazed at her bravery, her love of her daughter, her ability to articulate the most difficult thoughts in the world, and certainly her desire to overcome all challenges. Many times we asked Sandy to put her blogs into a book so that they could inspire, educate and comfort others.

Through her incredible blogs, we re-formed a strong emotional bond with Sandy. Today already, even as she struggles through difficult and trying times as her disease gets the better of her, we miss reading her weekly blogs. We know with heavy hearts that one day we will also miss Sandy. This woman is a shining example of bravery, of inspiration, of a mother's love for her daughter, of overcoming adversity and of all that the human spirit can deliver. We pray that when the time comes, Sandy's final wishes will come to fruition and that others will gain strength from Sandy's story.

We are so truly blessed and thankful to have Sandy back in our lives. We love you Sandy and everything that you stand for and believe in.

Kristee Lyle

I have been an avid follower of Sandy's blog since meeting her 4 years ago. I have learned so much about living from this amazing woman who is dying. I am always in awe at Sandy's ability to write about her life with such honesty and humility. Her words are her legacy and I am so proud to be able to call Sandy my friend.

Deborah Reiche

From the moment I met Sandy at work, I knew she was a good person. We had a few things in common, having previously worked in the travel industry for the same employer. As I got to know her better over the years, my admiration and respect grew for her as she became my boss and my friend. Ever since I've known her, Sandy has been dealing with health issues and misdiagnoses, until eventually it was determined she had Erdheim Chester, a very rare disease -- a difficult pill to swallow!

What has always struck me about Sandy, though, is her positive attitude throughout everything that life has thrown at her -- and it's been quite a bit! As per her usual modus operandi - - when life gives you lemons, make lemonade -- Sandy started a blog to document her journey with this illness, opening up her world for other people to see what it's really like to live with a debilitating disease, along with all the ups and downs in life. I have used her blog to stay in touch with her when we couldn't get together or chat. When I was having a bad day, I would read her blog and realize that I was so lucky to have my 'life.' I always told Sandy she should write a book about her life story and I am glad that her 'shining' spirit will live on in this book and help others. She leaves a wonderful legacy, not only in her beautiful daughter and the amazing photos she's produced, but also in her message to never give up hope and always take the high road. She will always be my 'shining' spirit!

Donna Henrikson
I've known Sandy for a long time, first as her family doctor, and then reconnected as a friend when her journey with ECD began. She had some challenging times then – both physically and personally – and she's certainly had plenty in the last few years. Her grace, her sense of humour, her generous spirit and her big heart have always defined her, even when her physical heart was giving her trouble!

The task of living with a terminal illness is always a hard one, and is harder still when you're a mother, and when you're young. Sandy has approached this time with openness, laughter, a willingness to continue learning, a desire for giving a voice to others in her position who are quiet...and her big heart. A heart which loves and laughs, and which also fears and hurts and gets angry, and is sad. She captures the essence of continuing to live as well as one can, in the face of an ever-approaching death, beautifully. It's not easy...and it's harder still to rise above challenging and frustrating circumstances and continue to laugh and love...but she does.

As a physician, who daily encounters people dealing with loss of all kinds, and particularly of loved ones or opportunities, and as one with a special interest in end-of-life care, I was thrilled to hear that her blog was becoming a book. Her words not only help those living close to the ends of their lives to feel understood, but their friends and family to understand. I, for one, will be recommending it widely!'

Kathy DeSantis
I met Sandy through 'Acclaim Health,', who contacted me because I run a volunteer meal delivery program called, "Pat's Food Train.". Unlike other recipients of our service, I came to know more about Sandy through her blog and my visits and naturally a friendship developed. Sandy is probably the most inspirational, courageous, and caring person that I've had the privilege to call a friend.

She is passionate, eloquent and even with all the challenges she's had to face, she has met them head on with fierce determination. Through her blog, she has educated and enriched our lives. She has been a staunch crusader in the ongoing debate of 'Dying with Dignity,' and has echoed the view that many of us share. It is our choice and our voice that should be heard and with Sandy's legacy, her voice will be heard forever.

Janet Miele
With humour, and grace, and resilience – this is how Sandy approaches each hurdle and speed bump she has faced with the progression of her illness. I've seen her in action, in the 'trenches' if you will, in the midst of some of her toughest and sometimes most frustrating battles. Through her writings, she has an amazing ability to peel away all the trivial stuff and focus on the true issue. With honesty, she shares her views, and her struggles.

This is her legacy to us all who know and love her: A life lived with purpose, (a lot of laughs in the mix) and integrity through all of the tough stuff. And always there is gratitude, and dignity in the end.

Deborah Bakti
I met Sandy through her blog in 2010 when I was researching Erdheim-Chester, as my husband had just been diagnosed with this disease. For a

disease that only had 400 diagnoses in the world, it was unbelievable we lived in the same city. We met the same day, talked for hours, and had an immediate connection as women, mothers, spouses, and as a result of this disease. We talk openly about its impact, and Sandy has been there for me as my husband's disease progressed to him living in a nursing home while she dealt with her own issues with her disease. The opportunity to meet Sandy, and experience the authenticity and deepness of our friendship is a gift that has come out of this disease. I am so grateful to Sandy for our friendship, and will always remember and cherish the deep and meaningful discussions and the laughter we've shared together.

Chris Oddy

Through random chance, an innocent game of Scrabble introduced me to this amazing lady. Never have I met a well person with such grace, consideration and spirit as Sandy, so to learn of her illness and her courage has changed me forever. To put it simply, she is everything good about this world and I love her for it. My words are simple and can never describe the impact Sandy has had on me. She is inspirational to all who know her and always will be. Sandy you're the best. I would consider it an amazing honour if my name could appear anywhere on what I know will be a fantastic and beautifully written book. Xxxxxxx

Judy Armstrong McKay
BA Psych; BA Sociology, MSW, RSW

I have had the honour and privilege to get to know Sandy through our conversations and her blog. I have developed great respect for this wonderful woman who is facing the end of her life way too soon. She is a testament to living one's life fully and being "present." Sandy's blog does not wallow, although she also does not hide her pain and her honesty.

Sandy lives her life through all of her senses and writes from this perspective. It reminds us all to pay attention; to truly be grateful and gracious in our lives every day. Sandy has given us all the gift of her presence and for those of us lucky enough to have shared her life, she leaves us all in a better place. Sandy, you will be missed. But thank you so much for leaving this piece of yourself behind for the rest of us who have much to learn!

Sandi Evelyn

Sandy, this is very hard for me to put into words as I feel an overwhelming sadness. I do not want my journey with you to end. You are my inspiration. Through your blogs I have realized how fortunate I am. How much I have to be thankful for. How strong you are. How amazing your daughter is. I have known you many years. You are in my life for a reason and I am blessed. Hugs and prayers.

Bert Hesselink

Since we first met in September 2012, we have very seldom communicated other than by hundreds of single word interactions on Words with Friends. Yet, through your well-articulated blog posts, I believe I've gotten to know you very well and feel we've developed a most wonderful friendship.

You are an amazingly gracious woman and I am truly honoured to be included with the few good men who restored your faith in men (October 31, 2012 post). To this day, I continue to be inspired by your courage in facing these very daunting and difficult circumstances.

> the very first time we met,
>> I remarked at how articulate you were,
>>> and then, you pointed me to your blog;
>
> and then later,
>> we sparred over many Words with Friends,
>>> just to while away your long, waking hours
>
> and now,
>> I marvel even more at the wonderful gift you are,
>>> sharing your beautiful spirit and soul
>
> and forever,
>> will be truly humbled and honoured to proclaim
>>> that I have only too briefly known you
>
> May the Peace of God be with you, my dear Friend

Erin Carroll

We met as kids, connected again on Facebook in 2010... I believe for a reason. And a damn good one. You have inspired me, challenged my thinking, and shaken me to the core. Woken me up!! I read about your day and realize how special my day was too. You show me the real person I long to be, with your humility and honesty and bravery. Some want to read Oprah or others that can arouse their "Ah-ha moments." Sandy you have done that for me time and time again.

Sheryl McKee

I wanted to write something for you, but I think you know words are my enemy. I can't seem to get what is in my heart and my head on to the keyboard.... I can try again, or you can take bits and pieces, rearrange, or fill in the blanks if something does not make sense. I'm not sure if this is what you are looking for, but here goes......

I met Sandy via email, through a mutual friend of ours last year. At that time, Sandy was asking people to share stories, photos, and anything they could spare about New York. I had only been there once, but thought Sandy would get a kick out of a silly story of me in my youth in the Big Apple.

I have never met someone so determined, focused, and yet caring at the same time. Sandy is such an inspiration to me by facing extreme health decline and still being concerned for others. I have gone through a very challenging year and when I read Sandy's blog it makes me realize that I too can take charge of my mental state. You really do have to find the positive in things and enjoy the people in your life that matter.

Sandy, I take my hat off to you. You are an inspiration to others and even now that you are in so much pain and unable to do so many physical things, you still can touch people's hearts. I wish I could take your pain and sorrow away, but I thank you for sharing your experience for others. My health issues are very minor, but I can only imagine with how much strength and dignity you have helped others with your writing. You are a very talented, gifted, and caring person and I am so glad that I have had the honour to have met you and I thank you for the strength you have given me. You are an inspiration and an educator, and have gone through so many struggles and disappointments with kindness, compassion and dignity.

Thanks lady.

Denise K. Rago
Sandy always dreamed of traveling to New York City with her daughter and then-husband Paul, whom I had met in an on-line writing workshop.

She hoped to see all the sights and photograph New York, yet when she could not travel there, she asked readers to share their experiences of New York City with her. I did and then we had the pleasure of speaking on the telephone about more of them. I have since shared my photographs on social media so she could experience more of New York City as well.

Though we have never met face to face, she has inspired me, not only through her photography but by her determination to live life on her terms. She is intelligent, positive, and one of the bravest people I have ever known.

I have a photograph, which she took and put on canvas, hanging in my home. It will forever remind me of her talent, vision, and spirit. It reminds me of the beauty in how people touch one another and influence one another's lives in such a positive way.

Thank you Sandy.

Pat McArthur
Sandy, your blog has been such an honest conversation of all that you have had to contend with over the past few years. Some posts are very difficult to read. I can only imagine how very, very hard it has been for you to live through and then write about all that has happened.

I respect and admire your choices and determination and I love your photography.

Debra Brault
Sandy, I pray comfort and peace for you. You are an inspiration and dearly loved by so many. Your light remains in your daughter and all the lives you've touched.

God bless xo

Dawna Halat

I met Sandy many years ago when our daughters were mutual friends in elementary school. Having lost touch for a number of years, her blog was brought to my attention by my daughter just this past summer. I have continued to be a faithful follower over the past months, always looking forward to a new post and captivated by her integrity and candid reflection.

Sandy's courage, honesty, wisdom, humour, insight, and strength are a true testament to the human spirit when faced with enduring difficult circumstances and health challenges. I have gained an immense respect and admiration for those suffering with a terminal illness through her poignant writings and it has most definitely resonated with me and made a difference in my life, for which I am grateful. This has allowed me to reflect upon my life, my views on end-of-life choices, and understanding those suffering with terminal illness. Her blog has touched many souls, as it has mine, and allowed me to pause and look at our existence on this earth with a renewed sense of appreciation and value and for this I am truly grateful.

Anne Sproull

Sandy and I were childhood and high school friends who lost touch for 30 years. We reconnected when I heard her name and voice on the radio, and learned of her struggles with both Erdheim-Chester disease and the Canadian medical system. Since that day - through her blog, in our personal conversations, and in her presence - I have witnessed highs and lows that go beyond what you think the human heart can withstand; I have witnessed miracles that have challenged and changed how I view my life and the nature of reality itself. In short, my understanding of what my life is -- and what it can be -- is altered for good. Sandy shows us all how to be human beyond belief.

Chantal Tranchemontagne

In following her blog, *Without a Manual*, and taking a journey to her life's end, Sandy gave me a great gift; a guide to living fully. A few lessons I will continue to embrace: Celebrate everything. Gripe with purpose. Move on.

Embrace help graciously. Be funny even when life isn't. Hug your friends. And finally, love with a capital L.

Heather Dekker

I've been thinking and praying for you and your daughter since the day I dropped off a meal. I stumbled on your blog through the Food Train coordinator, and spent an entire day, reading every single entry. It moved me to tears. I shared a couple of the entries with my husband, my parents, and my in-laws, and they were also moved, and have been praying for you as well.

Lisa Nemni

We all have a hero in life. Mine is not a fictional character, she does not come from a comic book or from a TV show...she is real and her name is Sandy Trunzer. Sandy Trunzer.

Sandy is stunning! Her big blue eyes and her gorgeous smile can be spotted miles away. When my husband and I bought our current house, who would have known that it was going to bring a gift into my life? Stopping by the house before the closing date to take measurements, we were greeted at the door by the owner with a warm and friendly smile. She was super nice and even showed us everything we needed to know about the house. I did notice she was running out of breath a bit when she was talking...at the end of our meeting she mentioned she was ill and that was one of the reasons she was moving. I did not know how serious her illness was until I found her blog.

I Googled Sandy's name because I learned that she was a professional photographer. I hoped we could meet to chat about photography, a passion of mine. I found her blog by accident and was shocked to learn of her serious illness. We decided to meet for a coffee. As I picked her up in my car, I remarked to myself how stunning she was, with no outward signs of being ill. Later I discovered that she had actually been very sick that day but she hid it very well.

Her blog has meant a lot to me. I'm an avid fan of her writing. Sandy has given me so many life lessons... lessons like, it is never too late to pursue a dream; always tell a loved one how much they mean to you; and never complain about meaningless things. I learned to stop at any moment during the day, close my eyes, and just breathe. I learned what insomnia really means and that I should not complain about mine. And, I learned we are never too old to be who we always wanted to be when growing up. My list goes on....

I just want Sandy and Suzi, and all the people that know them, to know that they have a very special purpose in life. They have changed the lives of others, including mine. They made me see, feel, and discover things about myself. We all have different personal reasons for wanting to follow her blog, these are mine. I want Sandy to know that meeting her has meant the world to me. A sense of peace comes over me every time at that wall where she placed her gift to me.

Today, I'm thanking God for giving me the privilege of allowing me to meet Sandy Trunzer, a real superhero in my eyes. Today and always in my heart, Sandy.

Bruce A. Krobusek
Farmington NY

I met Sandy at a photographic workshop in Savannah GA, in March of 2006. The workshop was designed to help the attendees overcome their creative fears, and to move outside of their comfort zones. As I got to know Sandy, I scratched my head wondering why she was in the workshop, for she was (and is) one of the most fearless people I know.

Our friendship continued as my wife and I would drive up to Sandy's area every fall for a car show. Somewhere along the line, I found her blog, and got to know her even better through reading it. What I found was a woman who has more strength and courage than anyone else I know. The problems she's had to deal with, and her ability to keep a positive outlook despite just about any drawback, is, to me, the stuff of legend. I despise the Fates for putting her through this gauntlet, but consider myself fortunate to know her and to have been even a remote and occasional companion on her journey. If ever I start feeling sorry for myself because of my own challenges, all I need do is remember how Sandy has dealt with her problems, and suddenly mine become minuscule by comparison.

Lorna Gurnell

I am not a blogger myself but I have been reading Sandy's blog for the past year or so that I have known her. What a wonderful way to connect with someone who is in a very difficult situation and is not always able to have face-to-face conversation due to her illness. I got insight into her views on so many topics. Also a wonderful way for Sandy to keep in contact with lots of people at once without having to send out of individual emails.

Vanessa McElroy

When I first met Sandy, what struck me so noticeably was how beautiful and calm her energy or aura was. She was the recipient of a meal from me through a small organization that cooks meals for people/families in need in the city of Burlington, ON, called Pat's Food Train. Afterwards, we ended up talking on the phone at length, coincidentally right after she'd had a difficult conversation with her doctor as to when her pacemaker would or could be turned off; a thought that has led her on a journey to where she is today. I have always been moved by Sandy's eloquent honesty in her blog writing and in speaking with her. She has a disease that is slowly taking the life out of her but she conducts herself with grace, integrity, bravery, and courage in a way that I've never come across, which will stay with me forever. I am honoured to be a part of the legacy she is leaving behind – you're an inspiration Sandy!

Laura Phillips Sears
Quispamsis, New Brunswick

Sandy was born brave. She was always 'Sandy,' never 'Sandra,' from the day we met at age thirteen. Extremely smart and kind, deliberate yet respectful – a fierce, quiet strength.

We shared our friendship through school and our first few apartments. I always felt, even as kids, that Sandy bore far more than her fair share of 'rain clouds.' She never had it easy but always knew how to make sense of the most unreasonable circumstances. She could make me cry with laughter.

Given life's unfortunate turn of events, Sandy is today as stoic and determined as ever. Her blog has enabled me to stay connected with my friend after so many years apart. Thank you for your candour Sandy! I still laugh and cry as I read. Something good will come of this. I love you.

Tracey Carr Snyder
Friend and Former Colleague of Sandy
Sandy is an inspiration to everyone who reads her blog. She continues to face uncertainty and negativity every day but still manages to speak positively and share the joy she has inside. Her blog has been a way for me to connect with her when I don't get the opportunity to see her in person as much as I'd like or when distance makes it impossible. In person, Sandy spends a lot of time asking about myself, my family and others and how they are doing; her blog is a way for Sandy to express <u>her</u> reality and what she's feeling or experiencing. I'm so very thankful that it has been turned into a publication so that others can share in her words of wisdom and kindness.

Lori Albrough
Sandy's blog allows us to share with her in the journey of having a rare disease. While no one would choose to be in Sandy's shoes, her grace, dignity, and humour as she allows us a glimpse into the realities of her world are simply inspiring and fill me with awe.

CPSIA information can be obtained at www.ICGtesting.com
Printed in the USA
LVOW07*1835150515

438599LV00003BA/4/P

9 781460 239469